Pandemic of Diabetes and Prediabetes: Prevention and Control

Editor

K.M. VENKAT NARAYAN

ENDOCRINOLOGY AND METABOLISM CLINICS OF NORTH AMERICA

www.endo.theclinics.com

Consulting Editor
ADRIANA G. IOACHIMESCU

September 2021 • Volume 50 • Number 3

ELSEVIER

1600 John F. Kennedy Boulevard • Suite 1800 • Philadelphia, Pennsylvania, 19103-2899

http://www.theclinics.com

**ENDOCRINOLOGY AND METABOLISM CLINICS OF NORTH AMERICA Volume 50, Number 3
September 2021 ISSN 0889-8529, ISBN 13: 978-0-323-80905-4**

Editor: Katerina Heidhausen
Developmental Editor: Jessica Cañaberal

Endocrinology and Metabolism Clinics of North America (ISSN 0889-8529) is published quarterly by Elsevier Inc., 360 Park Avenue South, New York, NY 10010-1710. Months of issue are March, June, September, and December. Periodicals postage paid at New York, NY and additional mailing offices. Subscription prices are USD 383.00 per year for US individuals, USD 1037.00 per year for US institutions, USD 100.00 per year for US students and residents, USD 454.00 per year for Canadian individuals, USD 1089.00 per year for Canadian institutions, USD 497.00 per year for international individuals, USD 1089.00 per year for international institutions, USD 100.00 per year for Canadian students/residents, and USD 245.00 per year for international students/residents. To receive student/resident rate, orders must be accompanied by name of affiliated institution, date of term, and the signature of program/residency coordinator on institution letterhead. Orders will be billed at individual rate until proof of status is received. Foreign air speed delivery is included in all *Clinics* subscription prices. All prices are subject to change without notice. **POSTMASTER:** Send address changes to *Endocrinology and Metabolism Clinics of North America*, Elsevier Health Sciences Division, Subscription Customer Service, 3251 Riverport Lane, Maryland Heights, MO 63043. **Customer Service: Telephone: 1-800-654-2452** (U.S. and Canada); **1-314-447-8871** (outside U.S. and Canada). **Fax: 1-314-447-8029. E-mail: journalscustomerservice-usa@elsevier.com (for print support); journalsonlinesupport-usa@elsevier.com (for online support)**.

Reprints. For copies of 100 or more, of articles in this publication, please contact the Commercial Rights Department, Elsevier Inc., 360 Park Avenue South, New York, NY 10010-1710; phone: +1-212-633-3874; fax: +1-212-633-3820; E-mail: reprints@elsevier.com.

Endocrinology and Metabolism Clinics of North America is covered in *MEDLINE/PubMed (Index Medicus), EMBASE/Excerpta Medica, Current Contents/Clinical Medicine, Current Contents/Life Sciences, Science Citation Index, ISI/BIOMED, BIOSIS,* and *Chemical Abstracts.*

Contributors

CONSULTING EDITOR

ADRIANA G. IOACHIMESCU, MD, PhD
Professor of Medicine (Endocrinology), Emory University School of Medicine, Atlanta, Georgia, USA

EDITOR

K.M. VENKAT NARAYAN, MD, MSc, MBA
Director, Emory Global Diabetes Research Center, Ruth and OC Hubert Chair of Global Health, Professor of Epidemiology and Medicine, Emory University, Atlanta, Georgia, USA

AUTHORS

ANN L. ALBRIGHT, PhD, RD
Division of Diabetes Translation, Centers for Disease Control and Prevention, Atlanta, Georgia, USA

YAMUNA ANA, MPH
Research Associate, Public Health Foundation of India (PHFI), Indian Institute of Public Health-Bangalore, Karnataka, India

GIRIDHARA R. BABU, PhD
Professor and Head, Lifecourse Epidemiology, Indian Institute of Public Health-Bangalore, Public Health Foundation of India (PHFI), Bangalore, Karnataka, India

ARLEEN F. BROWN, MD, PhD
Department of Medicine, Olive View-UCLA Medical Center, David Geffen School of Medicine at UCLA, Sylmar, California, USA

JAMES BUCKLEY, MPH
Department of Epidemiology and Biostatistics, School of Public Health, MRC Centre for Environment and Health, School of Public Health, Faculty of Medicine, Imperial College London, London, United Kingdom

MERYEM CICEK, MPH
Department of Primary Care and Public Health, School of Public Health, Imperial College London, London, United Kingdom

STEPHEN COLAGIURI, MD
Professor of Metabolic Health, Boden Collaboration, Charles Perkins Centre, The University of Sydney, Sydney, New South Wales, Australia

WINSTON CRASTO, MBBS, MRCP, MD
Department of Diabetes and Endocrinology, George Eliot Hospitals NHS Trust, Nuneaton, United Kingdom

DANA DABELEA, MD, PhD
Director, Lifecourse Epidemiology of Adiposity and Diabetes (LEAD) Center, Professor of Epidemiology and Pediatrics, Colorado School of Public Health, University of Colorado School of Medicine, Anschutz Medical Campus, Aurora, Colorado, USA

MELANIE J. DAVIES, CBE, MBChB, MD, FRCP, FRCGP, FMedSci
Professor, Diabetes Research Centre, College of Life Sciences, University of Leicester, Leicester General Hospital, Leicester, United Kingdom

GEORGIA M. DAVIS, MD
Division of Endocrinology, Emory University School of Medicine, Georgia, USA

RAVI DEEPA, PhD scholar
Research Associate, Indian Institute of Public Health-Bangalore, Public Health Foundation of India (PHFI), Bangalore, Karnataka, India

DAISY DUAN, MD
Division of Endocrinology, Diabetes and Metabolism, Department of Medicine, Johns Hopkins School of Medicine, Baltimore, Maryland, USA

JUSTIN B. ECHOUFFO-TCHEUGUI, MD, PhD
Division of Endocrinology, Diabetes and Metabolism, Department of Medicine, Johns Hopkins School of Medicine, Welch Prevention Center for Prevention, Epidemiology and Clinical Research, Johns Hopkins University, Baltimore, Maryland, USA

EDWARD W. GREGG, PhD
Professor, Department of Epidemiology and Biostatistics, School of Public Health, MRC Centre for Environment and Health, School of Public Health, Faculty of Medicine, Imperial College London, London, United Kingdom

ALFREDO DANIEL GUERRÓN, MD
Division of Metabolic and Bariatric Surgery, Duke University, Durham, North Carolina, USA

SARIA HASSAN, MD
Assistant Professor of Medicine, Hubert Department of Global Health, Rollins School of Public Health, Emory University, Department of Medicine, Emory University School of Medicine, Atlanta, Georgia, USA

ANNA R. KAHKOSKA, MD, PhD
Assistant Professor, Department of Nutrition, The University of North Carolina at Chapel Hill, Chapel Hill, North Carolina, USA

ANDRE P. KENGNE, MD, PhD
Non-Communicable Diseases Research Unit, South African Medical Research Council, Cape Town, South Africa

KAMLESH KHUNTI, FRCGP, FRCP, MD, PhD, FMedSci
Professor, Diabetes Research Centre, College of Life Sciences, University of Leicester, Leicester General Hospital, Leicester, United Kingdom

CHANG LIU, MPH
Department of Epidemiology, Emory University Rollins School of Public Health, Atlanta, Georgia, USA

VASANTI S. MALIK, MSc, ScD
Assistant Professor, Department of Nutritional Sciences, Temerty Faculty of Medicine, University of Toronto, Ontario, Canada; Adjunct Assistant Professor, Department of Nutrition, Harvard, T.H. Chan School of Public Health, Boston, Massachusetts, USA

NASSER MIKHAIL, MD
Chief, Endocrinology Division, Department of Medicine, Olive View-UCLA Medical Center, David Geffen School of Medicine at UCLA, Sylmar, California, USA

K.M. VENKAT NARAYAN, MD, MSc, MBA
Director, Emory Global Diabetes Research Center, Ruth and OC Hubert Chair of Global Health, Professor of Epidemiology and Medicine, Emory University, Atlanta, Georgia, USA

VINOD PATEL, BSc (Hons), MD, FRCP, DRCOG, MRCGP, FHEAA, RCPathME
Professor, Department of Diabetes and Endocrinology, George Eliot Hospitals NHS Trust, Nuneaton, United Kingdom; Warwick Medical School, University of Warwick, Coventry, United Kingdom

FRANCISCO J. PASQUEL, MD, MPH
Division of Endocrinology, Emory University School of Medicine, Georgia, USA

JONATHAN PEARSON-STUTTARD, FRSPH, MD
Department of Epidemiology and Biostatistics, School of Public Health, MRC Centre for Environment and Health, School of Public Health, Faculty of Medicine, Imperial College London, Health Analytics, Lane Clark & Peacock LLP, London, United Kingdom; Northumbria Healthcare NHS Foundation Trust, North Shields, United Kingdom

SHRIYAN PRAFULLA, MPH
Research Assistant, Public Health Foundation of India (PHFI), Indian Institute of Public Health-Bangalore, Karnataka, India

RAKALE QUARELLS, PhD
Associate Professor of Community Health and Preventative Medicine, Cardiovascular Research Institute, Morehouse School of Medicine, Atlanta, Georgia, USA

NAVEED SATTAR, MD, PhD, FMedSci
Professor of Metabolic Medicine, University of Glasgow, Institute of Cardiovascular and Medical Sciences, BHF Glasgow Cardiovascular Research Centre, Glasgow, United Kingdom

MEGHA SHAH, MD, MSc
Assistant Professor of Medicine, Department of Family and Preventive Medicine, Emory University School of Medicine, Atlanta, Georgia, USA

KAREN R. SIEGEL, PhD, MPH
Division of Diabetes Translation, Centers for Disease Control and Prevention, Hubert Department of Global Health, Rollins School of Public Health, Emory University, Atlanta, Georgia, USA

YAN V. SUN, PhD
Associate Professor, Department of Epidemiology, Emory University, Rollins School of Public Health, Atlanta, Georgia, USA; Atlanta VA Healthcare System, Decatur, Georgia, USA

MARIA G. TINAJERO, BSc
Department of Nutritional Sciences, Temerty Faculty of Medicine, University of Toronto, Toronto, Ontario, Canada

SOMA WALI, MD
Chair, Department of Medicine, Olive View-UCLA Medical Center, David Geffen School of Medicine at UCLA, Sylmar, California, USA

MARY BETH WEBER, MPH, PhD
Assistant Professor of Global Health, Hubert Department of Global Health, Rollins School of Public Health, Emory University, Atlanta, Georgia, USA

Contents

Diabetes diagnosis has important implications for individuals. Diagnostic criteria for fasting and 2-hour plasma glucose and HbA1c are universally agreed. Intermediate hyperglycemia/prediabetes is a risk factor for diabetes and cardiovascular disease. Because risk is a continuum, determining cut-point is problematic and reflected in significant differences in recommended fasting glucose and HbA1c criteria. Many types of diabetes are recognized. Diabetes classification systems are limited by a lack of understanding of etiopathogenetic pathways leading to diminished β-cell function. The World Health Organization classification system is designed to assist clinical care decisions. Newly recognized phenotypic clusters of diabetes might inform future classification systems.

Type 2 diabetes (T2D) is a public health burden associated with immense health care and societal costs, early death, and morbidity. Largely because of epidemiologic changes, including nutrition transitions, urbanization, and sedentary lifestyles, T2D is increasing in every region of the world, particularly in low-income and middle-income countries. This article highlights global trends in T2D and discusses the role of genes, early-life exposures, and lifestyle risk factors in the cause of T2D, with an emphasis on populations in current hotspots of the epidemic. It also considers potential impacts of the coronavirus disease 2019 pandemic and T2D prevention policies and action.

The number of adults living with diabetes has increased substantially globally over the past 40 years, driven by a combination of increased age-standardized prevalence, population growth, aging, and increases in obesity prevalence. Patients with diabetes in high-income countries are living longer, with large declines in vascular disease mortality rates. This appears to be resulting in a diversification of cause of death, complications, and comorbidities that those with diabetes live with. This has large implications for prevention and management approaches, which should be reviewed to update the breadth of conditions that patients with diabetes are at excess risk of throughout their life. These trends have not yet been seen in low- and middle-income countries, where evidence is also more scarce.

Overt type 2 diabetes mellitus (T2DM) is preceded by prediabetes and latent diabetes (lasts 9–12 years). Key dysglycemia screening tests are fasting plasma glucose and hemoglobin A_{1C}. Screen-detected T2DM benefits from multifactorial management of cardiovascular risk beyond glycemia. Prediabetes is best addressed by lifestyle modification, with the goal of preventing T2DM. Although there is no trial evidence of prediabetes/T2DM screening effectiveness, simulations suggest that clinic-based opportunistic screening of high-risk individuals is cost-effective. The most rigorous extant recommendations are those of the American Diabetes Association and US Preventive Services Task Force, which advise opportunistic 3-yearly screening.

The global diabetes burden is staggering, and prevention efforts are needed to reduce the impact on individuals and populations. There is strong evidence from efficacy trials showing that lifestyle interventions promoting increased physical activity, improvements in diet, and/or weight loss significantly reduce diabetes incidence and improve cardiometabolic risk factors. Implementation research assessing the feasibility, effectiveness, and cost-effectiveness of delivering these proven programs at the community level has shown success, but more research is needed to overcome barriers to implementation in different settings globally. New avenues of research should be considered to combat this public health issue.

Type 2 diabetes (T2DM) is increasingly considered an epidemic rooted in modern society as much as in individual behavior. Addressing the T2DM burden thus involves a dual approach, simultaneously addressing high-risk individuals and whole populations. Within this context, this article summarizes the evidence base, in terms of effectiveness and cost-effectiveness, for population-level approaches to prevent T2DM: (1) modifications to the food environment; (2) modifications to the built environment and physical activity; and (3) programs and policies to address social and economic factors. Existing knowledge gaps are also discussed.

Cardiovascular (CV) mortality in diabetes has declined substantially over the last 3 decades in high-income countries from a multifactorial approach targeting glucose, cholesterol, and blood pressure, and lower smoking rates. Additional CV gains may be achieved from large-scale weight loss, which ongoing trials are testing, and from delaying diabetes in those at highest risk. Finally, recent outcome trials support a role for (1) sodium/glucose cotransporter-2 inhibitors, which lower major adverse cardiovascular events but incident heart failure more strongly, and (2) glucagon-like peptide-1 receptor agonists, which lower atherothrombotic outcomes more consistently, including stroke and peripheral arterial disease.

Microvascular complications of diabetes present a significant challenge due to their diverse presentations, significant morbidity, and as strong predictors of cardiovascular disease. Prevention and management strategies should focus on lifestyle modification, education and awareness, systematic screening for early complications, and intensive management of modifiable risk factors. This review discusses the microvascular complications of diabetes, including diabetic retinopathy, diabetic kidney disease, and diabetic neuropathy, and provides best practice clinical care recommendations to guide health care professionals to better manage people with these conditions.

Remarkable advances in diabetes management have occurred since the discovery of insulin 100 years ago. Advances across a therapeutic spectrum, including pharmacotherapy, metabolic surgery, and diabetes technology, offer superior treatment options for diabetes management. New medication classes (glucagon-like peptide-1 receptor analogs and SGLT-2 inhibitors) have demonstrated cardiorenal benefits beyond glycemic control in type 2 diabetes mellitus, while evolving metabolic surgical interventions also help patients achieve diabetes remission. The use of artificial pancreas systems has shown consistent improvement in glycemic control in type 1 diabetes mellitus. It is time for policy changes to expand access to such advantageous therapies.

Diabetes disproportionably affects minorities in the United States. Substantial disparities exist in diabetes incidence, glycemic control, complications, mortality, and management. The most important biologic contributors to diabetes disparities are obesity, insulin resistance, and inadequate glycemic control. Providers and health systems must also recognize the behavioral, social, and environmental factors that promote and sustain racial/ethnic differences in diabetes and its complications. Metformin and sodium-glucose cotransporter 2 inhibitors are the most convenient drugs for treatment of diabetes in minority patients. Multilevel interventions at the patient, provider, health system, community, and policy levels are needed to reduce diabetes disparities in high-risk groups.

Diabetes is a common disease among pediatric populations in the United States and worldwide. The incidence of type 1 and type 2 diabetes is increasing, with disproportional increases in racial/ethnic subpopulations. As the prevalence of obesity continue to increase, type 2 diabetes now represents a major form of pediatric diabetes. The management of diabetes in youth centers on maintaining glycemic control to prevent acute and chronic complications. This article summarizes the epidemiology, etiology, management, and complications of type 1 and type 2 diabetes in youth, as well as future directions and opportunities.

We review the evidence available worldwide on the various challenges in the screening, management, prevention of gestational diabetes mellitus and diabetes in pregnancy. The use of multiple screening and diagnostic tests prescribed by numerous guidelines is challenging for practitioners. Also, sociocultural, demographic and economic challenges affect the prevention and care. Life-course perspectives need to be adopted, as well as an integrated approach in public health care is essential. Tackling these challenges at each phase of life-course, with development and adherence to the country-specific guidelines by practitioners can decrease the burden of gestational diabetes mellitus and diabetes in pregnancy.

Patients with type 2 diabetes mellitus (T2DM) often live with and develop multiple co-occurring conditions, namely multimorbidity, with diffuse impacts on clinical care and patient quality of life. However, literature characterizing T2DM-related multimorbidity patterns is limited. This review summarizes the findings from the emerging literature characterizing and quantifying the association of T2DM with multimorbidity clusters. The authors' findings reveal 3 dominant cluster types appearing in patients with T2DM-related multimorbidity, such as cardiometabolic precursor conditions, vascular conditions, and mental health conditions. The authors recommend that holistic patient care centers around early detection of other comorbidities and consideration of wider risk factors.

Precision diabetes is a concept of customizing delivery of health practices based on variability of diabetes. The authors reviewed recent research on type 2 diabetes heterogeneity and -omic biomarkers, including genomic, epigenomic, and metabolomic markers associated with type 2 diabetes. The emerging multiomics approach integrates complementary and inter-connected molecular layers to provide systems level understanding of disease mechanisms and subtypes. Although the multiomic approach is not currently ready for routine clinical applications, future studies in the context of precision diabetes, particular in populations from diverse ethnic and demographic groups, may lead to improved diagnosis, treatment, and management of diabetes and diabetic complications.

ENDOCRINOLOGY AND METABOLISM CLINICS OF NORTH AMERICA

SERIES OF RELATED INTEREST

Medical Clinics
https://www.medical.theclinics.com
Primary Care: Clinics in Office Practice
https://www.primarycare.theclinics.com/

VISIT THE CLINICS ONLINE!
Access your subscription at:
www.theclinics.com

Dedication

This special theme issue on diabetes is dedicated to the 100th anniversary of the discovery of insulin in the hope that it will catalyze the realization of the vision of Best, Banting, and Macleod to deliver best and affordable care to the hundreds of millions worldwide suffering from diabetes, and that it will also catapult global interdisciplinary research to prevent and cure the disease.

K.M. Venkat Narayan, MD, MSc, MBA
Emory Global Diabetes Research Center
Emory University
1518 Clifton Road NE
Atlanta, GA 30322, USA

E-mail address:
KNARAYA@emory.edu

Endocrinol Metab Clin N Am 50 (2021) xiii
https://doi.org/10.1016/j.ecl.2021.06.003
0889-8529/21/© 2021 Published by Elsevier Inc.

endo.theclinics.com

Foreword

A Population-Based Approach to Diabetes and Prediabetes

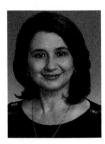

Adriana G. Ioachimescu, MD, PhD
Consulting Editor

The "Pandemic of Diabetes and Prediabetes: Prevention and Control" issue of the *Endocrinology and Metabolism Clinics of North America* is a fascinating journey through the epidemiology, prevention, and therapeutic advances of one of most prevalent and complex health care problems in twenty-first century. Dr K.M. Venkat Narayan, MD, MSc, MBA, Professor of Epidemiology and Medicine at Emory School of Medicine, the Director of Emory Global Diabetes Research Center, and the Ruth and O.C. Hubert Chair of Global Health kindly agreed to serve as our guest editor.

The issue includes a collection of sixteen excellent articles written by experts in the field. Some articles provide insight into the global magnitude of diabetes and its comorbidities and tackle important racial and ethnic disparities. Different body mass index thresholds in racial/ethnic minority populations with higher prevalence of diabetes represent one example; however, other important factors consist of behavioral, social, and health care system differences. Population-level approaches include environment and policy modifications to promote access to healthy foods and increase physical activity. The evidence for population-based programs to prevent type 2 diabetes is carefully examined. Recent changes in worldwide mortality in patients with diabetes and its main causes are presented. New studies supporting a clustering approach for risk stratification of patients with type 2 diabetes patients are presented; they suggest taking into consideration the metabolic, vascular, and mental health comorbidities as part of the health care delivery.

Screening for prediabetes is approached through a pragmatic lens, which emphasizes opportunities for clinic-based interventions that target early identification of both hyperglycemia and cardiovascular risk factors. For patients with prediabetes, the authors review the current evidence of lifestyle interventions to prevent diabetes across diverse communities and populations. Secondary prevention of microvascular

Endocrinol Metab Clin N Am 50 (2021) xv–xvi
https://doi.org/10.1016/j.ecl.2021.06.002
0889-8529/21/© 2021 Published by Elsevier Inc.

endo.theclinics.com

and macrovascular complications entails a multifactorial management of cardiovascular risk factors, including lifestyle changes and use of medications.

The short- and long-term consequences of diabetes diagnosed at a young age or during pregnancy call for timely preventative and therapeutic measures, which can only be successful if the specific sociocultural and economic environments are considered.

Important advances have occurred in the last decade with new drug classes with cardiorenal benefit, minimally invasive bariatric surgery options, continuous glucose monitoring systems, and automatic insulin delivery systems. However, the access to these beneficial clinical innovations is still limited, and policy changes are necessary to expand patient access. Emerging research in the field of epigenomics, metabolomics, and an integrative multi-omics approach at the population level increases our understanding of disease heterogeneity and gives hope for implementation of precision medicine in this field.

I found this issue of the *Endocrinology and Metabolism Clinics of North America* informative and inspiring. I thank Dr Venkat Narayan for guest-editing this very exciting issue and the authors for their excellent contributions. I would like to also recognize the Elsevier editorial staff for their support.

Adriana G. Ioachimescu, MD, PhD
Emory University School of Medicine
1365 B Clifton Road, Northeast, B6209
Atlanta, GA 30322, USA

E-mail address:
aioachi@emory.edu

Preface

Untamed Pandemic of Diabetes: 100 years After the Discovery of Insulin

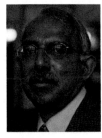

K.M. Venkat Narayan, MD, MSc, MBA
Editor

One hundred years ago in 1921, in one of science's great breakthroughs, Best, Banting, and Macleod discovered insulin, and it was subsequently purified by James Collip.[1] In those days, children with diabetic ketoacidosis (DKA) lay in crowded dark wards, comatose and dying, while family members, helpless in grief, watched the young die before their eyes. One dramatic day in 1922, Banting, Best, and Collip walked from bed to bed in one of these wards at the University of Toronto and injected purified insulin into several children dying of DKA. Within minutes, the children injected earlier were waking from their coma. The tears of joy and momentary exuberance in the room still resonate, and a "cure" for diabetes seemed to have arrived.

One hundred years later, and in the midst of a fast and furious COVID-19 pandemic, diabetes rages like a creeping tsunami in the background as a slow and silent killer. Diabetes remains a chronic condition, and no single act/intervention has yet turned that around. All of the interventions in our armamentarium require dedicated and long-standing behavior change and commitment by the person affected. The disease already affects 463 million worldwide, 80% of who live in resource-challenged low- and middle-income countries (LMIC), tolling a huge burden on health, and costing human societies worldwide $760 billion annually. It is also significant that a high proportion of those suffering the complications of COVID-19, the pandemic we are in, are people with diabetes, and high blood glucose levels, even in those without diabetes, have emerged as one of the strongest prognostic predictors of adverse COVID-19 outcomes.[2]

In the past several decades, we have witnessed much progress in our knowledge about diabetes, including its pathophysiology, possibility of prevention, and

Endocrinol Metab Clin N Am 50 (2021) xvii–xix
https://doi.org/10.1016/j.ecl.2021.06.001
0889-8529/21/© 2021 Published by Elsevier Inc.

remarkable technological advances in its diagnosis and treatment. Several efficacious interventions now exist to delay diabetes onset in those at high risk and to prevent diabetes complications in those with the disease. However, the translation of this scientific progress into clinical and public health practice and policy remains largely abysmal, disproportionately affecting socioeconomically and otherwise disadvantaged people in high-income countries (HIC), and the vast majority of people residing in LMICs.

Diabetes in 50% of people worldwide remains undetected; access to affordable health care and essential medications (including insulin) remains elusive to a substantial majority, especially in LMICs, and outcomes of care vary widely. On the one hand, in many HICs, death rates and incidence of major complications among people with diabetes have been improving during the past 2 decades. But, on the other hand, these positive trends accruing from better organized and affordable health care have not yet reached the poorer people in HICs and the majority with diabetes in LMICs.

In this annual issue of *Endocrinology and Metabolism Clinics of North America*, we have assembled a collection of sixteen articles, each written by experts in the field, covering the gamut of topics relevant to the practicing physician and public health professional dealing with diabetes. Authoritatively written, the articles span epidemiology, prevention, quality of care, advances in therapeutics, diabetes in special populations, and emerging areas, including genomics and precision medicine, and population-based approaches that can complement improved delivery of diabetes prevention and treatment to individuals.

One hopes that this 100th anniversary of the discovery of insulin will remind us all of how far we have yet to travel to realize the vision of Best, Banting, and Macleod to deliver the best-quality care at affordable costs to every one suffering from diabetes. Perhaps, we might redeem ourselves by using the 100th anniversary of the monumental discovery of insulin as a rallying cry to catalyze greater investment in and attention to diabetes research and programs for the hundreds of millions of people with diabetes worldwide. We need to seriously commit ourselves to implement what we know well and support patients in preventing or delaying bad outcomes and in the discovery process that might still hold much hope in terms of one day "curing" diabetes.

ACKNOWLEDGMENTS

K.M. Venkat Narayan was supported in parts by grants P30DK11102 and Radx-UP P30DK111024-05S1 from the National Institute of Diabetes, Digestive, and Kidney Diseases of the National Institutes of Health.

K.M. Venkat Narayan, MD, MSc, MBA
Emory Global Diabetes Research Center
Emory University
1518 Clifton Road NE
Atlanta, GA 30322, USA

E-mail address:
KNARAYA@emory.edu

REFERENCES

1. Available at: https://www.diabetes.org.uk/about_us/news_landing_page/first-use-of-insulin-in-treatment-of-diabetes-88-years-ago-today#:~:text=Insulin%20was%20discovered%20by%20Sir,than%20a%20year%20or%20two.
2. Lazarus G, Audrey J, Wangsaputra VK, et al. High admission blood glucose independently predicts poor prognosis in COVID-19 patients: a systematic review and dose-response meta-analysis. Diabetes Res Clin Pract 2021;171:108561. https://doi.org/10.1016/j.diabres.2020.108561.

Definition and Classification of Diabetes and Prediabetes and Emerging Data on Phenotypes

Stephen Colagiuri, MD

KEYWORDS

- Diagnosis • Classification • Diabetes • Prediabetes • Intermediate hyperglycemia

KEY POINTS

- Diagnostic criteria for diabetes are universally agreed.
- Definitions for intermediate hyperglycemia/prediabetes for fasting plasma glucose and HbA1c are not universally agreed.
- Diabetes classification systems are limited by understanding of etiopathogenetic pathways to β-cell destruction or diminished function.
- The new World Health Organization classification system is based on guiding clinical care decisions.
- Information on new distinct phenotypic clusters of diabetes is emerging.

The term "diabetes mellitus" describes a heterogeneous group of disorders that have in common hyperglycemia in the absence of treatment. Although pathogenetic pathways to hyperglycemia include defects in insulin secretion, insulin action, or both, dysfunction or destruction of pancreatic β-cells is the underlying characteristic common to all forms of diabetes. Mechanisms leading to β-cell decline include genetic abnormalities, epigenetic processes, insulin resistance, autoimmunity, inflammation, and environmental factors.

Diagnosing and classifying diabetes are important steps to appropriate treatment to reduce the risk or progression of long-term complications. Although diabetes may present with characteristic symptoms or severe clinical manifestations such as ketoacidosis, many adults with diabetes will be asymptomatic, and diagnosis relies on biochemical testing for hyperglycemia.

DIAGNOSIS OF DIABETES

Four biochemical tests are universally accepted for diagnosing diabetes (**Table 1**).[1,2]

Boden Collaboration, Charles Perkins Centre, The University of Sydney, Sydney, New South Wales 2006, Australia
E-mail address: Stephen.Colagiuri@sydney.edu.au

Endocrinol Metab Clin N Am 50 (2021) 319–336
https://doi.org/10.1016/j.ecl.2021.06.004
0889-8529/21/© 2021 Elsevier Inc. All rights reserved.

endo.theclinics.com

Table 1 Diagnostic criteria for diabetes	
Diagnostic Test	**Result Diagnostic of Diabetes**
Fasting plasma glucose	$\geq$ 7.0 mmol/L (140 mg/dL)
Plasma glucose 2-h post 75 g oral glucose load (OGTT)	$\geq$ 11.1 mmol/L (200 mg/dL)
Glycated hemoglobin (HbA1c)	$\geq$ 6.5% (48 mmol/mol)
Random glucose in the presence of diabetes symptoms and signs	$\geq$ 11.1 mmol/L (200 mg/dL)

A diagnosis of diabetes has significant implications for an individual, not only for their health but also for the potential impact on employment opportunities, health and life insurance, driving status, social opportunities, and cultural, ethical, and human rights consequences. Therefore, it is important that abnormal values in an asymptomatic individual be confirmed with repeat testing, preferably with the same test, as soon as practicable on a subsequent day.[2] This is different to defining diabetes for epidemiologic purposes where repeat testing is rarely performed. When repeat testing is performed, only 75% of people with diabetes diagnosed in epidemiologic studies are confirmed to have clinical diabetes.[3,4]

Deriving Diabetes Diagnostic Cut-Points

Plasma glucose (PG) or a plasma glucose surrogate (glycated hemoglobin [HbA1c]) remain the most specific biological marker for defining diabetes. Debate continues as to whether diabetes represents the upper end of a continuous distribution of glucose or a discrete entity. Two sets of information have been used to derive diagnostic cut-points for diabetes—glycemic levels associated with risk of diabetes-specific microvascular complications, particularly retinopathy, and the population distribution of glycemia. Data examining the relationship between glycemia and prevalence of retinopathy detect a glycemic decile range at which risk of retinopathy increases, and this has been used as the diagnostic cut-point for diabetes. Several studies have shown a bimodal distribution of PG and describe 2 separate but overlapping curves with the point at which the 2 curves intersect used to separate abnormal from normal. A bimodal distribution of PG was first described in a 1971 study in Pima Indians[5] and subsequently in other populations with high prevalence of diabetes.[1] However, this is not observed in all populations, with the DETECT-2 study finding a bimodal distribution for fasting PG (FPG) in 5 of 27 populations and for 2-hour PG (2-h PG) in 8 of 26 populations.[6]

Diagnostic Cut-Point for 2-Hour Plasma Glucose

The diagnostic cut-point of 11.1 mmol/L (200 mg/dL) for 2-h PG following a 75 g oral glucose tolerance (OGTT) has been used by the American Diabetes Association (ADA) since 1979[7] and by World Health Organization (WHO) since 1985.[8] This cut-point was originally adopted because 11.1 mmol/L (200 mg/dL) was the approximate cut-point separating the 2 components of the bimodal distribution of 2-h PG in Pima Indians. It also represents the point at which prevalence of retinopathy increased sharply.[9] This cut-point has remained unchanged for many years because there has been no new data suggesting a more appropriate value, and considerable clinical and epidemiologic data are based on this cut-point.

Diagnostic Cut-Point for Fasting Plasma Glucose

The diagnostic cut-point of 7.0 mmol/L (126 mg/dL) for FPG has been used by the ADA since 1997[9] and by WHO since 1999.[10] Before this diabetes was defined by an FPG greater than or equal to 7.8 mmol/L (140 mg/dL), but this represents more severe hyperglycemia than a 2-h PG greater than or equal to 11.1 mmol/L (200 mg/dL).[11]

The reduction in FPG to 7.0 mmol/L (126 mg/dL) was intended to ensure both tests reflected a similar degree of hyperglycemia and risk of adverse outcomes and that most people diagnosed with diabetes by the 2-h postload PG would be identified by the simpler FPG without the need for an OGTT. However, the equivalent FPG to a 2-h PG is slightly lower than 7.0 mmol/L (126 mg/dL), and fewer people will be diagnosed with an FPG than by an OGTT.[9]

Diagnostic Cut-Point for Glycated Hemoglobin

Glycated hemoglobin (HbA1c) for diabetes diagnosis was adopted by the ADA in 2010[12] and by WHO in 2011,[2] followed by the 2009 recommendation by an International Expert Committee (IEC) supporting HbA1c as a diagnostic test for diabetes.[13]

The globally accepted cut-point for HbA1c for diagnosing diabetes is greater than or equal to 6.5% (48 mmol/mol). This cut-point was derived from DETECT-2 study data that examined the relationship between HbA1c levels and occurrence of diabetes-specific retinopathy.[14] A recent systematic review and meta-analysis confirmed increased prevalence of nephropathy and moderate retinopathy with HbA1c values greater than or equal to 6.5% (48 mmol/mol) and the high specificity of this value for diagnosing diabetes.[15]

Using HbA1c to diagnose diabetes requires balancing potential advantages and limitations. Although HbA1c is more convenient and does not require fasting or a glucose challenge, it is unavailable in many countries and is more costly. The accuracy and precision of HbA1c assays have improved and are comparable to glucose assays. Indeed, the inaccuracies of glucose measurement are often not appreciated by clinicians. Both fasting and 2-h PG have a higher within-person variability than HbA1c.[16,17] HbA1c can be affected by genetic, hematologic and illness-related factors. The most common important global factors (depending on the assay used) are hemoglobinopathies, certain anemias, and disorders associated with accelerated red cell turnover such as malaria.[2]

These considerations are encapsulated in the WHO recommendation, which states *"HbA1c can be used as a diagnostic test for diabetes providing that stringent quality assurance tests are in place and assays are standardised to criteria aligned to the international reference values, and there are no conditions present which preclude its accurate measurement."*[2]

Racial and ethnic differences in glycated hemoglobin

Several studies have examined racial differences in HbA1c. A systematic review and meta-analysis by Cavagnolli and colleagues investigated the effect of ethnicity on HbA1c levels in individuals without diabetes. Mean HbA1c was significantly higher in people of African descent by 0.26%, Asians by 0.24%, and Latinos by 0.08% compared with white people.[18] Khosla and colleagues reported a more complex relationship finding overdiagnosis of diabetes and prediabetes with HbA1c compared with OGTT in African Americans but underdiagnosis in Afro-Caribbean and Africans living in the United States.[19] An analysis of 3819 individuals with IGT from the Diabetes Prevention Program found increased mean HbA1c in Hispanics, Asians, American Indians, and Afro-Americans compared with white people after adjustment for several factors.[20] However, Butler and colleagues found an increased risk of retinopathy in

African-Americans at HbA1c less than 6.5%.[15] The potential impact of these small differences on HbA1c-diagnosed diabetes in some ethnic populations remains unclear.

Concordance of the fasting, 2-h plasma glucose, and HbA1c to diagnose diabetes. It is well documented that the 3 diabetes diagnostic tests do not result in the same population prevalence of diabetes, with some individuals having diabetes by one measure but not another. The US NHANES data showed a substantially lower prevalence of diabetes based on HbA1c, which detected only 30% of undiagnosed diabetes, compared with 2-h PG, which detected 90% of undiagnosed diabetes. In addition, 19% of undiagnosed diabetes was detected by both FPG and 2-h PG but not by HbA1c. HbA1c alone identified 0.3% of undiagnosed diabetes, FPG alone 0.2%, and 2-h PG alone 2.5%.[21] Data from 16,381 participants without known diabetes in the DETECT-2 study who had all 3 glycemic measures showed that the proportion with newly diagnosed diabetes was 7.7% for FPG, 13.9% for 2-h PG, and 5.7% for HbA1c.[14] Data from 96 populations reported 2% to 6% higher diabetes prevalence with FPG or 2-h PG compared with FPG alone. HbA1c-based prevalence was lower than FPG-based prevalence in 42·8% and higher in another 41·6% and similar in the other 15·6%. Participants' age accounted for some of the variation across studies.[22]

Overall HbA1c-based definition alone identifies substantially less previously undiagnosed people who would be diagnosed with diabetes using a glucose-based test. This incongruence affects population estimates of diabetes but more importantly has implications for the diagnosis of diabetes in an individual. Whether these biomarkers identify individuals with a different risk profile for diabetes complications is not known. Another contentious issue is what criterion should serve as the gold standard for diabetes diagnosis. Although this gold standard has been traditionally the 2-h postload PG, this has been questioned given the greater inherent variability of glucose measurements compared with HbA1c.

Other potential diagnostic tests. There has been increasing interest in the 1-hour PG (1-h PG) during the OGTT as a diagnostic criterion for type 2 diabetes mellitus (T2DM). A recent meta-analysis assessed the optimum cut-off of 1-h PG for detection of T2DM using the 2-h PG as the gold standard.[23] The analysis included 35,551 participants, 2705 with newly detected diabetes based on 2-h PG during OGTT. Three cut-offs of 1-h PG, (10.6 mmol/L, 11.6 mmol/L, and 12.5 mmol/L) were considered, with the 11.6 mmol/L (209 mmol/L) cut-off assessed as the most appropriate having a sensitivity of 92% and specificity of 91%, and detected 92% of cases of T2DM while missing 8% based on the 2-h PG result. However, 55% of individuals classified as having diabetes by this 1-h PG did not have diabetes according to the 2-h PG. This means that using the 1-h PG as an additional diagnostic criterion would further exacerbate the incongruence of currently accepted criteria. Although statistical parameters can be used to establish cut-point equivalence, the more accepted approach is to determine criterion by prediction of diabetes-related complications. Data on this approach for 1-h PG are currently not available.

INTERMEDIATE HYPERGLYCEMIA/PREDIABETES

Lesser degrees of hyperglycemia less than the diagnostic thresholds for diabetes are associated with increased risk of developing diabetes and cardiovascular disease (CVD). Intermediate hyperglycemia/prediabetes are not clinical entities but risk markers for future diabetes and/or adverse outcomes. Although there is an increased risk of progressing to diabetes, many will not progress or will revert to normal, even without intervention.

Intermediate hyperglycemia/prediabetes includes 3 categories:
- Impaired glucose tolerance (IGT)
- Impaired fasting glycaemia (IFG)
- Intermediate glycated hemoglobin (HbA1c)

There are important differences in the definition and terminology recommended by WHO and ADA. WHO uses the term "intermediate hyperglycemia" and discourages the term "prediabetes" because it implies inevitable progression to diabetes without intervention and can stigmatize individuals. The differences in criteria are summarized in **Table 2**.

IMPAIRED GLUCOSE TOLERANCE

IGT was introduced in 1979 by the US National Diabetes Data Group[7] and featured in the 1980 WHO report[24] to denote a state of increased risk of progressing to diabetes. IGT is associated with muscle insulin resistance and defective insulin secretion, resulting in less efficient disposal of glucose during the OGTT.[25] The 2-h PG of 7.8 to 11.1 mmol/L (140–199 mg/dL) following a 75 g OGTT used to define IGT was derived primarily from Pima Indian data and the risk of incident diabetes.[26]

A population prevalence of IGT greater than 10% is common, increases with age, and is more common in women than men. Data from Mauritius indicate that over an 11-year period, 30% of people with IGT at baseline revert to normal, 35% remain as IGT, 5% change to IFG, and 30% develop diabetes.[27] The reproducibility of IGT with retesting within 6 weeks is only moderate, with the proportion of people classified with IGT on the first OGTT and on retesting ranging from 33% to 48% and 39% to 46% being reclassified as normal and 6% to 13% as having diabetes on repeat testing.[28] The pooled cumulative incidence of diabetes in people with IGT ranged from 13% after 1 year to 60% after 20 years. The incidence rate ratio for risk of developing diabetes was 4.48 for IGT compared with a normal 2-h PG.[29]

Cai and colleagues evaluated the association between IGT and all-cause mortality and incident cardiovascular disease.[30] The relative risk was 1.25 for all-cause mortality, 1.23 for composite CVD, 1.21 for coronary heart disease, and 1.30 for stroke. Gujral and colleagues also reported clinical outcomes in people with IGT.[31] The hazard ratio (HR) for IGT and all-cause mortality was 1.19, cardiovascular mortality 1.21, CVD 1.18, coronary heart disease 1.13, and stroke 1.24.

Table 2
Differences in World Health Organization and American Diabetes Association criteria for intermediate hyperglycemia/prediabetes

	WHO	ADA
Impaired Glucose Tolerance		
Fasting Plasma Glucose	<7.0 mmol/L (126 mg/dL)	Not required
2-h Plasma Glucose	and ≥7.8 and < 11.1 mmol/L	≥7.8 and < 11.1 mmol/L
Following 75 g OGTT	(140–199 mg/dL)	(140–199 mg/dL)
Impaired Fasting Glucose		
Fasting Plasma Glucose	6.1–6.9 mmol/L (110–125 mg/dL)	5.6–6.9 mmol/L
2-h Plasma Glucose	Not required but if measured	(100–125 mg/dL)
following 75g OGTT	≥7.8 and < 11.1 mmol/L	Not required
	(140–199 mg/dL)	
Intermediate HbA1c	Not specified	5.7%–6.4%
		39–47 mmol/mol

Impaired Fasting Glucose

IFG was introduced in 1997 by the ADA to describe an intermediate state of FPG between the upper limit of normal and the lower limit of the diabetic FPG, which was intended to be analogous to IGT.[9] In 1999 WHO endorsed IFG as a new category of intermediate hyperglycaemia.[10] Initially both ADA and WHO defined IFG by an FPG 6.1 to 6.9 mmol/L (110–125 mg/dL) but in 2003 the ADA lowered the IFG range to 5.6 to 6.9 mmol/L (100–125 mg/dL).[32] WHO reviewed its criteria in 2006 and recommended continuing with a level of 6.1 to 6.9 mmol/L (110–125 mg/dL) for IFG.[1]

IFG is also a risk factor for future diabetes and adverse outcomes. It is associated with impaired insulin secretion and impaired suppression of hepatic glucose output. IFG $_{6.1-6.9}$ prevalence rates of 5% or more are common, is typically more common in men than in women, and generally increases with age, although in some populations prevalence decreases in the very elderly. Over an 11-year follow-up period in people with IFG $_{6.1-6.9}$ at baseline, 40% reverted to normal, 15% remained as IFG, 20% changed to IGT, and 25% developed diabetes.[27] Reproducibility of IFG with retesting within 6 weeks showed that the proportion of people classified as IFG on the first test and on retesting was approximately 60%, with the majority being reclassified as normal and less than 10% as having diabetes.[28]

The 2003 ADA decision to change the lower cut-point for IFG to 5.6 mmol/L (100 mg/dL) was based on ROC curve analyses of baseline FPG, which maximized sensitivity and specificity for predicting diabetes.[32] In 2006 WHO expressed reservations about using incident diabetes as the only end point for recommending a cut-point for IFG and concluded that other factors should be considered, especially clinical and public health considerations.[1]

Neither the WHO nor ADA IFG criteria require a 2-h PG measurement that has implications for the correct categorization of glucose tolerance because some people with IFG will have diabetes or IGT. The DECODE study showed that in Europeans with IFG$_{6.1-6.9mmol}$, 64.8% had IFG only, 28.6% also had IGT, and 6.6% had diabetes.[33] For Asians with IFG$_{6.1-6.9mmol}$, 45.9% had IFG alone, 35.2% also had IGT, and 18.9% had diabetes.[34]

Prevalence of IFG is increased 2- to 3-fold with ADA IFG$_{5.6-6.9}$ compared with WHO IFG$_{6.1-6.9}$. In the DETECT-2 study the prevalence of IFG increased from 11.8% to 37.6% in Denmark, from 10.6% to 37.6% in India, and from 9.5% to 28.5% in the United States, with the ADA IFG$_{5.6-6.9}$ compared with WHO IFG$_{6.1-6.9}$. In absolute terms India would have 13 million more and China 20 million more with ADA IFG$_{5.6-6.9}$ compared with WHO IFG$_{6.1-6.9}$.[35]

The prognostic value of ADA IFG $_{5.6-6.9}$ and WHO IFG $_{6.1-6.9}$ for predicting T2DM was examined in a systematic review.[29] The cumulative incidence of diabetes for ADA IFG $_{5.6-6.9}$ was 2% at 2 years and 31% at 12 years and HR for developing diabetes was 4.3. For WHO IFG$_{6.1-6.9}$, cumulative incidence of diabetes was 11% at 2 years and 31% at 12 years, and the HR for developing diabetes was 5.5. Both were associated with increased diabetes risk with WHO IFG$_{6.1-6.9}$ having a higher, but not statistically significant, risk compared with ADA IFG$_{5.6-6.9}$.

Cai and colleagues evaluated the association between IFG and outcomes.[30] ADA IFG$_{5.6-6.9}$ was associated with a relative risk of 1.07 for all-cause mortality, 1.09 for composite CVD, 1.09 for coronary heart disease, and 1.06 for stroke, whereas corresponding risks for WHO IFG$_{6.1-6.9}$ were 1.13 for all-cause mortality, 1.20 for composite CVD, 1.17 for coronary heart disease, and 1.18 for stroke. A comparison of risk associated with FPG 5.6 to 6.05 mmol/L (100–109 mg/dL) and 6.1 to 6.9 mmol/L (110–126 md/dL) showed no increase in risk for the lower range for all-cause mortality, composite CVD, and stoke, indicating that risk was driven by the higher PG range.

Gujral and colleagues also examined the ADA and WHO criteria and clinical outcomes.[31] ADA IFG$_{5.6-6.9}$ was associated with an HR for all-cause mortality of 1.22, CVD mortality 1.14, CVD 1.15, coronary heart disease 1.10, and chronic kidney disease (CKD) 1.09. The HRs for WHO IFG$_{6.1-6.9}$ were 1.17 for all-cause mortality, 1.20 for CVD mortality, 1.21 for CVD, 1.14 for coronary heart disease, and 1.22 for stroke.

Unlike IGT, there are limited data on interventions to prevent diabetes in people with isolated IFG, and results have been generally negative. The largest study recruited 641 overweight Japanese people aged 30 to 60 years with an FPG 5.6 to 6.9 mmol/L (100–126 mg/dL) who were randomly assigned to an intervention group that received lifestyle modification or a control group. Although the overall HR for T2DM was 0.56 (95% confidence interval [CI] 0.36–0.87) in favor of the intervention group, a subgroup analysis of individuals with isolated IFG showed no reduction in diabetes risk.[36]

One reason the ADA lowered the IFG cut-point was to increase concordance of IFG with IGT. Data from the Danish INTER-99 study[37] showed that the percentage of people with IGT who also have IFG increases from 25% using the WHO IFG$_{6.1-6.9}$ criteria to 60% with ADA IFG$_{5.6-6.9}$. However, the overall percentage of people who have IGT decreases from 25% with WHO IFG$_{6.1-6.9}$ to 20% with ADA IFG$_{5.6-6.9}$.

The considerably higher prevalence with ADA IFG$_{5.6-6.9}$ compared with WHO IFG$_{6.1-6.9}$ has implications for all health system but especially in countries struggling to cope with the care of people with diabetes. Implementing unproven prevention interventions in a larger proportion of the population with IFG might reduce resources for effective prevention programs for people with IGT.

INTERMEDIATE GLYCATED HEMOGLOBIN

There is a continuum of risk for the development of diabetes with increasing levels of HbA1c.[38] Similar to glucose, there is no specific cut-point where diabetes risk clearly increases although risk increases closer to the diabetes diagnostic threshold. In 2009 an International Expert Committee (IEC) recommended individuals with HbA1c levels 6.0% to 6.4% (42–47 mmol/mol) be considered a very high-risk group that should receive counseling to prevent diabetes.[13]

In 2010 the ADA reviewed the IEC recommendation and concluded that an HbA1c 6.0% to 6.4% (42–47 mmol/mol) fails to identify a substantial number of people who have IFG and/or IGT. US NHANES data indicated an HbA1c between 5.5% (40 mmol/mol) and 6.0% (47 mmol/mol) most accurately identifies people with IFG or IGT. Although acknowledging that determining a lower limit for intermediate HbA1c was somewhat arbitrary, ADA recommended an HbA1c range of 5.7% to 6.4% (39–47 mmol/mol) for identifying individuals at high risk for future diabetes for inclusion in the prediabetes category based on ROC analyses of NHANES data.[12]

In 2011 WHO endorsed the use of HbA1c for the diagnosis of diabetes but did not endorse the use of HbA1c to identify intermediate hyperglycemia on the grounds of insufficient evidence.[2] WHO is in the process of reviewing its guidelines for intermediate hyperglycemia but is yet to publish its findings and recommendations.

Prevalence of intermediate HbA1c is substantially higher with ADA compared with IEC criteria. ADA HbA1c$_{5.7-6.4}$ typically more than double the prevalence of high-risk individuals compared with IEC HbA1c$_{6.0-6.4}$. In the Whitehall II cohort, prevalence of ADA HbA1c$_{5.7-6.4}$ was 10.5% compared with 4.1% for IEC HbA1c$_{6.0-6.4}$.[39] In the ARIC study, prevalence of ADA HbA1c$_{5.7-6.4}$ was 18.9% compared with 9.0% with IEC HbA1c$_{6.0-6.4}$.[40] A study in China reported a high prevalence of intermediate HbA1c of 36% in adults using ADA HbA1c$_{5.7-6.4}$.[41]

Richter and colleagues reported the cumulative diabetes incidence for $HbA1c_{5.7-6.4}$ was 14% at 4 year and 31% at 10 years, whereas the HR for developing diabetes was 5.55. For $HbA1c_{6.0-6.4}$ the cumulative diabetes incidence was 7% at 3 years and 29% at 15 years, whereas the HR for developing diabetes was 10.10.[29] A more recent study reported similar HRs for incident diabetes for $HbA1c_{5.7-6.4}$ ($6\cdot9$) and $HbA1c_{6.0-6.4}$ ($7\cdot2$) over a mean 3.7-year period.[42]

Cai and colleagues evaluated the association of $HbA1c_{5.7-6.4}$ and $HbA1c_{6.0-6.4}$ and diabetes-related outcomes.[30] $HbA1c_{5.7-6.4}$ was associated with a risk ratio (RR) of 1.09 for all-cause mortality, 1.17 for composite CVD, 1.30 for coronary heart disease, and 1.25 for stroke, whereas for corresponding risks for $HbA1c_{6.0-6.4}$ were 1.21 for all-cause mortality, 1.15 for composite CVD, 1.76 for coronary heart disease, and 1.94 for stroke. Gujral and colleagues also examined these 2 ranges of HbA1c and clinical outcomes.[31] $HbA1c_{5.7-6.4}$ was associated with CVD HR 1.15, coronary heart disease 1.28, stroke 1.23, and CKD 1.32, whereas $HbA1c_{6.0-6.4}$ was associated with all-cause mortality of 1.30, CVD 1.32, and CKD 1.50.

There is a lack of evidence on the effect lifestyle or pharmaceutical interventions to reduce diabetes with intermediate HbA1c. One randomized controlled trial in India and the United Kingdom assessed mobile phone SMS lifestyle modifications messages in people with intermediate HbA1c ($\geq6.0\%$ and $\leq6.4\%$ [≥42 and ≤47 mmol/mol]). The study included 1031 subjects in the control and 1031 in the intervention group. After 2 years the HR for developing T2DM was 0.89 (95% CI 0.74, 1.07; $P = .22$), indicating no significant reduction in T2DM.[43]

Both $HbA1c_{5.7-6.4}$ and $HbA1c_{6.0-6.4}$ predict the development of diabetes, mortality, and diabetes-related complications although studies on outcomes were limited. Arguments in favor of the higher more specific rather than the lower more sensitive range include the significantly lower prevalence of intermediate hyperglycemia and a somewhat stronger association with diabetes and diabetes-related complications.

CONGRUENCE OF INTERMEDIATE HYPERGLYCEMIA DEFINITIONS

The equivalence of the various forms of intermediate hyperglycemia is unclear. Although some individuals will have intermediate hyperglycemia by more than one criterion, others will only be positive by one.

A systematic review and meta-analysis assessed diagnostic accuracy of screening tests for prediabetes. Five studies compared prevalence of prediabetes for all 3 tests. Using IEC and current WHO criteria, 27% had prediabetes by one of the tests (of whom 48% had a raised HbA1c alone). Using the ADA criteria for HbA1c, 49% had prediabetes (of whom 71% had a raised HbA1c alone). There was low agreement between the 3 tests on which individuals were classified with prediabetes.[44]

This incongruence of definitions has implications for predicting diabetes. The ELSA-Brazil study reported prevalences of intermediate hyperglycemia of $20\cdot0\%$ for IGT, 43.5% for ADA-IFG, 10.2% for WHO-IFG, 9.0% for IEC-HbA1c, and 20.5% for ADA-HbA1c. IFG based on WHO criteria and IGT predicted diabetes progression better than the other 3 definitions of intermediate hyperglycemia, but sensitivity was low. IFG based on ADA criteria has better sensitivity than the others but classified almost half of adults as having intermediate hyperglycemia and poorly predicts diabetes.[42]

Other Potential Diagnostic Tests

An isolated elevated 1-h postglucose load PG in people with otherwise normal glucose tolerance on an OGTT has been proposed as a criterion for intermediate hyperglycaemia[45] with a value of greater than or equal to 8.6 mmol/L (155 mg/dL) as the proposed cut-point. This value is predictive of progression to T2DM, microvascular and macro-vascular complications, and mortality. Analysis of the STOP DIABETES study showed the effectiveness of interventions in reducing future risk of T2DM in people with an isolated elevated 1-h PG greater than or equal to 8.6 mmol/L (155 mg/dL).[46]

The introduction of a new criterion for intermediate hyperglycemia raises similar consideration as for diabetes diagnosis. Broadening the pool of people with intermediate hyperglycemia and increasing incongruence of current criteria have implications for diabetes prevention and care especially in struggling health systems.

Classification of Diabetes

The first WHO guidance on the classification of diabetes was published in 1965[47] and updated in 1980,[24] 1985,[8] and 1999.[10]

Classification of diabetes has traditionally been based around 2 main types—type 1 diabetes mellitus (T1DM) and T2DM. The distinction between T1DM and T2DM is increasingly difficult due to increasing overweight and obesity in young people with T1DM and increasing occurrence of T2DM in young people, making assigning diabetes type, especially at diagnosis, problematic.[48–50]

There have been calls to review and update the classification system for diabetes and consider new approaches. A recent proposal suggested a classification system centered on the β-cell.[51] Considering that all forms of diabetes have abnormal pancreatic β-cell function as the final common denominator, 11 distinct pathways were suggested for β-cell stress, dysfunction, or loss, including direct β-cell loss/dysfunction, altered incretin effect, altered α-cell activity, adipose tissue, muscle or liver insulin resistance, altered brain, colon/biome, stomach/intestine or kidney activity, and immune dysregulation/inflammation. These specific mediating pathways of hyperglycemia could be targeted with specific treatment in a given patient. This proposal expands on an earlier model describing 8 core defects of diabetes.[52]

In 2017 WHO convened a technical advisory group to review the evidence on classification of diabetes and develop recommendations, which were published in 2019.[53]

Classification systems for diabetes are designed with 3 broad aims:

- Guiding clinical care decisions
- Stimulating research into etiopathology
- Providing a basis for epidemiologic studies

An ideal classification framework would achieve all 3 aims but this is currently not possible because of significant knowledge gaps and available resources. Consequently, the updated WHO classification of diabetes prioritizes clinical care to guide health professionals choose appropriate treatments, particularly at the time of diagnosis.

A clinically based classification system relies on readily available clinical parameters and should be easily applied in a range of clinical settings with varying resources. Although centers in some countries can supplement clinical parameters with measurement of C-peptide, autoantibodies, and genotyping, these are not universally available. Reliance on these tests would limit the global applicability of a diabetes classification system.[53] The WHO 2019 classification of diabetes is shown in **Box 1** and schematically in **Fig. 1**.

The differences between the WHO 2019 and 1999 classification systems are as follows:

- The removal of subtypes of T1DM and T2DM
- The introduction of 2 new types of diabetes

> **Box 1**
> **WHO classification of diabetes**
>
> Type 1 diabetes
>
> Type 2 diabetes
>
> Hybrid forms of diabetes
> • Slowly evolving immune-mediated diabetes of adults
> • Ketosis prone type 2 diabetes
>
> Other specific types
> • Monogenic diabetes
>   ○ Monogenic defects of β-cell function
>   ○ Monogenic defects of insulin action
> • Diseases of the exocrine pancreas
> • Endocrine disorders
> • Drug- or chemical-induced
> • Infections
> • Uncommon forms of Immune-mediated diabetes
> • Other genetic syndromes sometimes associated with diabetes
>
> Unclassified diabetes
>
> Hyperglycemia first detected during pregnancy
> • Diabetes mellitus in pregnancy
> • Gestational diabetes mellitus
>
> *Adapted from* World Health Organization World Health Organization. Classification of diabetes mellitus. Geneva: World Health Organization; 2019. Licence: CC BY-NC-SA 3.0 IGO.

   ○ Hybrid types of diabetes
   ○ Unclassified diabetes

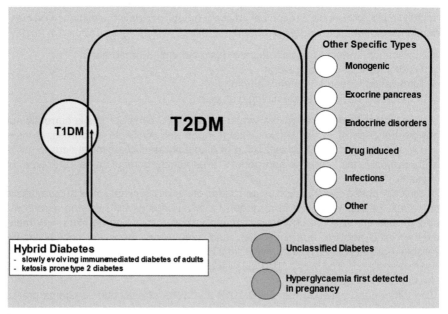

Fig. 1. WHO types of diabetes. (*Data from* World Health Organization World Health Organization. Classification of diabetes mellitus. Geneva: World Health Organization; 2019. Licence: CC BY-NC-SA 3.0 IGO.)

- Updated nomenclature for diabetes due to genetic defects
- Updated categories of hyperglycemia first diagnosed during pregnancy

In addition, practical guidance is provided to clinicians for assigning a type of diabetes at diagnosis.

Readers should refer to the 2019 WHO publication for a detailed description of the diabetes subtypes.[53] Some key points are summarized in the following sections.

Type 1 diabetes

The incidence of childhood T1DM is increasing by 3% to 4% in many high-income countries. T1DM decreases life expectancy by approximately 13 years but prognosis is far worse in countries with limited access to affordable insulin. Approximately 85% of people living with T1DM are adults, with an estimated 40% occurring after the age of 30 years and accounts for 5% of all diabetes diagnosed between ages 31 and 60 years in Europeans.

Seventy to ninety percent of people with T1DM at diagnosis have β-cell autoantibodies against GAD65, IA-2, ZnT8 transporter, or insulin. In Europeans, most of the genetic associations is with HLA DQ8 and DQ2. The pathogenesis of T1DM in those without immune features is unclear. These 2 groups of T1DM were previously been referred to as type 1A (autoimmune) and type 1B (nonimmune) diabetes but these terms are not frequently used nor clinically helpful. Consequently, the 2019 WHO classification refers only to T1DM without subtypes.

Fulminant type 1 diabetes is a form of acute-onset T1DM in adults accounting for approximately 20% of acute-onset T1DM in Japan but is rare in Europeans. It is characterized by an abrupt onset with very short duration of hyperglycemic symptoms, frequent flulike and gastrointestinal symptoms before onset, ketoacidosis at diagnosis, virtually no C-peptide secretion, mostly negative for islet autoantibodies, and increased levels of serum pancreatic enzymes.

Type 2 diabetes

T2DM accounts for 90% to 95% diabetes with the highest proportions in low- and middle-income countries. Although most common in adults the numbers in children and adolescents are increasing.

Most people with T2DM are overweight or obese or have visceral adiposity. Although β-cell dysfunction is required to develop T2DM, in some populations (South Asians) β-cell dysfunction may play a greater role in diabetes development.[54]

Young-onset T2DM is a particularly severe phenotype of diabetes. Compared with T1DM of similar duration complications are more common and mortality rates and cardiovascular disease risk factors are higher. The response to oral blood glucose lowering medications is often poor.

Hybrid forms of diabetes

This new subtype of diabetes is referred to as "hybrid" because clinically these types of diabetes have features between those of T1DM and T2DM. This subtype includes 2 conditions:

- Slowly evolving immune-mediated diabetes of adults
- Ketosis-prone type 2 diabetes

Slowly evolving immune-mediated diabetes of adults. Slowly evolving immune-mediated diabetes occurs mostly in adults who present clinically with T2DM but who have autoantibodies, usually glutamic acid decarboxylase (GAD). Insulin is not required at diagnosis, but progress to requiring insulin occurs more rapidly than people with typical T2DM. Previously referred to as "latent autoimmune diabetes in adults" (LADA), the term "latent" was used to distinguish slow-onset cases and classic T1DM. The appropriateness of this name has been recently questioned. WHO recommends the term "slowly evolving immune-mediated diabetes of adults" instead of LADA.

Diagnosis of this form of diabetes is hampered by the lack of universally agreed criteria but 3 are often used including age older than 35 years at diagnosis, the presence of GAD autoantibodies, and the lack of insulin treatment in the first 6 to 12 months after diagnosis. Whether slowly evolving immune-mediated diabetes represents a separate clinical subtype or is merely a stage in the process leading to T1DM is debated.

Ketosis-prone type 2 diabetes. This unusual form of ketosis-prone diabetes was first reported in young African-Americans in Flatbush, USA and subsequently described in sub-Saharan Africans. It typically presents with ketosis and evidence of severe insulin deficiency but later goes into remission and does not require insulin treatment. Further ketotic episodes occur in 90% of individuals within 10 years. It has been observed in all populations but is least common in Europeans. Although it presents with DKA, the subsequent clinical course resembles T2DM. The pathogenesis is unclear but there are no genetic markers or markers of autoimmunity.

Other specific types of diabetes

These include a wide range of diabetes subtypes (**Table 3**). It is important that clinicians consider the possibility of these at the time of diagnosis and take an appropriate history and perform a detailed clinical examination.

Monogenic diabetes. The most common forms of monogenic diabetes result from defects in β-cell function. A new nomenclature system has been adopted using the

---

Table 3
Age at diagnosis as a guide to type of diabetes

Age at Diagnosis	Type of Diabetes	Comments
< 6 mo	Monogenic neonatal diabetes	T1DM extremely rare in this age group
6 mo–<10 y	Type 1 diabetes Monogenic diabetes Type 2 diabetes	Monogenic diabetes rare before puberty (except for neonatal) T2DM rare before puberty
10 y– < 25 y	Type 1 diabetes Type 2 diabetes Monogenic diabetes	Should be considered equally in this age group although will differ by ethnic group T2DM predominant form in some Asian populations Monogenic diabetes peak age 15–20 y
25 y–50 y	Type 2 diabetes Slowly evolving immune-mediated Type 1 diabetes	Consider non-T2DM in normal weight adults Slowly evolving diabetes mostly after age 35 y T1DM 5% of all diabetes in age group 30–60 y
> 50 y	Type 2 diabetes Slowly evolving immune-mediated Type 1 diabetes	T1DM less likely in this age group

symbol of the mutated gene followed by the clinical syndrome. For example, a child with permanent neonatal diabetes (PNDM) due to mutation KCNJ11 would be classified as KCNJ11 PNDM.

The commonest forms of monogenic diabetes are maturity-onset diabetes of the young (MODY), PNDM, and transient neonatal diabetes. MODY is a dominantly inherited early onset familial form of diabetes with onset usually when younger than 25 years, and individuals are not usually dependent on insulin treatment. However, phenotype and treatment responses vary. The most frequent mutations occur in the glucokinase (GCK MODY) and hepatonuclear factor genes (HNF1A and HNF4A MODY).

Unclassified diabetes

Subtyping diabetes is increasingly complex, and it is not always possible to classify all newly diagnosed cases of diabetes into a specific category. Therefore, a new category of "unclassified diabetes" has been introduced by WHO. For most individuals this will be a temporary category, as it is usually possible to assign diabetes subtype at some point after diagnosis. If diabetes type is uncertain, treatment decisions must be made based on clinical need and reassessed over time.

Hyperglycemia first detected in pregnancy

In 2013 WHO updated its definition and diagnostic criteria for hyperglycemia first detected at any time during pregnancy and described 2 categories of diabetes[55]:

- Diabetes mellitus in pregnancy
- Gestational diabetes mellitus

Assigning diabetes type

The WHO classification includes practical guidance for assigning diabetes type. Because most clinics throughout the world do not have access to laboratory investigations to measure C-peptide or antibodies or do genetic studies, the guidance is based on clinical parameters.

Decisions should be made using the following key steps:
- Confirm the diabetes diagnosis in an asymptomatic individual
- Consider and exclude secondary causes of diabetes
- Consider the following to differentiate subtypes:
  - Age at diagnosis
  - Family history
  - Physical findings, especially presence of obesity
- Note presence or absence of ketosis or ketoacidosis
- Perform additional tests if available (autoantibodies, C-peptide)

Age at diagnosis as a guide to diabetes type

Although the aforementioned factors and other clinical and biochemical markers should be considered, age at diagnosis can be used to narrow possible diabetes subtypes at diagnosis as summarized in **Table 3**.

Emerging phenotypes

Recent studies have identified a variety of diabetes phenotypes using data-driven cluster analysis and modeling. Ahlqvist and colleagues[56] identified clusters based on 6 variables (GAD antibodies, age at diagnosis, body mass index [BMI], HbA1c, and HOMA 2 estimates of β-cell function and insulin resistance) in individuals with newly diagnosed diabetes. Five replicable clusters were identified with significantly different characteristics and risk of diabetic complications:

- *Severe autoimmune diabetes* accounted for 6% of diabetes and featured anti-GAD antibodies, low insulin secretion, and poor metabolic control. This was considered to equate to T1DM and latent-autoimmune diabetes.
- *Severe insulin-deficient diabetes (SIDD)* accounted for 18% of diabetes and featured low insulin secretion, poor metabolic control, and increased risk of retinopathy and nephropathy.
- *Severe insulin-resistant diabetes* accounted for 15% of diabetes and featured insulin resistance, obesity, late onset, and increased risk of nephropathy and fatty liver.
- *Mild obesity-related diabetes* accounted for 22% of diabetes and featured obesity and early onset.
- *Mild age-related diabetes (MARD)* accounted for 39% of diabetes and featured late onset and low risk of complications.

The latter 4 clusters equated to forms of T2DM. These clusters have also been observed in a US and Chinese population, although with differences in cluster distribution.[57]

The INSPIRED study used cluster analysis to determine subtypes of T2DM in Asian Indians. Cluster analysis was performed using age at diagnosis, BMI, waist circumference, HbA1c, serum triglycerides, serum HDL cholesterol, and C peptide (fasting and stimulated). Four clusters of T2DM were identified that differed in phenotypic characteristics and outcomes:

- SIDD—accounted for 27%
- Insulin-resistant obese diabetes (IROD)—accounted for 30%
- Combined insulin-resistant and deficient diabetes (CIRDD)—accounted for 8%
- MARD—accounted for 35%

Although SIDD and MARD were similar to previously reported clusters, IROD and CIRDD were novel. The coexistence of insulin deficiency and insulin resistance seemed peculiar to the Asian Indian population and was associated with an increased risk of microvascular complications.[58] It should be noted that there is overlap between reported clusters, which has implications for subtyping of individuals.

The clinical utility of cluster-based subgrouping diabetes types for predicting outcomes was compared with a strategy of developing models for each outcome using simple patient characteristics. Subjects in the ADOPT study were separated into the 5 clusters described by Ahlqvist and colleagues.[56] Differences between clusters in glycemic and renal progression were compared with stratification based on age at diagnosis for glycemic progression and baseline renal function for renal progression. Although clusters showed differences in glycemic progression, a model using age at diagnosis alone explained a similar amount of variation in progression. Estimated glomerular filtration rate at baseline was a better predictor of time to CKD than the incidence of CKD between clusters. Overall simple clinical features outperformed clusters to select therapy for individual patients. This study suggests that precision medicine in T2DM is likely to have most clinical utility when based on using specific phenotypic measures to predict specific outcomes, rather than assigning patients to cluster driven subgroups.[59]

Subphenotyping of intermediate hyperglycemia has also been reported. Six distinct clusters were identified, 3 with increased glycaemia, but only individuals in 2 clusters had imminent diabetes risk. Another cluster had moderate risk of T2DM but an increased risk of kidney disease and all-cause mortality.[60]

Future diabetes classification systems

Ongoing research will advance understanding of etiopathologic pathways and mechanisms that lead to β-cell destruction or diminished function and hyperglycemia and should lead to more accurate delineation of diabetes types, which in turn should improve clinical decision-making, prediction of complication risk at diagnosis, and ultimately targeted personalized treatment.

Implementing more elaborate classification systems will be challenging in many settings as long as the measurement of nonclinical variables (autoantibodies, C-peptide, genetic typing) remains routinely unavailable in clinics around the world.

CLINICS CARE POINTS

- Confirm diagnosis of diabetes in an asymptomatic individual.
- Treatment at diagnosis should be based on clinical need, especially use of insulin.
- Consider type of diabetes, as this will guide ongoing treatment.
- Be prepared to reconsider type of diabetes if uncertain at the time of diagnosis.
- Recommend preventive interventions in people with intermediate hyperglycemia/ prediabetes.

DISCLOSURE

The author has nothing to disclose.

REFERENCES

1. Definition and diagnosis of diabetes mellitus and intermediate hyperglycaemia. Geneva: World Health Organization; 2006.
2. Report of a World Health Organization consultation. Use of glycated haemoglobin (HbA1c) in the diagnosis of diabetes mellitus. Diabetes Res Clin Pract 2011;93: 299–309.
3. Mooy JM, Grootenhuis PA, de Vries H, et al. Intra-individual variation of glucose, specific insulin and proinsulin concentrations measured by two oral glucose tolerance tests in a general Caucasian population: the Hoorn study. Diabetologia 1996;39:298–305.
4. Christensen JO, Sandbæk A, Lauritzen T, et al. Population-based stepwise screening for unrecognised Type 2 diabetes is ineffective in general practice despite reliable algorithms. Diabetologia 2004;47:1566–73.
5. Rushforth NB, Bennett PH, Steinberg AG, et al. Diabetes in the Pima Indians: evidence of bimodality in glucose tolerance distributions. Diabetes 1971;20: 756–65.
6. Vistisen D, Colagiuri S, Borch-Johnsen K, for the DETECT-2 Collaboration. Bimodal distribution of glucose is not universally useful for diagnosing diabetes. Diabetes Care 2009;32:397–403.
7. National Diabetes Data Group. Classification and diagnosis of diabetes mellitus and other categories of glucose intolerance. Diabetes 1979;28:1039–57.
8. World Health Organization. Diabetes mellitus: report of a WHO study group. Geneva: World Health Organization; 1985 (Tech. Rep. Ser., no. 727).
9. The Expert Committee on the Diagnosis and Classification of Diabetes Mellitus: Report of the expert committee on the diagnosis and classification of diabetes mellitus. Diabetes Care 1997;20:1183–97.

10. World Health Organization. Definition, diagnosis and classification of diabetes mellitus and its complications: report of a WHO Consultation.Part 1: diagnosis and classification of diabetes mellitus. Geneva: World Health Organization; 1999.

11. Harris MI, Hadden WC, Knowler WC, et al. Prevalence of diabetes and impaired glucose tolerance and plasma glucose levels in the U.S. population aged 20–74 yr. Diabetes 1987;36:523–34.

12. American Diabetes Association. Diagnosis and classification of diabetes mellitus. Diabetes Care 2010;33(Suppl 1):S62–9 [Erratum, Diabetes Care 2010; 33(4): e57.

13. Nathan DM, Balkau B, Bonora E, et al. International Expert Committee report on the role of the A1C assay in the diagnosis of diabetes. Diabetes Care 2009;32: 1327–34.

14. Colagiuri S, Lee CMY, Wong TY, et al. the DETECT-2 Collaboration Writing Group. Glycemic Thresholds for Diabetes-Specific Retinopathy. Diabetes Care 2011;34: 145–50.

15. Butler AE, English E, Kilpatrick ES, et al. Diagnosing type 2 diabetes using Hemoglobin A1c: a systematic review and meta-analysis of the diagnostic cutpoint based on microvascular complications. Acta Diabetol 2021;58:279–300.

16. Gambino R. Glucose: a simple molecule that is not simple to quantify. Clin Chem 2007;53:2040–1.

17. Chai JH, Ma S, Heng D, et al. Impact of analytical and biological variations on classification of diabetes using fasting plasma glucose, oral glucose tolerance test and HbA1c. Sci Rep 2017;7(1):13721.

18. Cavagnolli G, Pimentel AL, Freitas PAC, et al. Effect of ethnicity on HbA1c levels inindividuals without diabetes: Systematic review and meta-analysis. PLoS One 2017. https://doi.org/10.1371/journal.pone.0171315.

19. Khosla L, Bhat S, Fullington LA, et al. HbA1c Performance in African Descent Populations in the United States With Normal Glucose Tolerance, Prediabetes, or Diabetes: A Scoping Review. Prev Chronic Dis 2021;18:200365.

20. Herman WH, Ma Y, Uwaifo G, et al. Differences in A1C by Race and Ethnicity Among Patients With Impaired Glucose Tolerance in the Diabetes Prevention Program. Diabetes Care 2007;30:2453–7.

21. Cowie CC, Rust KF, Byrd-Holt DD, et al. Prevalence of Diabetes and High Risk for Diabetes Using A1C Criteria in the U.S. Population in 1988–2006. Diabetes Care 2010;33:562–8.

22. NCD Risk Factor Collaboration (NCD-RisC). Effects of diabetes definition on global surveillance of diabetes prevalence and diagnosis: a pooled analysis of 96 population-based studies with 331288 participants. Lancet Diabetes Endocrinol 2015;3:624–37.

23. Ahuja V, Aronen P, Pramodkumar TA, et al. Accuracy of 1-Hour Plasma Glucose During the Oral Glucose Tolerance Test in Diagnosis of Type 2 Diabetes in Adults: A Meta-analysis. Diabetes Care 2021;44:1062–9.

24. World Health Organization. Expert Committee on diabetes mellitus. Geneva: World Health Organization; 1980 (Tech. Rep. Ser., no. 646).

25. Abdul-Ghani MA, Jenkinson CP, Richardson DK, et al. Insulin secretion and action in subjects with impaired fasting glucose and impaired glucose tolerance. Results from the Veterans Administration Genetic Epidemiology Study. Diabetes 2006;55:1430–5.

26. Bennett PH, Knowler WC, Pettitt DJ, et al. Longitudinal studies of the development of diabetes in the Pima Indians. In: Eschwege E, editor. Advances in

diabetes Epidemiology. Amsterdam, The Netherlands: Elsevier Biomedical Press; 1982. p. 65–74.

27. Soderberg S, Zimmet P, Tuomilehto J, et al. High incidence of type 2 diabetes and increasing conversion rates from impaired fasting glucose and impaired glucose tolerance to diabetes in Mauritius. J Intern Med 2004;256:37–47.

28. McMaster University Evidence Based Practice Center. Diagnosis, prognosis and treatment of impaired glucose tolerance and impaired fasting glucose. Evidence report 128. Available at: www.ahrq.gov. Accessed May 2, 2021.

29. Richter B, Hemmingsen B, Metzendorf MI, et al. Development of type 2 diabetes mellitus in people with intermediate hyperglycaemia. Cochrane Database Syst Rev 2018;29. 10:CD012661.

30. Cai X, Zhang Y, Li M, et al. Association between prediabetes and risk of all cause mortality and cardiovascular disease: updated meta-analysis. BMJ 2020;370: m2297.

31. Gujral UP, Jagannathan R, He S, et al. Association between varying cut-points of intermediate hyperglycaemia and risk of mortality, cardiovascular events and chronic kidney disease: a systematic review and meta-analysis. BMJ Open Diab Res Care 2021;9:e001776.

32. The Expert Committee on the Diagnosis and Classification of Diabetes Mellitus. Follow-up Report on the Diagnosis of Diabetes Mellitus. Diabetes Care 2003; 26:3160–7.

33. DECODE Study Group. Age- and sex-specific prevalences of diabetes and impaired glucose regulation in 13 European Cohorts. Diabetes Care 2003; 26:61–9.

34. DECODA Study Group. Age- and sex-specific prevalence of diabetes and impaired glucose regulation in 11 Asian Cohorts. Diabetes Care 2003;26: 1770–80.

35. Borch-Johnsen K, Colagiuri S, Balkau B, et al. Creating a pandemic of prediabetes: the proposed new diagnostic criteria for impaired fasting glycaemia. Diabetologia 2004;47:1396–402.

36. Saito T, Watanabe M, Nishida J, et al, Zensharen Study for Prevention of Lifestyle Diseases Group. Lifestyle modification and prevention of type 2 diabetes in overweight Japanese with impaired fasting glucose levels: a randomized controlled trial. Arch Intern Med 2011;171:1352–60.

37. Glümer C, Jørgensen T, Borch-Johnsen K. Prevalence of diabetes and impaired glucose regulation in a Danish population—The Inter99 study. Diabetes Care 2003;26:2335–40.

38. Little RR, England JD, Wiedemeyer HM, et al. Glycated haemoglobin predicts progression to diabetes mellitus in Pima Indians with impaired glucose tolerance. Diabetologia 1994;37:252–6.

39. Vistisen D, Witte DR, Brunner EJ, et al. Risk of Cardiovascular Disease and Death in Individuals With Prediabetes Defined by Different Criteria: The Whitehall II Study. Diabetes Care 2018;41(4):899–906.

40. Warren B, Pankow JS, Matsushita K, et al. Comparative prognostic performance of definitions of prediabetes: a prospective cohort analysis of the Atherosclerosis Risk in Communities (ARIC) study. Lancet Diabetes Endocrinol 2017;5(1):34–42.

41. Wang L, Gao P, Zhang M, et al. Prevalence and Ethnic Pattern of Diabetes and Prediabetes in China in 2013. J Am Med Assoc 2017;317(24):2515–23.

42. Schmidt MI, Bracco PA, Yudkin JS, et al. Intermediate hyperglycaemia to predict progression to type 2 diabetes (ELSA-Brasil): an occupational cohort study in Brazil. Lancet Diabetes Endocrinol 2019;7(4):267–77.

43. Nanditha A, Thomson H, Susairaj P, et al. A pragmatic and scalable strategy using mobile technologyto promote sustained lifestyle changes to prevent type 2 diabetes in India and the UK: a randomised controlled trial 2. Diabetologia 2020;63:486–96.
44. Barry E, Roberts S, Oke J, et al. Efficacy and effectiveness of screen and treat policies in prevention of type 2 diabetes: systematic review and meta-analysis of screening tests and interventions. BMJ 2017;356:i6538.
45. Bergman M, Manco M, Sesti G, et al. Petition to replace current OGTT criteria for diagnosing prediabetes with the 1-hour post-load plasma glucose $\geq$ 155 mg/dl (8.6 mmol/L). Diabetes Res Clin Pract 2018;146:18–33.
46. Armato JP, DeFronzo RA, Abdul-Ghani M, et al. Successful treatment of prediabetes in clinical practice using physiological assessment (STOP DIABETES). Lancet Diabetes Endocrinol 2018. https://doi.org/10.1016/S2213-8587(18)30234-1.
47. World Health Organization. Diabetes mellitus: report of a WHO Expert Committee. Geneva: World Health Org.; 1965 (Tech. Rep. Ser., no. 310.
48. Leslie RD, Palmer J, Schloot NC, et al. Diabetes at the crossroads: relevance of disease classification to pathophysiology and treatment. Diabetologia 2016;59: 13–20.
49. Kahn SE, Cooper ME, del Prato S. Pathophysiology and treatment of type 2 diabetes: perspectives on the past, present, and future. Lancet 2014;383:1068–83.
50. Skyler JS, Bakris GL, Bonifacio E, et al. Differentiation of diabetes by pathophysiology, natural history, and prognosis. Diabetes 2017;66:241–55.
51. Schwartz SS, Epstein S, Corkey BE, et al. The time is right for a new classification system for diabetes: rationale and implications of the β-cell-centric classification schema. Diabetes Care 2016;39:179–86.
52. Defronzo RA. Banting Lecture. From the triumvirate to the ominous octet: a new paradigm for the treatment of type 2 diabetes mellitus. Diabetes 2009;58:773–95.
53. World Health Organization World Health Organization. Classification of diabetes mellitus. Geneva: World Health Organization; 2019. Licence: CC BY-NC-SA 3.0 IGO.
54. Narayan KMV, Kondal D, Daya N, et al. Incidence and pathophysiology of diabetes in South Asian adults living in India and Pakistan compared with US blacks and whites. BMJ Open Diab Res Care 2021;9:e001927.
55. Diagnostic criteria and classification of hyperglycaemia first detected in pregnancy: a World Health Organization Guideline. Diabetes Res Clin Pract 2014; 103:341–63.
56. Ahlqvist E, Storm P, Käräjämäki A, et al. Novel sub-groups of adult-onset diabetes and their association with outcomes: a data-driven cluster analysis of six variables. Lancet Diabetes Endocrinol 2018;6(5):361–9.
57. Zou X, Zhou X, Zhu Z, et al. Novel subgroups of patients with adult-onset diabetes in Chinese and US populations. Lancet Diabetes Endocrinol 2019;7:9–11.
58. Anjana RM, Baskar V, Nair ATN, et al. Novel subgroups of type 2 diabetes and their association with microvascular outcomes in an Asian Indian population: a data-driven cluster analysis: the INSPIRED study. BMJ Open Diab Res Care 2020;8:e001506.
59. Dennis JM, Shields BM, Henley WE, et al. Disease progression and treatment response in data-driven subgroups of type 2 diabetes compared with models based on simple clinical features: an analysis using clinical trial data. Lancet Diabetes Endocrinol 2019;7:442–51.
60. Wagner R, Heni M, Tabák AG, et al. Pathophysiology-based sub-phenotyping of individuals at elevated risk for type 2 diabetes. Nat Med 2021;27:1–9.

An Update on the Epidemiology of Type 2 Diabetes: A Global Perspective

Maria G. Tinajero, BSc[a], Vasanti S. Malik, MSc, ScD[a,b,*]

KEYWORDS

- Type 2 diabetes • Obesity • Diet quality • Plant-based diets • Carbohydrate quality
- Developmental origins of health and disease

KEY POINTS

- The prevalence of type 2 diabetes (T2D) has been increasing globally over the last 4 decades; most dramatically in countries undergoing rapid epidemiologic transitions, particularly in Asia, the Middle East, and North Africa.
- The increases in T2D have been largely attributed to changes in living environments and lifestyles, which have led to declines in nutritional quality and increases in sedentary behaviors, giving rise to overweight and obesity in regions that were once predominately burdened by undernutrition.
- T2D and obesity manifest differently across ethnic groups, primarily because of differences in patterns of body fat accumulation, which may be driven in part by gene-environment interactions occurring during early development in conjunction with the adoption of unhealthy lifestyles later in life.
- Diet, including the increased consumption of red and processed meat, and low-quality carbohydrates, including refined grains and sugary beverages, coupled with inadequate intake of healthful plant-based foods, is an important contributor to the T2D epidemic.
- Lifestyle modifications are critical for curbing T2D; this is magnified by the coronavirus disease 2019 pandemic, which has been worsened by obesity, highlighting the urgency for global prevention efforts.

INTRODUCTION

Type 2 diabetes (T2D) is a chronic health condition that has reached alarming rates across the globe. A little more than 2 decades ago, the International Diabetes Federation (IDF) published the first ever Diabetes Atlas, which estimated that 151 million adults had T2D worldwide.[1] This estimate increased to 463 million in 2019, indicating

[a] Department of Nutritional Sciences, Temerty Faculty of Medicine, University of Toronto, 1 King's College Circle, 5th Floor, Toronto, ON M5S 1A8, Canada; [b] Department of Nutrition, Harvard T.H. Chan School of Public Health, Boston, MA, USA
* Corresponding author. Department of Nutritional Sciences, Temerty Faculty of Medicine, University of Toronto, 1 King's College Circle, 5th Floor, Toronto, ON M5S 1A8, Canada.
E-mail address: vasanti.malik@utoronto.ca

Endocrinol Metab Clin N Am 50 (2021) 337–355
https://doi.org/10.1016/j.ecl.2021.05.013
0889-8529/21/© 2021 Elsevier Inc. All rights reserved.

endo.theclinics.com

a tripling in the global burden over this time.[2] Along with the increase in prevalence, there has also been a staggering increase in economic costs to health systems attributable to T2D. In 2007, the amount of direct health care expenditures caused by T2D was estimated to be US$232 billion, whereas, in 2019, it increased to an estimated US$760 billion.[2] The health consequences of T2D are severe and debilitating, being frequent causes of early death and reduced work productivity. At present, approximately 80% of T2D cases occur in low-income and middle-income countries (LMICs), and projections suggest that the steepest increases will continue to occur in these regions in upcoming decades.[2] Curbing the worldwide increase of T2D is of the utmost importance to mitigate economic costs and improve the health and well-being of individuals and populations.

The cause of T2D is complex and is known to be influenced by numerous risk factors; some of which are nonmodifiable, such as age and genetics, and others that are modifiable through lifestyle changes, such as following healthful dietary patterns and adequate physical activity levels. The surge in T2D that has occurred over recent years has been largely attributed to lifestyle changes. Since the start of the twenty-first century, several regions, particularly those in which T2D has escalated most rapidly, have undergone major structural adjustments through the implementation of free trade agreements and widespread urbanization, which have affected food and built environments.[3] The Western dietary pattern, characterized by high intakes of red and processed meats, refined carbohydrates, and free sugars (primarily sugar sweetened beverages [SSBs]), has become increasingly popular worldwide and has been strongly linked to T2D risk.[3] Through increases in motorized transportation and sedentary occupations, physical activity levels have also decreased across populations.[4] The combination of these factors, in conjunction with other socioeconomic and cultural influences, has led to increases in overweight and obesity, a well-established risk factor for T2D.[5]

Clearly, the dynamics of T2D have changed considerably over the last few decades. Although previous research on T2D was focused predominantly on Western or European populations, with emerging evidence on T2D from across the world, it has become evident that T2D manifests differently across ethnicities, suggesting that a one-size-fits-all approach may not be optimal when assessing risk factors. Accumulating evidence also suggests that dietary patterns that have been adopted across the globe, including the Western dietary pattern, are not only contributing to increased risk of T2D and related comorbidities but also pose a threat to environmental sustainability. In the coming years, the dynamics of the T2D epidemic are expected to change further in light of increasing prevalence in global obesity, the aging population, and infectious disease pandemics such as coronavirus disease 2019 (COVID-19); therefore, continued monitoring of T2D trends, particularly through an equity lens, will be critical to prevention efforts. This article highlights global trends in T2D prevalence and discusses the role of genes, early-life exposures, and lifestyle risk factors in the cause of T2D with an emphasis on populations in current hotspots of the epidemic. It also considers potential impacts of the COVID-19 pandemic and directions for T2D prevention policies and action.

Global Trends of Type 2 Diabetes

The prevalence of T2D has increased throughout all world regions during the last 3 decades (**Fig. 1**). According to Global Burden of Disease (GBD) data, the age-standardized global prevalence of T2D was approximately 6.0% in men and 5.0% in women in 2019, reflecting a considerable increase since 1990, when it was estimated to be 3.9% in men and 3.5% in women.[6] The incidence of T2D increases with age, and global pooled estimates suggest that it occurs most commonly around

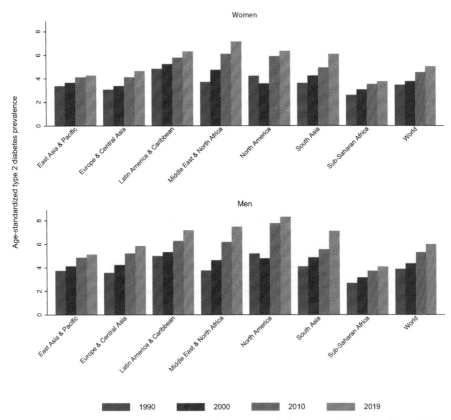

Fig. 1. Trends in age-adjusted prevalence of T2D across different world regions from 1990 to 2019. Age-adjusted prevalence of T2D across different world regions in 1990 (*blue bars*), 2000 (*red bars*), 2010 (*green bars*), and 2019 (*yellow bars*). Top panel shows data for women and bottom panel shows data for men. (*Data from* Global Health Data Exchange. Global Burden of Disease (GBD) Study. Results for 1990, 2000, 2010 and 2019. Available at http://ghdx.healthdata.org/gbd-results-tool?params=gbd-api-2019-permalink/3b8da1b28ce2fce970ae3aeb1ec80875. Accessed April 26, 2021.)

55 to 59 years, on average manifesting slightly earlier in men than in women.[7] No major shifts in the global age distribution of T2D incidence or prevalence have been observed during the last 3 decades[7]; however, with the increasing obesity epidemic, it is expected that increases in T2D among younger age groups will occur.[2]

Most recently, the highest percentage increases in age-standardized prevalence of T2D have occurred in the Middle East and North Africa (MENA) and in South Asia[6]; regions that have undergone rapid epidemiologic transitions such as urbanization, declines in nutritional quality, and increased sedentary behaviors over the last few decades.[8,9] Notably, the MENA region is increasingly being recognized as an emerging hotspot of the T2D epidemic.[10] Women living in MENA have shown the highest age-standardized prevalence of T2D worldwide for the last decade, whereas estimates from 2019 suggest that men living in MENA had the second highest age-standardized prevalence of T2D.[6]

South Asia and East Asia Pacific have also been widely recognized as hotspots of the T2D epidemic.[3] The countries with the highest age-standardized prevalence of

T2D, namely the Marshall Islands and Kiribati, are located in the East Asia Pacific.[2] This region also has the highest number of T2D-attributed deaths worldwide.[2] In contrast, China and India have the highest number of adults with T2D worldwide, with an estimated 116.4 million and 77.0 million people affected in 2019, respectively.[2] Several high-quality reviews have discussed in detail the T2D epidemic in Asia[8,11–13]; overall, the increasing numbers have been attributed to not only the epidemiologic transitions occurring in Asian countries but also to the increased epigenetic risk of T2D shown by individuals of Asian, and particularly South Asian, ethnicity. Populations of South Asian descent have been shown to develop T2D at a younger age and lower body mass index (BMI) compared with other populations.[12]

The most recently published data from the IDF estimated that, by 2045, the number of people affected by T2D worldwide will increase to 700 million.[14] Although it is likely that the regions described here will remain as the T2D hotspots, it is also important to note that the most recent predictions for future T2D prevalence were made before the emergence of the COVID-19 pandemic. In a short time, COVID-19 has affected the health and lifestyles of populations, the global economy, and health care systems. Evidence regarding the impacts of the COVID-19 pandemic on T2D and cardiometabolic health is just emerging, but early data suggest that services to treat noncommunicable diseases, including T2D, have been compromised in response to the heightened efforts needed to manage COVID-19.[15] Whether the increases in sedentary behaviors caused by lockdowns, changes to the diet, and worsening food insecurity linked to COVID-19[16,17] will affect T2D incidence and severity of complications will be of great interest to monitor, particularly in regions that are already disproportionally affected by T2D.

RISK FACTORS

T2D is a complex disease influenced by a multitude of risk factors, some of which are nonmodifiable (such as age, ethnicity, and genetics) and others that are modifiable by lifestyle changes (including diet, physical activity levels, and tobacco use) (**Fig. 2**). The Diabetes prevention programs have shown the efficacy of lifestyle modification to manage body weight in reducing T2D risk in the long term compared with insulin-sensitizing drugs.[18–20] This article focuses next on some key risk factors for T2D that may be putative drivers of global epidemiologic transitions and those that can be modified through lifestyle changes. Emphasis is also given to how T2D risk factors may manifest differently across ethnicities.

Obesity: One Size Does Not Fit All

Overweight and obesity, characterized by high body adiposity, particularly around the central depots, are well-established risk factors for T2D. Globally, approximately 2 billion adults had overweight in 2016, and, among these, 650 million had obesity.[21] Like T2D, obesity prevalence has been increasing rapidly across all world regions.[5] Given the strong links with adiposity, T2D trends tend to follow those for obesity. However, it has been observed that in some regions where the most rapid increases in T2D prevalence have occurred, such as in India, obesity prevalence has remained paradoxically low (**Fig. 3**). For instance, in 2014, the respective obesity prevalence among men and women was approximately 3% and 5% in South Asia, but 28% and 29% in high-income Western countries.[22] In contrast, T2D prevalence was highest among men and women in South Asia, with respective estimates of approximately 10% and 9%, whereas prevalence in high-income Western countries was estimated to be 7% in men and 5% in women.[22] Similar patterns of low obesity prevalence, but high T2D prevalence, have been observed in East and South East Asia and the high-income Asia Pacific.[22]

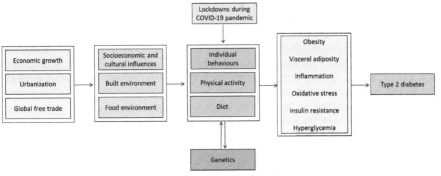

Fig. 2. Major drivers of the current T2D epidemic. Economic growth, urbanization, and global free trade (*blue boxes*) represent macrolevel forces that influence built environments, food environments, and socioeconomic and cultural factors (*green boxes*). These forces can influence modifiable risk factors such as diet, physical activity levels, and other individual behaviors (*orange boxes*), which interact with genes through gene-environment interactions (*purple box*), contributing to the emergence of risk factors for T2D (*yellow boxes*), and ultimately to the development of clinical T2D (*pink box*). The COVID-19 pandemic is also influencing behavioral risk factors through lockdowns, which may affect diet and physical activity levels (*gray box*).

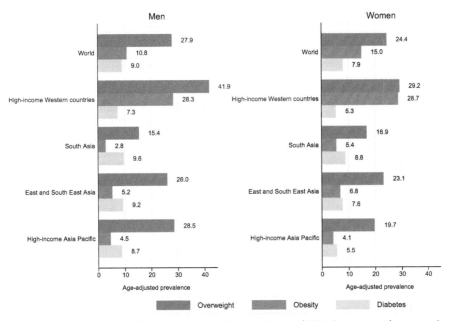

Fig. 3. Age-adjusted prevalence of overweight, obesity, and T2D in men and women in different world regions in 2014. Age-adjusted prevalence of overweight (*blue bars*), obesity (*brown bars*), and diabetes (*light blue bars*) in men (*left panel*) and women (*right panel*) in 2014 in different world regions. Compared with high-income Western countries, South Asia and East and Southeast Asia have higher T2D prevalence, but lower prevalence of overweight and obesity. (*Data from* Non-communicable Disease (NCD) Collaboration. NCD Risk Factor Database. Diabetes: Evolution of diabetes over time. Results for 2014. Available at https://ncdrisc.org/data-downloads-diabetes.html. Accessed April 5, 2021 and Non-communicable Disease (NCD) Collaboration. NCD Risk Factor Database. National adult body-mass index: Evolution of BMI over time. Results for 2014. Available at https://ncdrisc.org/data-downloads-adiposity.html. Accessed April 5, 2021.)

This paradox can be attributed in part to ethnic differences in the associations between BMI and body adiposity.[23] In 1998, the World Health Organization (WHO) developed BMI categories to define underweight, normal weight, overweight, and obesity based on chronic-disease data stemming from predominantly European populations.[24] However, since that time it has been consistently observed that T2D and other cardiometabolic conditions tend to manifest differently across ethnic groups. For example, at the same BMI level, South Asians tend to possess higher body fat percentages and visceral adiposity, but lower lean muscle mass, compared with Europeans.[25,26] This metabolically obese or thin-fat phenotype has been linked to increased insulin resistance and dyslipidemia, and in turn higher risk of T2D, at lower BMIs. In contrast, individuals of African ethnicity have been observed to possess lower body fat percentages and visceral adiposity, but higher lean muscle mass, for a given BMI level compared with Europeans.[23] Although this phenotype is expected to result in more favorable lipid profiles and lower insulin resistance, Africans still have a higher incidence of T2D compared with Europeans living in Europe and North America.[27,28] These disparities may be explained by differences in the social determinants of health, resulting from systemic racism, which unjustly affect African populations, making them vulnerable to chronic health conditions.

Overall, there is strong evidence that a one-size-fits-all approach is not appropriate to define obesity across ethnicities. As a result of the higher incidence of T2D occurring among Asian populations at lower BMIs, in 2004 the WHO suggested lowering the BMI cutoffs to define overweight and obesity among Asian populations.[26] Given that Asian subgroups are highly heterogenous, and that differences in BMI-adiposity associations have been observed across these subgroups, it was recommended that Asian countries independently develop cut points for their own populations. Whether specific cutoffs to define overweight and obesity should be developed for Asian adults living outside of Asia remains under debate; however, the American Diabetes Association recommends that T2D screening should be considered for all Asian American adults with a BMI greater or equal to 23 kg/m^2.[29] To achieve better surveillance of obesity and risk of T2D, further research is necessary to establish whether different BMI cutoffs are necessary for other ethnic groups besides Asians. Current recommendations also suggest that measures of visceral adiposity, such as waist circumference or waist-to-height ratio, should be considered along with BMI when screening for T2D and other cardiometabolic conditions, because these have been suggested to be better predictors of risk across ethnic groups.[30]

Paralleling the global increase in obesity and T2D has been an unprecedented increase in the prevalence of gestational diabetes mellitus (GDM), a transient state of glucose intolerance with onset during pregnancy. It has been estimated that GDM affects, ~14% of pregnancies worldwide, representing ~18 million births annually. Approximately 60% of women with GDM develop T2D later in life.[31] GDM can also lead to long-term cardiometabolic complications for offspring through fetal metabolic programming. Children born to mothers with GDM have almost double the risk of developing obesity in childhood and have an increased risk of future T2D and CVD.[31] Women in LMICs are prone to developing GDM because of being born with a low birth weight combined with excess gestational weight gain during pregnancy.[32] Screening should be integrated into standard obstetric care, and policies to support healthy gestational weight gain should be prioritized by regional public health units.

Genetic Susceptibility

Large-scale genome-wide association studies (GWASs) have elucidated that T2D is a polygenic disease; influenced by more than 400 genetic variants.[33,34] However, compared with other traditional risk factors such as obesity, sedentary lifestyles, and unhealthy diets, these variants seem to have only a modest predictive value of the development of T2D.[34–36] Further, although differences in the location and frequency of T2D risk alleles have been observed across ethnic groups, to date there is limited evidence that these variations explain ethnic differences in T2D risk.[33] However, most large-scale GWASs have been conducted among predominantly European populations, which may impair the identification of variants that are not common in Europeans but are common in other populations.[33] To further understand differences in genetic risk, additional GWASs are being conducted across multiple populations; however, the evidence is just emerging, and further large-scale studies are needed to reach more reliable conclusions.[37–39]

Despite scientific interest in genetic risk, the current evidence suggests that it is unlikely to be genetics alone that places certain individuals or populations at higher risk of T2D. Interactions between genetic, behavioral, and environmental factors may play a more prominent role.[40] In particular, there is a growing interest in how gene-environment interactions that take place during early development, including in utero, may influence the risk of cardiometabolic diseases in adulthood. This question is in keeping with the developmental origins of health and disease (DOHaD) framework, which has been implicated in the development of T2D and other noncommunicable diseases.[41]

Early-life Risk Factors

According to DOHaD, in response to adverse events during critical stages of development, the fetus adapts to optimize the chances of immediate survival. Although these adaptations are effective in the short to medium term, they may increase the risk of cardiometabolic diseases in adulthood, particularly when exposed to certain environmental triggers.[42] Consistent associations observed between maternal undernutrition and low birthweight with higher risk of T2D and other cardiometabolic conditions in adulthood provide important but indirect evidence for a role of early-life environment on future disease risk.[43–45] In a recent meta-analysis of observational studies, a J-shaped association between birthweight and T2D risk in adulthood was observed.[43] Specifically, among infants born with low birthweights, a 22% reduction in T2D risk was observed per 1-kg increase in weight (odds ratio [OR], 0.78; 95% confidence interval [CI], 0.70 to 0.87), whereas macrosomic infants (>4.5 kg) had a 19% higher risk of T2D compared with the reference group (4.0–4.5 kg) (OR, 1.19; 95% CI, 1.04–1.36).[43] In other meta-analyses, significant associations between exposure to famine during gestation and early infancy and T2D risk in adulthood have been observed.[46,47]

Although the underlying mechanisms are not completely understood, it is thought that nutritional deprivation during in utero development promotes a so-called thrifty phenotype, which results in glucose intolerance caused by a reduction in pancreatic β-cell populations and impaired islet function.[42] It is suggested that this adaptation, in conjunction with overnutrition later in life, places individuals at increased risk of T2D. It has also been hypothesized that these occurrences are mediated by epigenetic modifications of the genome, through processes such as DNA methylation and histone modification, which ultimately result in changes in gene expression.[42,48]

DOHaD has been considered a key factor in the rapid increase of T2D in regions undergoing epidemiologic transitions, such as India and China, where undernutrition was once rampant but now coexists with increasing overnutrition.[49,50] The Great Chinese Famine (1959–61), for example, has been described as an important contributor to China's current T2D epidemic.[41,47] Adults that were exposed to the Chinese famine during gestation have been found to have higher rates of T2D than nonexposed adults.[51] Adults exposed to the Chinese famine during gestation have also been observed to have significantly higher waist-to-height ratios compared with nonexposed Chinese adults.[52] Women that were exposed to the famine during gestation and childhood were also observed to have significantly higher visceral adiposity, although no differences were observed in men.[53] More recently, an analysis in the Shanghai Women's Health Study and the Shanghai Men's Healthy study showed that although low birthweight was associated with lower BMI and smaller waist circumference in adulthood, it was also associated with larger waist-to-hip and waist-to-height ratios, which have been suggested to be better predictors of T2D risk among Chinese individuals.[54] These observations are intriguing because they may provide some insight into why individuals of Asian ethnicity tend to have higher visceral adiposity patterns than Europeans at lower BMIs.

Diet

Diet quality is a major driver of the obesity and T2D epidemics. Several LMICs, once burdened primarily by undernutrition, have faced rapid changes in food production, processing, and distribution, which have shifted diets toward the other end of the spectrum, promoting overnutrition.[55,56] Referred to as the nutrition transition, the major shifts being observed include increased consumption of high-calorie foods low in nutritional quality, characterized by refined grains, animal fat and protein, added sugar, sodium and trans fat.[55] At the same time, the consumption of legumes, whole grains, vegetables, and fruits has decreased considerably, with concurrent declines in physical activity.[57] This combination of low-quality dietary patterns and low physical activity levels, often termed the Western lifestyle, has been adopted in many LMICs, including those considered hotspots for T2D. In addition to being detrimental to human health, diets rich in highly processed foods and animal products have also been deemed unsustainable for the environment because of their intensive resource needs and production impacts posing a threat to planetary health and the well-being of future generations.[58–60]

Plant-based Diets

A particular component of the Western diet that has gained considerable attention over recent years, because of its negative impacts on health and the environment, is the consumption of red and processed meats.[58,61,62] In 2019, the EAT-Lancet Commission on Healthy Diets from Sustainable Food Systems published a new universal healthy reference diet, which aims to both promote human health and environmental sustainability.[60] The proposed diet is primarily plant based, placing particular emphasis on consuming minimal amounts animal products, especially red and processed meats.[60]

Meta-analyses of randomized controlled trials (RCTs) and prospective cohort studies have provided strong evidence to suggest that intake of red and processed meat is associated with higher risk of T2D, whereas high-quality plant-based diets are protective.[63,64] An umbrella review of meta-analyses evaluating associations between dietary factors and T2D risk concluded that there was very strong evidence linking consumption of red meat, processed meat, and bacon to higher risk of T2D.[64] In contrast, some meta-analyses of RCTs have shown that red meat intake does not affect cardiometabolic risk.[65,66] However, these inconsistencies are likely attributed to differences in diets consumed by comparison groups.[63] A recent meta-analysis of 36 RCTs including 1803 participants found no significant differences in changes in blood lipids, apolipoproteins, and blood pressure between red meat intake and all comparison groups combined. However, when red meat intake was analyzed by specific comparison diets, relative to high-quality plant protein sources, red meat lead to less favorable changes in total cholesterol (weighted mean difference [WMD], 0.264 mmol/L; 95% CI, 0.14–0.38) and low-density lipoprotein (WMD, 0.20 mmol/L; 95% CI, 0.065–0.033).[63] Although the magnitude of the differences was small, they are expected to yield meaningful differences when translated to the population level. The benefits of replacing red meat with plant-based foods has been further supported by evidence from observational studies on plant-based diets. In a meta-analysis of 9 prospective cohort studies with 307,099 participants, adherence to a plant-based dietary pattern (defined as plant-based dietary indices, and vegetarian or vegan diets) was significantly associated with lower risk of T2D (relative risk [RR], 0.77; 95% CI, 0.71–84).[67] The association was further strengthened when only studies that considered a healthful plant-based dietary index, rather than an overall plant-based dietary index, were included in the analysis (RR, 0.70; 95% CI, 0.62–79).

Several potential mechanisms have been suggested to explain the adverse impacts of meat consumption on T2D risk. Red and processed meats have been linked to weight gain, which is a potent risk factor for T2D,[68] and also contain high levels of saturated fat, heme iron, and dietary cholesterol, constituents that have been linked to T2D risk through exasperating oxidative stress, systemic inflammation, and insulin sensitivity.[69] In contrast, lower consumption of meat may make room for healthful plant-based foods such as fruits, vegetables, nuts, legumes, and whole grains, which contain fiber, antioxidants, and unsaturated fatty acids. These constituents have been shown to have beneficial effects on T2D through improvements in insulin sensitivity, blood pressure, and systemic inflammation, while also reducing long-term weight gain.[67] Red meat products have also been found to contain high amounts choline and carnitine; precursors for trimethylamine-N-oxide (TMAO), a metabolite produced by the gut microbiota that has been strongly associated with T2D risk.[70] In a recent crossover trial comparing the consumption of plant-based and animal products during 8-week periods, it was observed that mean serum concentrations of TMAO were significantly lower in the plant-based phase compared with the animal phase.[71] However, this was observed only among participants who were randomized to receive the animal intervention first; participants who consumed plant-based products first did not show increases in TMAO levels when they shifted to the animal phase. An explanation for these results requires further investigation, but it is possible that following a vegetarian diet for 8 weeks altered the microbiome to prevent the production of TMAO during the subsequent animal phase. This study was also one of the first to assess the potential impacts of plant-based alternative meats on cardiometabolic health. Although these products are becoming increasingly common in the global market,[72] their impacts on health remain narrowly explored. Further research on these products is needed as they continue to enter the food supply in response to plant-based diet recommendations.

Although previous reports have suggested that intake of animal-based protein in India, particularly from dairy products, has increased over recent years, data from a representative sample that participated in the Consumption Expenditure Survey in India reported that, in 2011 to 2012, most Indian households consumed low amounts of both animal and plant-based proteins.[73] Although this deficit was most pronounced among rural low-income groups, it was common among all sectors, regions, and income groups, including high-income households. At the same time, this survey also suggested that a healthy plant-based diet, comprising fruits, vegetables, and legumes, is also not followed in India.[73] Therefore, although high consumption of red and processed meat does not seem to be a major contributor to the increase in

T2D in India, the consumption of refined grains and highly processed foods coupled with low intake of high-quality plant-based products may be playing an important role. This situation may also be the case for other countries in Asia where the diet is largely based on refined carbohydrate staples.

Carbohydrate Quality

Another dietary factor that has been strongly implicated with T2D risk is carbohydrate quality. Although much attention has been given to the quantity of carbohydrates consumed, a large body of evidence has shown that the type or quality of carbohydrate plays an equally or more important role in population health.[74–76]

Several studies have shown that fiber intake is protective against T2D. Whole grains, which are high in fiber as well as other nutrients, have also been observed to have a protective role. In a recently published series of systematic reviews and meta-analyses of cohort studies, a significant dose-response association was observed between the intake of whole grains and dietary fiber and the risk of T2D, whereby every 15-g/d increase in whole grains and every 8-g/d increase in total dietary fiber was associated with a 12% (RR, 0.88; 95% CI, 0.81–0.95) and 15% (RR, 0.85; 95% CI, 0.82–0.89) lower risk, respectively.[77] In addition, a meta-analysis of RCTs found that high intakes of fiber and whole grains resulted in significantly lower body weights, systolic blood pressure, and total cholesterol compared with low levels of intake.[77] Although this meta-analysis did not compare insoluble fiber with viscous soluble fiber, results from previous meta-analyses of trials have suggested that improvements of intermediate T2D risk factors are more consistently linked with sources of viscous soluble fiber compared with sources of insoluble fiber.[78–80] However, these distinctions have not been observed in meta-analyses of prospective cohort studies, which have suggested that high fiber intake is associated with lower risk of T2D, independent of its source or type.[81,82] Although it is true that observational studies may be vulnerable to residual confounding, the impacts of insoluble fiber remain of clinical interest and merit further investigation. Recently, it has been suggested that the benefits of insoluble fiber may be explained by its impacts on the gut microbiome, which has been identified as an important environmental factor in the development of T2D.[83] In contrast, the protective effects of viscous soluble fiber are thought to occur through improved glycemic control, lipid levels, blood pressure, and reduced body weight.[84]

Carbohydrates have also been linked to T2D risk through their potential to increase blood glucose level after ingestion. The glycemic index (GI) is a standardized index to rank different carbohydrate-containing foods based on the glycemic response they elicit after consumption, whereas the glycemic load (GL) also accounts for the quantity of available carbohydrate in the food. Mechanistically, high-GL diets may result in increased demand for insulin and, in the long term, lead to β-cell exhaustion. Whole grains and fiber-rich foods tend to have low GI and GL values. Previous meta-analyses on the associations between GI and GL and the risk of T2D have yielded conflicting findings.[77,85–88] A meta-analysis by Reynolds and colleagues[77] observed an 11% lower risk of T2D among individuals who consumed low-GI compared with high GI-diets (RR, 0.89; 95% CI, 0.82–0.97). The investigators concluded that the quality of the evidence linking GI and GL to T2D risk was very low; however, several methodological errors complicate interpretation of the findings.[89,90] More recently, Livesey and colleagues[89] published an updated meta-analysis where they observed a 27% higher risk of T2D per 10-unit increase in GI (RR, 1.27; 95% CI, 1.15–1.40) and a 26% higher risk of T2D per 80 g of daily GL (RR, 1.26; 95% CI, 1.15–1.37). Livesey and colleagues[90] also conducted a critical evaluation of observational and trial evidence, where they identified GI and GL as probable causal factors contributing to the risk of T2D. These findings were also consistent across world regions, suggesting that there is sufficient evidence to incorporate GI and GL considerations into future dietary guidance for T2D prevention. The metabolic effects of high-GL diets have been shown to be greater among individuals with central adiposity who are more likely to have increased insulin secretion in response to carbohydrate intake; thus, reducing dietary GL among this group may have the most pronounced benefits.[91] This consideration is important for many LMICs where obesity is increasing and dietary staples are predominately refined carbohydrates such as white rice that contribute to a high dietary GI and GL. Intake of white rice has been linked to higher risk for T2D, whereas intake of brown rice, a whole grain, has been inversely associated, suggesting that brown rice could be a healthful alternative.[92–94]

Intake of added or free sugars is another important dimension of carbohydrate quality that has been linked to risk of T2D. The largest source of added sugars in the diet stems from the consumption of SSBs, which have been strongly linked to weight gain, T2D, and other chronic health conditions.[95–97] In a recent meta-analysis of prospective cohort studies, a linear dose-response association was observed whereby every 250-mL increase in daily SSB consumption was significantly associated with a 12% higher risk of obesity (RR, 1.12; 95% CI, 1.05–1.19) and a 19% higher risk of T2D (RR, 1.19; 95% CI, 1.05–1.19).[97] Weight gain, caused by excess consumption of liquid calories, as well as the contribution to a high dietary GL and metabolic effects of fructose from constituent sugars, are considered important contributors to the increased risk of T2D caused by SSB consumption.[3] Studies have also shown that SSB consumption is associated with higher visceral adiposity in both adults and children of predominantly European ethnicity, although this remains narrowly explored among other ethnic groups.[98–100] Few studies have assessed the impacts of SSBs on T2D risk specifically in Asian populations,[101] which is of great public health interest given that there was a 145% increase in sales of SSBs between 2005 and 2018 in South Asia.[102]

Physical Activity and Sedentary Behaviors

It is well documented that maintaining a physically active lifestyle decreases the risk of T2D. A large meta-analysis found that engaging in high levels of cardiorespiratory fitness, occupational activity, and walking resulted in 55% (RR, 0.45; 95% CI, 0.29–0.70), 15% (RR, 0.85; 95% CI, 0.79–0.92), and 15% (RR, 0.85; 95% CI, 0.79–0.91) lower risk of T2D, respectively, compared with low levels.[103] Another large meta-analysis showed that higher daily sitting time was associated with a statistically significant 13% higher risk of T2D (RR, 1.13; 95% CI, 1.04–1.22), before adjusting for physical activity levels, and a 11% higher risk after adjusting for physical activity levels (RR, 1.11; 95% CI, 1.01–1.19).[104]

The associations between physical activity, sedentary time, and the risk of T2D seem to be largely mediated by reduced adiposity.[103] Physical activity expends energy and also tends to take the place of sedentary behavior, which is often accompanied by increased energy intake. Moreover, partaking in physical activity has been suggested to have beneficial effects on insulin sensitivity and glucose homeostasis, which may be driven by increased translocation of the GLUT4 (glucose transporter type 4) transporter to the skeletal muscle cell membranes.[103,105]

Worldwide estimates from 2016 found that more than 80% of adolescents and approximately 27.5% adults were not meeting physical activity recommendations.[4,106] With widespread lockdowns to prevent the spread of COVID-19 in many countries with extended periods of stay-at-home orders and limited opportunities for physical activity, there is growing concern that sedentary behaviors are increasing worldwide now more than ever.[107,108] Since 2019, several governments have implemented lockdowns with the aim of reducing infection spread. In a recent systematic review of 41 observational studies, it was reported that COVID-19 confinements were associated with weight gain among 7.2% to 72.4% of study participants, with those that were already overweight, obese, and of lower socioeconomic status being particularly prone to weightgain.[109] These weight increases were attributed to several factors, in particular decreased energy expenditure, (caused by reductions of activities that used take place outside the home), as well as increased food intake (including increased snacking and consumption of highly processed foods), inadequate sleep, stress, increased alcohol consumption, and increased smoking.[109] This comprehensive review included studies from several regions, including the United States, China, and India, as well as several countries in Europe and the MENA, suggesting that this phenomenon is occurring worldwide. Taken together, these data suggest that, to diminish the potential long-term effects of the COVID-19 pandemic on cardiometabolic health, governments should encourage individuals to partake in at-home physical activity when possible and create safe spaces and infrastructure to promote active living.

TYPE 2 DIABETES PREVENTION POLICIES

In response to the growing burden of T2D, several jurisdictions worldwide have implemented policies aiming to improve weight management, diet quality, and screening practices for pre-T2D and GDM. Since the early 2000s, about 40 countries have implemented taxes on SSBs to reduce excess intake of free sugars and calories.[110] A recent meta-analysis showed that taxation has resulted in decreases in sales and consumption of SSBs,[111] but whether these effects will continue in the long term, and whether they will translate into improvements in health, will need to be evaluated in the coming years. Some governments have also explored implementing taxes for other unhealthy foods; for instance, in 2016, Kerala became the first state in India to apply a 14.5% tax on fast food items sold in branded restaurants.[112] Although the impacts of this policy are yet to be evaluated, it has been suggested that its benefits will be maximized only if coupled with other public health strategies, such as public health awareness campaigns and increasing accessibility of healthy foods.[112] Other noteworthy strategies that have been gaining global momentum include front-of-package labeling (such as traffic light labeling, Nutri-Score, or star labeling), restriction of marketing of unhealthy foods and beverages to children, and banning the sales of unhealthy items in schools. In 2016, Chile was the first country to implement a Law of Food Labeling and Advertising, a set of policies that encompassed a combination of these 3 strategies. An early evaluation of this policy revealed that household purchases of high-in-sugar beverages decreased by 23.7% per day following its implementation.[113] This reduction is higher compared with changes in purchases following the implementation of stand-alone policies, such as SSB taxation, in other regions,[113] supporting the notion that a combination of several strategies is necessary to achieve meaningful differences in consumption patterns.

SUMMARY

T2D is a public health problem of great magnitude that has been increasing globally over the last 4 decades. Countries undergoing rapid epidemiologic transitions, particularly in Asia and MENA, have experienced some of the most rapid increases in this disease. This increase has been largely attributed to changes in living environments and lifestyles, which have led to declines in nutritional quality and increases in sedentary behaviors. As a result, increases in overweight and obesity are being seen in regions that were once predominantly burdened by undernutrition. The evidence also suggests that the relation between T2D and obesity manifests differently across ethnic groups, primarily because of differences in patterns of body fat accumulation. This process may be driven in part by gene-environment interactions occurring during early development, in conjunction with the adoption of unhealthy lifestyles later in life. Diet, including the increased consumption of red and processed meat, and low-quality carbohydrates, including refined grains and sugary beverages, coupled with inadequate intake of healthful plant-based foods, is an important contributor to the T2D epidemic. At the same time, data suggest that a large proportion of the population, both youth and adults, do not engage in sufficient physical activity. Policy strategies are needed across all sectors of society that prioritize obesity and T2D prevention through diet and lifestyle modification. Improving carbohydrate quality by reducing intake of refined grains and added sugar and increasing intakes of whole grains and more healthful plant-based foods are important steps in improving overall diet quality that could have a meaningful impact on weight management and improving cardiometabolic health. The importance of lifestyle modification is magnified by the COVID-19 pandemic and has been worsened by obesity, highlighting the urgency for global prevention efforts.

DISCLOSURE

V.S.M. is on a pro bono retainer for expert support for litigation related to SSBs and has served as a consultant for the City of San Francisco for a case related to health warning labels on soda. V.S.M. has received funding from the Canada Research Chairs Program and the Canadian Foundation for Innovation. M.G.T. is supported by a Canadian Institutes of Health Research fellowship. There are no other financial or personal conflicts of interest to disclose that are related to the contents of this article.

CLINICS CARE POINTS

- Among groups at higher risk for T2D (eg, people of South and East Asian ethnicity), screening for prediabetes (oral glucose tolerance test ≥140 mg/dL, fasting blood glucose ≥100 mg/dL) should begin earlier in life (≥30 years of age) and at lower BMI levels (BMI ≥ 23 kg/m^2).

- Measures of visceral adiposity, such as waist circumference (WC), should also be incorporated into screening practices for T2D, and ethnic-specific cutoffs for these should be considered (eg, WC ≥ 90 cm for South Asian men vs WC ≥ 94 cm for European men).

- Pregnant women should be screened for GDM early in the second trimester (24–28 weeks' gestation), and women in high-risk groups should be screened even earlier. Throughout pregnancy, emphasis should be placed on achieving healthy gestational weight gain by maintaining healthy diets and engaging in safe levels of physical activity.

- When providing dietary guidance for patients with prediabetes or GDM, recommendations should emphasize incorporating healthy plant-based proteins and high-quality sources of carbohydrates (high in fiber, low GI and GL) into the diet, and limiting the intake of added sugars, refined carbohydrates, and red and processed meats.

- To promote healthy diets and lifestyles, health literacy should be incorporated into clinical practice, or patients should be directed to dieticians for health literacy education. Prescriptions for diets and exercise should also be considered.

REFERENCES

1. International Diabetes Federation. IDF diabetes atlas. 1st edn. Brussels, Belgium: International Diabetes Federation; 2000. Available at: https://www.diabetesatlas.org.
2. International Diabetes Federation. IDF diabetes Atlas. 9th edn. Brussels, Belgium: International Diabetes Federation; 2019. Available at: https://www.diabetesatlas.org.
3. Hu FB. Globalization of diabetes: the role of diet, lifestyle, and genes. Diabetes Care 2011;34(6):1249–57.
4. Guthold R, Stevens GA, Riley LM, et al. Worldwide trends in insufficient physical activity from 2001 to 2016: a pooled analysis of 358 population-based surveys with 1·9 million participants. Lancet Glob Health 2018;6(10):e1077–86.
5. Malik VS, Willet WC, Hu FB. Nearly a decade on — trends, risk factors and policy implications in global obesity. Nat Rev Endocrinol 2020;16(11):615–6.
6. Exchange GHD. Age-adjusted prevalence of type 2 diabetes 1990-2019. Available at: http://ghdx.healthdata.org/. [Accessed 5 May 2021].
7. Khan MAB, Hashim MJ, King JK, et al. Epidemiology of type 2 diabetes – global burden of disease and forecasted trends. J Epidemiol Glob Health 2020;10:1.
8. Hills AP, Arena R, Khunti K, et al. Epidemiology and determinants of type 2 diabetes in South Asia. Lancet Diabetes Endocrinol 2018;6(12):966–78.
9. Sherif S. Economic development and diabetes prevalence in MENA countries: Egypt and Saudi Arabia comparison. World J Diabetes 2015;6(2):304.
10. Khan Y, Hamdy O. Type 2 diabetes in the Middle East and North Africa (MENA). Diabetes mellitus in developing countries and underserved communities. New York, NY: Springer International Publishing; 2017. p. 49–61.
11. Nanditha A, Ma RCW, Ramachandran A, et al. Diabetes in Asia and the Pacific: implications for the global epidemic. Diabetes Care 2016;39(3):472–85.
12. Chan JCN, Malik V, Jia W, et al. Diabetes in Asia. JAMA 2009;301(20):2129.
13. Wolf RM, Nagpal M, Magge SN. Diabetes and cardiometabolic risk in south Asian youth: a review. Pediatr Diabetes 2021;22(1):52–66.
14. Federation ID. IDF Atlas: 9th edition 2019: Demographic and geographic outline 2019.
15. Chudasama YV, Gillies CL, Zaccardi F, et al. Impact of COVID-19 on routine care for chronic diseases: a global survey of views from healthcare professionals. Diabetes Metab Syndr Clin Res Rev 2020;14(5):965–7.
16. Stefan N, Birkenfeld AL, Schulze MB. Global pandemics interconnected — obesity, impaired metabolic health and COVID-19. Nat Rev Endocrinol 2021;17(3):135–49.
17. Ghosal S, Arora B, Dutta K, et al. Increase in the risk of type 2 diabetes during lockdown for the COVID19 pandemic in India: a cohort analysis. Diabetes Metab Syndr Clin Res Rev 2020;14(5):949–52.
18. Haw JS, Galaviz KI, Straus AN, et al. Long-term sustainability of diabetes prevention approaches. JAMA Intern Med 2017;177(12):1808.
19. Ramachandran A, Snehalatha C, Mary S, et al. The Indian Diabetes Prevention Programme shows that lifestyle modification and metformin prevent type 2 diabetes in Asian Indian subjects with impaired glucose tolerance (IDPP-1). Diabetologia 2006;49(2):289–97.
20. Long-term effects of lifestyle intervention or metformin on diabetes development and microvascular complications over 15-year follow-up: the Diabetes Prevention Program Outcomes Study. Lancet Diabetes Endocrinol 2015;3(11):866–75.

21. Obesity and overweight. Geneva: World Health Organization; 2020. Available at: https://www.who.int/news-room/fact-sheets/detail/obesity-and-overweight. Accessed June 16, 2021.
22. Age-adjusted prevalence of type 2 diabetes, overweight and obesity. 2014. Non-communicable Disease (NCD) Risk Factor Collaboration. Available at: https://ncdrisc.org/data-downloads.html. Accessed June 16, 2021.
23. Deurenberg P, Yap M, Van Staveren W. Body mass index and percent body fat: a meta analysis among different ethnic groups. Int J Obes 1998;22(12): 1164–71.
24. Obesity: preventing and managing the global epidemic. Report of a WHO consultation on obesity. Geneva: World Health Organization; 1998. Available at: https://apps.who.int/iris/handle/10665/42330. Accessed June 16, 2021.
25. Unnikrishnan R, Gupta PK, Mohan V. Diabetes in South Asians: phenotype, clinical presentation, and natural history. Curr Diab Rep 2018;18(6):30.
26. Appropriate body-mass index for Asian populations and its implications for policy and intervention strategies. Lancet 2004;363(9403):157–63.
27. Meeks KAC, Freitas-Da-Silva D, Adeyemo A, et al. Disparities in type 2 diabetes prevalence among ethnic minority groups resident in Europe: a systematic review and meta-analysis. Intern Emerg Med 2016;11(3):327–40.
28. Cheng YJ, Kanaya AM, Araneta MRG, et al. Prevalence of diabetes by race and ethnicity in the United States, 2011-2016. JAMA 2019;322(24):2389.
29. Hsu WC, Araneta MRG, Kanaya AM, et al. BMI cut points to identify at-risk Asian Americans for type 2 diabetes screening: Table 1. Diabetes Care 2015;38(1): 150–8.
30. Ross R, Neeland IJ, Yamashita S, et al. Waist circumference as a vital sign in clinical practice: a Consensus Statement from the IAS and ICCR Working Group on Visceral Obesity. Nat Rev Endocrinol 2020;16(3):177–89.
31. Plows JF, Stanley JL, Baker PN, et al. The pathophysiology of gestational diabetes mellitus. Int J Mol Sci 2018;19(11):3342.
32. Goldenberg RL, McClure EM, Harrison MS, et al. Diabetes during pregnancy in low- and middle-income countries. Am J Perinatol 2016;33(13):1227–35.
33. Cole JB, Florez JC. Genetics of diabetes mellitus and diabetes complications. Nat Rev Nephrol 2020;16(7):377–90.
34. Meigs JB. The genetic epidemiology of type 2 diabetes: opportunities for health translation. Curr Diab Rep 2019;19(8):62.
35. Fuchsberger C, Flannick J, Teslovich TM, et al. The genetic architecture of type 2 diabetes. Nature 2016;536(7614):41–7.
36. Ahmed SAH, Ansari SA, Mensah-Brown EPK, et al. The role of DNA methylation in the pathogenesis of type 2 diabetes mellitus. Clin Epigenetics 2020; 12(1):104.
37. Batool H, Mushtaq N, Batool S, et al. Identification of the potential type 2 diabetes susceptibility genetic elements in South Asian populations. Meta Gene 2020;26:100771.
38. Spracklen CN, Sim X. Progress in defining the genetic contribution to type 2 diabetes in individuals of East Asian ancestry. Curr Diab Rep 2021;21(6):17.
39. Chen J, Sun M, Adeyemo A, et al. Genome-wide association study of type 2 diabetes in Africa. Diabetologia 2019;62(7):1204–11.
40. Dietrich S, Jacobs S, Zheng JS, et al. Gene-lifestyle interaction on risk of type 2 diabetes: a systematic review. Obes Rev 2019;20(11):1557–71.
41. Hanson MA, Gluckman PD. Early developmental conditioning of later health and disease: physiology or pathophysiology? Physiol Rev 2014;94:1027–76.

42. Stein AD, Obrutu OE, Behere RV, et al. Developmental undernutrition, offspring obesity and type 2 diabetes. Diabetologia 2019;62(10):1773–8.

43. Knop MR, Geng TT, Gorny AW, et al. Birth weight and risk of type 2 diabetes mellitus, cardiovascular disease, and hypertension in adults: a meta-analysis of 7 646 267 participants from 135 studies. J Am Heart Assoc 2018;7(23): e008870.

44. De Mendonça ELSS, De Lima Macêna M, Bueno NB, et al. Premature birth, low birth weight, small for gestational age and chronic non-communicable diseases in adult life: a systematic review with meta-analysis. Early Hum Dev 2020;149: 105154.

45. Mi D, Fang H, Zhao Y, et al. Birth weight and type 2 diabetes: a meta-analysis. Exp Ther Med 2017;14(6):5313–20.

46. Liu L, Wang W, Sun J, et al. Association of famine exposure during early life with the risk of type 2 diabetes in adulthood: a meta-analysis. Eur J Nutr 2018;57(2): 741–9.

47. Li C, Lumey L. Exposure to the Chinese famine of 1959–61 in early life and long-term health conditions: a systematic review and meta-analysis. Int J Epidemiol 2017;46(4):1157–70.

48. Loh M, Zhou L, Ng HK, et al. Epigenetic disturbances in obesity and diabetes: epidemiological and functional insights. Mol Metab 2019;27S(Suppl):S33–41.

49. Su C, Zhao J, Wu Y, et al. Temporal trends in dietary macronutrient intakes among adults in rural China from 1991 to 2011: findings from the CHNS. Nutrients 2017;9(3):227.

50. Krishnaveni GV, Srinivasan K. Maternal nutrition and offspring stress response—implications for future development of non-communicable disease: a perspective from India. Front Psychiatry 2019;10:795.

51. Li Y, He Y, Qi L, et al. Exposure to the Chinese famine in early life and the risk of hyperglycemia and type 2 diabetes in adulthood. Diabetes 2010;59:2400–6.

52. Meng R, Lv J, Yu C, et al. Prenatal famine exposure, adulthood obesity patterns and risk of type 2 diabetes. Int J Epidemiol 2018;47(2):399–408.

53. Chen C, Zhao L, Ning Z, et al. Famine exposure in early life is associated with visceral adipose dysfunction in adult females. Eur J Nutr 2019;58(4):1625–33.

54. Xia Q, Cai H, Xiang Y-B, et al. Prospective cohort studies of birth weight and risk of obesity, diabetes, and hypertension in adulthood among the Chinese population. J Diabetes 2019;11(1):55–64.

55. Popkin BM, Adair LS, Ng SW. Global nutrition transition and the pandemic of obesity in developing countries. Nutr Rev 2012;70(1):3–21.

56. Ley SH, Hamdy O, Mohan V, et al. Prevention and management of type 2 diabetes: dietary components and nutritional strategies. Lancet 2014;383(9933): 1999–2007.

57. Popkin BM. Nutrition transition and the global diabetes epidemic. Curr Diab Rep 2015;15(9):64.

58. Vega Mejía N, Ponce Reyes R, Martinez Y, et al. Implications of the western diet for agricultural production, health and climate change. Front Sustain Food Syst 2018;2:88. https://doi.org/10.3389/fsufs.2018.00088.

59. Tilman D, Clark M. Global diets link environmental sustainability and human health. Nature 2014;515(7528):518–22.

60. Willett W, Rockström J, Loken B, et al. Food in the Anthropocene: the EAT–Lancet Commission on healthy diets from sustainable food systems. Lancet 2019;393(10170):447–92.

61. Lynch J, Pierrehumbert R. Climate Impacts of Cultured Meat and Beef Cattle. Front Sustain Food Syst 2019;3:5. https://doi.org/10.3389/fsufs.2019.00005.

62. Climate change and land: summary for policy makers. Geneva: Intergovernmental Panel on Climate Change; 2019.

63. Guasch-Ferré M, Satija A, Blondin SA, et al. Meta-analysis of randomized controlled trials of red meat consumption in comparison with various comparison diets on cardiovascular risk factors. Circulation 2019;139(15):1828–45.

64. Neuenschwander M, Ballon A, Weber KS, et al. Role of diet in type 2 diabetes incidence: umbrella review of meta-analyses of prospective observational studies. BMJ 2019;366:l2368.

65. O'Connor LE, Kim JE, Campbell WW. Total red meat intake of ≥0.5 servings/d does not negatively influence cardiovascular disease risk factors: a systemically searched meta-analysis of randomized controlled trials. Am J Clin Nutr 2017;105(1):57–69.

66. Maki KC, Van Elswyk ME, Alexander DD, et al. A meta-analysis of randomized controlled trials that compare the lipid effects of beef versus poultry and/or fish consumption. J Clin Lipidol 2012;6(4):352–61.

67. Qian F, Liu G, Hu FB, et al. Association between plant-based dietary patterns and risk of type 2 diabetes. JAMA Intern Med 2019;179(10):1335.

68. Mozaffarian D, Hao T, Rimm EB, et al. Changes in diet and lifestyle and long-term weight gain in women and men. N Engl J Med 2011;364(25):2392–404.

69. Micha R, Michas G, Mozaffarian D. Unprocessed red and processed meats and risk of coronary artery disease and type 2 diabetes – an updated review of the evidence. Curr Atheroscler Rep 2012;14(6):515–24.

70. Zhuang R, Ge X, Han L, et al. Gut microbe–generated metabolite trimethylamine N-oxide and the risk of diabetes: A systematic review and dose-response meta-analysis. Obes Rev 2019;20(6):883–94.

71. Crimarco A, Springfield S, Petlura C, et al. A randomized crossover trial on the effect of plant-based compared with animal-based meat on trimethylamine-N-oxide and cardiovascular disease risk factors in generally healthy adults: Study With Appetizing Plantfood—Meat Eating Alternative Trial (SWAP-ME. Am J Clin Nutr 2020;112(5):1188–99.

72. Ismail I, Hwang Y-H, Joo S-T. Meat analog as future food: a review. J Anim Sci Technol 2020;62(2):111–20.

73. Sharma M, Kishore A, Roy D, et al. A comparison of the Indian diet with the EAT-Lancet reference diet. BMC Public Health 2020;20(1):812.

74. Sievenpiper JL. Low-carbohydrate diets and cardiometabolic health: the importance of carbohydrate quality over quantity. Nutr Rev 2020;78(Supplement_1):69–77.

75. Ludwig DS, Hu FB, Tappy L, et al. Dietary carbohydrates: role of quality and quantity in chronic disease. BMJ 2018;361:k2340.

76. Korsmo-Haugen H-K, Brurberg KG, Mann J, et al. Carbohydrate quantity in the dietary management of type 2 diabetes: a systematic review and meta-analysis. Diabetes Obes Metab 2019;21(1):15–27.

77. Reynolds A, Mann J, Cummings J, et al. Carbohydrate quality and human health: a series of systematic reviews and meta-analyses. Lancet 2019;393(10170):434–45.

78. Jovanovski E, Khayyat R, Zurbau A, et al. Should viscous fiber supplements be considered in diabetes control? Results from a systematic review and meta-analysis of randomized controlled trials. Diabetes Care 2019;42(5):755–66.

79. Ho HVT, Sievenpiper JL, Zurbau A, et al. The effect of oat β-glucan on LDL-cholesterol, non-HDL-cholesterol and apoB for CVD risk reduction: a systematic review and meta-analysis of randomised-controlled trials. Br J Nutr 2016;116(8):1369–82.

80. Ho HVT, Jovanovski E, Zurbau A, et al. A systematic review and meta-analysis of randomized controlled trials of the effect of konjac glucomannan, a viscous soluble fiber, on LDL cholesterol and the new lipid targets non-HDL cholesterol and apolipoprotein B. Am J Clin Nutr 2017;105(5):1239–47.

81. Dietary fibre and incidence of type 2 diabetes in eight European countries: the EPIC-InterAct Study and a meta-analysis of prospective studies. Diabetologia 2015;58(7):1394–408.

82. Yao B, Fang H, Xu W, et al. Dietary fiber intake and risk of type 2 diabetes: a dose–response analysis of prospective studies. Eur J Epidemiol 2014;29(2):79–88.

83. Davison KM, Temple NJ. Cereal fiber, fruit fiber, and type 2 diabetes: explaining the paradox. J Diabetes Complications 2018;32(2):240–5.

84. Weickert MO, Pfeiffer AFH. Metabolic effects of dietary fiber consumption and prevention of diabetes. J Nutr 2008;138(3):439–42.

85. Greenwood DC, Threapleton DE, Evans CEL, et al. Glycemic index, glycemic load, carbohydrates, and type 2 diabetes: systematic review and dose-response meta-analysis of prospective studies. Diabetes Care 2013;36(12):4166–71.

86. Barclay AW, Petocz P, Mcmillan-Price J, et al. Glycemic index, glycemic load, and chronic disease risk—a meta-analysis of observational studies. Am J Clin Nutr 2008;87(3):627–37.

87. Bhupathiraju SN, Tobias DK, Malik VS, et al. Glycemic index, glycemic load, and risk of type 2 diabetes: results from 3 large US cohorts and an updated meta-analysis. Am J Clin Nutr 2014;100(1):218–32.

88. Dong J-Y, Zhang L, Zhang Y-H, et al. Dietary glycaemic index and glycaemic load in relation to the risk of type 2 diabetes: a meta-analysis of prospective cohort studies. Br J Nutr 2011;106(11):1649–54.

89. Livesey G, Taylor R, Livesey HF, et al. Dietary glycemic index and load and the risk of type 2 diabetes: a systematic review and updated meta-analyses of prospective cohort studies. Nutrients 2019;11(6):1280.

90. Livesey G, Taylor R, Livesey HF, et al. Dietary glycemic index and load and the risk of type 2 diabetes: assessment of causal relations. Nutrients 2019;11(6):1436.

91. Ebbeling CB, Feldman HA, Steltz SK, et al. Effects of sugar-sweetened, artificially sweetened, and unsweetened beverages on cardiometabolic risk factors, body composition, and sweet taste preference: a randomized controlled trial. J Am Heart Assoc 2020;9(15):e015668.

92. Hu EA, Pan A, Malik V, et al. White rice consumption and risk of type 2 diabetes: meta-analysis and systematic review. BMJ 2012;344:e1454.

93. Sun Q. White rice, brown rice, and risk of type 2 diabetes in US men and women. Arch Intern Med 2010;170(11):961.

94. Bhavadharini B, Mohan V, Dehghan M, et al. White rice intake and incident diabetes: a study of 132,373 participants in 21 countries. Diabetes Care 2020; 43(11):2643–50.

95. Imamura F, O'Connor L, Ye Z, et al. Consumption of sugar sweetened beverages, artificially sweetened beverages, and fruit juice and incidence of type 2 diabetes: systematic review, meta-analysis, and estimation of population attributable fraction. BMJ 2015;351:h3576.

96. Malik VS, Popkin BM, Bray GA, et al. Sugar-sweetened beverages, obesity, type 2 diabetes mellitus, and cardiovascular disease risk. Circulation 2010;121: 1356–64.

97. Qin P, Li Q, Zhao Y, et al. Sugar and artificially sweetened beverages and risk of obesity, type 2 diabetes mellitus, hypertension, and all-cause mortality: a dose–response meta-analysis of prospective cohort studies. Eur J Epidemiol 2020; 35(7):655–71.

98. Yi S-Y, Steffen LM, Terry JG, et al. Added sugar intake is associated with peri-cardial adipose tissue volume. Eur J Prev Cardiol 2020;27(18):2016–23.

99. Ma J, Mckeown NM, Hwang S-J, et al. Sugar-sweetened beverage consumption is associated with change of visceral adipose tissue over 6 years of follow-up. Circulation 2016;133(4):370–7.

100. Gallagher C, Moschonis G, Lambert KA, et al. Sugar-sweetened beverage con-sumption is associated with visceral fat in children. Br J Nutr 2021;125(7): 819–27.

101. Neelakantan N, Park SH, Chen G-C, et al. Sugar-sweetened beverage con-sumption, weight gain, and risk of type 2 diabetes and cardiovascular diseases in Asia: a systematic review. Nutr Rev 2021. https://doi.org/10.1093/nutrit/nuab010.

102. Eaton J. Country level sales of ultra-processed foods and sugar-sweetened bev-erages predict higher BMI and increased prevalence of overweight in adult and youth populations. Curr Dev Nutr 2020;4(Supplement_2):825.

103. Aune D, Norat T, Leitzmann M, et al. Physical activity and the risk of type 2 dia-betes: a systematic review and dose–response meta-analysis. Eur J Epidemiol 2015;30(7):529–42.

104. Bailey DP, Hewson DJ, Champion RB, et al. Sitting time and risk of cardiovascu-lar disease and diabetes: a systematic review and meta-analysis. Am J Prev Med 2019;57(3):408–16.

105. Flores-Opazo M, McGee SL, Hargreaves M. Exercise and GLUT4. Exerc Sport Sci Rev 2020;48(3):110–8.

106. Guthold R, Stevens GA, Riley LM, et al. Global trends in insufficient physical ac-tivity among adolescents: a pooled analysis of 298 population-based surveys with 1·6 million participants. Lancet Child Adolesc Health 2020;4(1):23–35.

107. Katsoulis M, Pasea L, Lai AG, et al. Obesity during the COVID-19 pandemic: both cause of high risk and potential effect of lockdown? A population-based electronic health record study. Public Health 2021;191:41–7.

108. Rundle AG, Park Y, Herbstman JB, et al. COVID-19–related school closings and risk of weight gain among children. Obesity 2020;28(6):1008–9.

109. Khan MA, Menon P, Govender R, et al. Systematic review of the effects of pandemic confinements on body weight and their determinants. Br J Nutr 2021;1–74.

110. Popkin BM, Ng SW. Sugar-sweetened beverage taxes: lessons to date and the future of taxation. PLoS Med 2021;18(1):e1003412.

111. Teng AM, Jones AC, Mizdrak A, et al. Impact of sugar-sweetened beverage taxes on purchases and dietary intake: systematic review and meta-analysis. Obes Rev 2019;20(9):1187–204.

112. Krishnamoorthy Y, Ganesh K, Sakthivel M. Fat taxation in India: a critical appraisal of need, public health impact, and challenges in nationwide imple-mentation. Health Promotion Perspect 2020;10(1):8–12.

113. Taillie LS, Reyes M, Colchero MA, et al. An evaluation of Chile's Law of Food La-beling and Advertising on sugar-sweetened beverage purchases from 2015 to 2017: a before-and-after study. PLoS Med 2020;17(2):e1003015.

The Changing Nature of Mortality and Morbidity in Patients with Diabetes

Jonathan Pearson-Stuttard, FRSPH, MD[a,b,c,d,*],
James Buckley, MPH[a,b], Meryem Cicek, MPH[e],
Edward W. Gregg, PhD[a,b]

KEYWORDS

- Diabetes epidemiology • Diversification of mortality • Diversification of morbidity
- Multimorbidity • Chronic diseases

KEY POINTS

- The number of adults living with diabetes globally has increased substantially over the past 40 years.
- Death rates in high-income countries have reduced, driven in part by large declines in vascular disease mortality.
- There is evidence of a diversification of cause of death and complications in patients with diabetes.
- This has implications for prevention and management approaches targeting those with diabetes across the life course, which should reflect the breadth of conditions that these patients are at excess risk from.

BACKGROUND

The number of adults living with diabetes mellitus (DM) has increased globally over the past 40 years from 108 million to 422 million[1] owing to a rise in age-standardised prevalence, population growth, and aging. DM, therefore, represents a substantial challenge to individuals, health-care systems, and economies.

Individuals with DM are generally living longer, but an increasing portion of life lived is with DM,[2] which is likely to impact their morbidity profile. The high risk for those with

[a] Department of Epidemiology and Biostatistics, School of Public Health, Imperial College London, Norfolk Place, London W2 1PG, UK; [b] MRC Centre for Environment and Health, Imperial College London, Norfolk Place, London W2 1PG, UK; [c] Health Analytics, Lane Clark & Peacock LLP, 95 Wigmore Street, London W1U 1DQ, UK; [d] Northumbria Healthcare NHS Foundation Trust, North Shields NE27 0QJ, UK; [e] Department of Primary Care and Public Health, School of Public Health, Imperial College London, St Dunstan's Road, London W6 8RP, UK
* Corresponding author. Department of Epidemiology and Biostatistics, School of Public Health, Imperial College London, London W2 1PG, UK.
E-mail address: j.pearson-stuttard@imperial.ac.uk

Endocrinol Metab Clin N Am 50 (2021) 357–368
https://doi.org/10.1016/j.ecl.2021.05.001
0889-8529/21/© 2021 The Authors. Published by Elsevier Inc. This is an open access article under the CC BY license (http://creativecommons.org/licenses/by/4.0/).
endo.theclinics.com

DM of developing and subsequently dying from vascular disease has been well characterized, and the accompanying high risk of ischemic heart disease (IHD),[3] stroke,[3,4] and renal[5] and neuropathic complications[6] has led to widely implemented specific secondary prevention guidelines for these traditional DM complications.[7]

However, there is now evidence that the spectrum of complications of diabetes is far more diverse than that portrayed by traditional complications. This diversification is likely due to several complex factors including increased longevity, changing risk factors, and changing treatment profiles. Exploring and quantifying these trends will be crucial to ensure that both policy and clinical care directed at those living with DM accurately reflects the breadth of health challenges they face and how this continues to evolve. We aim to review the evidence of this proposed diversification and outline the current knowledge in order to identify what this means for persons with DM and the public health efforts needed.

DISCUSSION
Trends in All-Cause Mortality

Estimating trends in all-cause and cause-specific mortality among those with diabetes provides insight into factors driving longevity, conditions contributing to excess risk of death in those with diabetes compared with those without to inform secondary prevention, and care pathway approaches. Despite the importance of this, only a few studies assess these trends in large diabetes populations.

Over the past two decades, all-cause mortality rates have generally declined steadily in persons with type 2 DM (T2DM) in populations across the United States (US),[8] Australia,[9] Canada,[9] and England,[10,11] with declines of between 30% and 35% over approximately 20-year periods in both US and England populations.[8,11] Similarly, a general reduction in the absolute gap in all-cause mortality rates between those with and without DM has also been found.[8] In the United States, the excess mortality in those with DM almost halved from 11.3 to 5.9 per 1000 person years in 1994 and 2015, respectively.[8] While similarly large declines in excess risk of mortality were found in Canada and the United Kingdom,[10] the reduction in excess risk was much more modest in men in England, with around a 10% decline from 12.3 to 11.1 deaths per 1000 from 2001 to 2018,[11] compared with a decline in excess risk from 14.5 to 10.8 per 1000 per year in women over the same time period.

Mixed Trends in Cause-Specific Mortality

The well-established association between diabetes and increased incidence of coronary heart disease (CHD) and stroke led[12] to wide implementation of specific secondary prevention guidelines for these traditional DM complications.[7] These efforts have likely contributed to large consistent declines in cardiovascular disease (CVD) mortality in those with DM across populations. Improvements in cancer mortality rates in those with DM, however, have generally been much more modest, compared with improvements in CVD mortality and compared with cancer mortality in those without DM. In women in England, for example, the average 10-year absolute change in mortality rates improved in vascular diseases by 6.6 deaths per 1000 people compared with no improvement (−0.1 deaths per 1000 people) in cancer mortality rates.[11] Death rates appear to be increasing in two specific causes in those with DM. Dementia mortality rates have increased several-fold in those with DM and at a worse rate than those without DM, whereas liver disease death rates worsened by approximately 23% in England DM populations compared with small declines in US populations.[8,11]

Diversification of Cause of Death

Alongside this decline in all-cause mortality, there has been a diversification in the causes of death in those with diabetes. This is reflected in the proportional contribution of different causes to the total. As the mortality burden attributed to vascular disease[8,9,11] has declined substantially over the past 30 years,[8,9,11] from 48% to 34% of all deaths in patients with DM in the United States and, with even larger reductions, from 44% to 24% in those with DM in England, other causes now take up a much larger proportional share (**Fig. 1**). The portion of deaths due to cancer has remained stable in US DM populations, with nonvascular, noncancer causes of death increasing, whereas deaths due to cancer increased in England from 22% to 28% over an 18-year period, with similar findings in Australia. Most striking in England is that this transition of mortality burden away from vascular diseases led to cancers being both the leading cause of death and the leading contributor to excess mortality risk in those with DM compared with those without,[11] with an excess cancer mortality risk of 4.5 per 1000 per year compared with an excess vascular of mortality risk 3.2 per 1000 per year in 2018.

There are only limited estimates of trends in causes of death in DM populations, and those that exist tend to be from high-income countries, with much fewer data on mortality trends in low- and middle-income countries (LMICs), which now bear the majority of the global diabetes burden. New data, however, are increasingly suggest that as individuals are living longer with DM, they are experiencing a diversification in cause of death away from traditional complications of DM such as IHD and stroke. This suggests that secondary prevention measures that have targeted vascular risk factors over past decades, along with population improvements in some key behavioral risk factors such as trans fats, blood pressure, and cholesterol, have been effective. However, in order to reduce the DM-related excess mortality risk further, we must widen the targeted preventative measures for those with DM to reflect the spectrum of conditions they are at increased risk of dying from and developing throughout the life course.

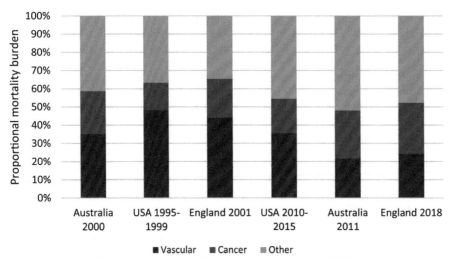

Fig. 1. Proportional mortality burden in those with diabetes attributable to vascular disease, cancers, or other disease in the United States, Australia, and England at time points over the past 25 years. (*Data from* Refs.[8,9,11])

DYNAMICS AND DIVERSIFICATION IN DIABETES-RELATED COMPLICATIONS

Diabetes complications have been traditionally classified into microvascular complications (eg, nephropathy, neuropathy, retinopathy), macrovascular complications (eg, stroke, CHD, peripheral vascular disease), and based on acute and chronic complications.[13] However, data from clinical settings have regularly shown that diabetes has far more diverse and wide-ranging effects on multiple organ systems than reflected in traditional complications. Furthermore, many of the most serious outcomes, such as lower extremity amputation (LEA), result from multiple simultaneous etiologic pathways.

Long-Term Trends in Incidence

There is now evidence from several population-based studies that the changing aspects of mortality among diabetes populations described previously are accompanied by, and possibly contributors to, changes in the spectrum of diabetes complications. In the United States, the incidence of diabetes-related complications as a whole declined by about half over 20 years, from 1990 to 2010.[6,14] Although there were reductions across a wide range of acute and chronic complications, the magnitude of decline was far greater for macrovascular diseases, particularly acute myocardial infarction (AMI), with decline by more than two-thirds over 2 decades, and stroke, hyperglycemic death, and LEAs, which declined by about half. The magnitude of decline was more modest, but still significant for end-stage renal disease (ESRD), which declined by about 30%. Importantly, the declines in diabetes-related complications were largely driven by older adults (aged >65 years) and only modest in young adults. This differential narrowed the age-related difference and the relative risk of most complications associated with age.

The differential trends in diabetes complications as per age and type have had three important effects on the character of population-wide diabetes-related complications in the United States. First, the age distribution of those with diabetes-related morbidity has shifted downward, such that persons younger than 65 years now account for about 90% of acute complication events, half of all events of microvascular complications, and 40% of all events of macrovascular disease.[6] Middle-aged adults now account for a third of strokes and more than half of amputations. Second, renal disease now takes up a greater proportion of all complications. This may also be true for microvascular disease complications in general, except that the lack of population-based data on incidence of retinopathy and neuropathy leaves this overall status of diabetes-related microvascular disease in the population unclear. A third by-product is that the combination of declining macrovascular disease complications and all-cause mortality, and perhaps a broader range of comorbid conditions, is permitting individuals with DM to live longer and develop second events. In the United States, rates of infections and cancers have not declined, and rates of other conditions not traditionally associated with diabetes, including chronic pulmonary disease and liver disease, have increased.[8] Furthermore, there is no clear evidence that levels of physical disability have declined.[14]

Similar trends in the incidence of LEA, CVD, and CVD mortality have been observed in several other countries of the world, most notably in Northern Europe.[15] A scoping review of international trends in diabetes complications revealed similar declines as those seen in the United States, Sweden, and South Korea and slightly more modest changes in Spain and the United Kingdom.[15] The review of the trends in LEAs has revealed declines in more than a dozen countries globally of varying magnitude both stronger and weaker than that seen in the United States. Reviews of ESRD have observed steady increases in several countries of the world but are based on a denominator of the general population, which partly reflects the growth in prevalence. There were no discernible variation in the magnitude of differences by region or specific country that could be inferred from these reviews because of the different metrics and population character-istics and because intervening factors are generally not assessed in surveillance-based analyses. However, it is noteworthy that virtually all the population-based studies of DM-related complications have been conducted in high-income countries of Europe, North America, or Asia. We are not aware of published population-based studies that provided comparative rates of complications in other major high-risk regions of the world for diabetes, including the Middle East/North Africa, India, China, or Latin America.

The factors driving trends are unclear because direct analyses to identify driving factors have not been conducted. Concurrent surveillance data revealed steady im-provements in HbA1c levels, blood pressure, and lipid levels in the general population in the United States and other countries, accompanying a general proliferation of integrated care to deliver preventive care practices and early screening for complica-tions. However, the factors that affect trends in the population are largely speculative because direct analyses have not been conducted. Most importantly, however, even at the time of the lowest overall rates of diabetes complications in the United States—around 2012—only a small minority of patients get all recommended preventive care practices, indicating there is an enormous opportunity to reduce diabetes-related morbidity through better implementation of evidence-based practices.

A recent update of rates from 2010 to 2018 raised concern about a potential resur-gence of diabetes complications, particularly in young adult populations with T2DM.[16] After the year 2010, rates of LEA and acute hyperglycemia increased by almost 50% among young patients (aged 20–44 years) along with smaller increases in rates of ESRD, AMI, and stroke. Increases in LEA, acute hyperglycemia, and stroke also increased in middle-aged (aged 45–64 years) US adults. Although rates of complications did not increase in older adults, the long-term improvements in all complications stalled after 2010. The explanations for this apparent reversal remain unclear, as to whether they are being paralleled by other countries. These findings paralleled other observations of increases in hospitalizations for infections and acute hyperglycemia.[17–19] Increasing duration of disease, stalled improvements in preventive care practices, and socioeco-nomic disparities related to the great recession seem to be the most likely factors.

DIABETES-RELATED MULTIMORBIDITY
Future of Diabetes-Related Multimorbidity

Improvements in secondary and tertiary prevention and related declines in mortality, combined with the diversification of complications, have driven a concern and emphasis in the diabetes-related multimorbidity. Multimorbidity is the coexistence of two or more chronic conditions that often produce cumulative adverse health effects. Multimorbidity is commonly quantified as descriptive estimations of disease combinations, using severity-weighted indices such as Charlson and Elixhauser indices, or as clusters. The commonest comorbidities in those with DM are hypertension, depression, coronary heart disease, asthma, and chronic kidney disease (CKD).[20] As age and relative depri-vation are the leading drivers of multimorbidity,[21] there is concern that continued aging of the population will lead to an expansion of diabetes-related multimorbidity over the next decade[22] and that this is likely to be felt most intensely in LMICs.[23] Despite the increasing awareness of multimorbidity as an increasingly urgent challenge, there is currently sparse detail to inform specific measures to address this.

Traditional, Emerging, and Other Complications

DM-related multimorbidity can be categorized into three general groups; traditional (concordant) complications, emerging complications, and other (discordant) comorbidities. Traditional complications—acute metabolic decompensation (hypo-glycemic and hyperglycemic episodes/crises), macrovascular conditions, and micro-vascular conditions—have been established for some time, and there are specific secondary prevention measures[7] in place for those with DM in order to mitigate this excess risk. Incidence of most of these traditional complications has declined, whereas hosptilizations for hypoglycaemic episodes have increased in young and middle-aged adults over recent decades.[24] Other vascular conditions such as heart failure are common in the T2DM population, with prevalence estimates of 2.7% to 3.6% at diagnosis.[20] There are several emerging conditions that have an increasing body of evidence to suggest a causal association with DM. Those with DM tend to have an increased risk of both signal[25] and common infections,[26] liver disease,[27] de-mentia,[28] and some site-specific cancers. Those with DM are estimated to have be-tween a 1.5- and 2.5 times as high risk of dementia than those without DM, while associations are increasingly clear for six common cancers—breast, endometrial, liver, colorectal, pancreas, and gallbladder.[29] Although this is estimated to account for nearly 300,000 cancer cases annually,[30] the etiological mechanism remains unclear; hence, there are no specific prevention measures in place to reduce this excess risk.

In addition to these traditional and emerging complications, whereby an etiological link with DM is proposed, there are other conditions that appear to be more prevalent in those with DM, even if there are no proposed etiological links. This other group includes a much broader set of discordant conditions that have a considerable impact on quality of life, physical functioning, and independence later in life. These conditions include mental ill-nesses such as depression and anxiety,[15] respiratory conditions,[31,32] and musculoskel-etal disorders.[33]

Depression is a very common discordant diabetes comorbidity that is illustrative of the increasing coprevalence of physical and mental health chronic conditions with onset in young and middle-aged adults. The primary link between diabetes and depression may be through common but distant third-degree factors such as corre-lated hormonal effects and inflammation. Depression is associated with lower quality of life and premature mortality in those with DM,[34,35] with an increasing consensus that this increased risk should be reflected in clinical care pathways.[35–38] However, similar to those emerging complications, we currently lack granular detail about the epidemi-ology of these comorbidities to inform specific action.

Who is at Risk of Diabetes Multimorbidity?

Age and relative deprivation are the leading drivers of multimorbidity in the general pop-ulation, and the same appears to be true in those with DM. Although the burden of comorbidities appears similar across sex groups, age affects both the likelihood and types of multimorbidity. The number of comorbidities accumulated increases in those with DM as individuals age and as the duration of DM increases[12] with clear age-related comorbidity profiles, such as gastritis and duodenitis (18- to 39-year-olds), tuberculosis and hepatitis (30- to 49-year-olds), frailty and dementia ($\geq$80-year-olds), and diversity of clusters increasing with age.[39] As traditional DM complications are more common among people with lower socioeconomic status,[40,41] it is perhaps unsur-prising that multimorbidity is higher in more deprived DM groups.[20] In such groups, CHD and asthma were more prevalent, which is suggestive of the role of behavioral risk fac-tors such as smoking or alcohol consumption in comorbidity profiles in those with DM.[20,35] Ethnicity is likely to impact risk and patterns of comorbidity in those with DM too. While there is scarce evidence currently estimating this, Black and Asian individuals are 2.36 and 1.1 times more likely to have poor glycemic control than white individuals in the United Kingdom,[41] which could be expected to impact the risk of vascular comorbidities and events. Similarly, early evidence suggests that non-Hispanic blacks and Hispanics bear the greatest burden of multimorbidity in the United States.[42–44]

Understanding How Conditions Cluster in Individuals with Diabetes

Disease surveillance systems can be leveraged to understand the network of nonrandom predictable clusters that comprise multimorbidity in wider populations and those with specific index chronic conditions such as DM.[45,46] Some of the emerging research in this relatively new field has used prevalence-driven pairwise techniques, and disease pairs that show co-occurrence frequencies, which are higher than predicted in the population, are considered connected.[47–49] Hypertension was the single most common condition among multimorbid patients with T2DM in a large UK cohort, with a higher prevalence among women than among men (45.8% vs 42.8%).[20] Musculoskeletal conditions, obesity, and hyperlipidemia made up the top 5 most common coprevalent conditions.[47,49] In the DM population, hypertension and CKD have the highest age-standardized coprevalence rate, with 12.1% at the time of diagnosis, increasing to 21.5% 9 years later[20] (**Fig. 2**). When considering three comorbid conditions concurrently, CVD, hypertension, and arthritis were the most prevalent ones found in 9.9% of patients with T2DM.[47] Hypertension is consistently found in the majority of T2DM-multimorbidity clusters of 2,[20,39,47,48] 3,[47,48] 4[50], and 5[50] comorbidities in several studies. However, the temporal sequence of multimorbidity in these T2DM populations is not well characterized.

Approaches such as latent class analyses, agglomerative, divisive hierarchical clustering,[39,50–52] and network and graph theory[53–55] have begun to identify patterns of comorbidities and trajectories of patient outcomes within specific subgroups. Some initial findings are perhaps expected, such as middle-aged men with T2DM and disorders of lipid metabolism being at a higher risk of major macrocardiovascular conditions, suggesting that dyslipidemia control is particularly important.[39] However, among older patients with long T2DM duration, there were more novel findings, identifying a cluster of conditions comprising depression, dementia, and end-stage organ complications.[35,56] This aligns with the American Diabetes Association guidelines for depression and dementia screening in elderly patients.[57]

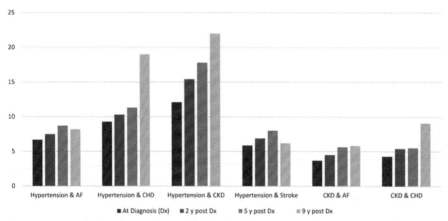

Fig. 2. Age-standardized prevalences of comorbidity combinations in those with diabetes at diagnosis and at 2, 5, and 9 years after diagnosis. (*Data from* Nowakowska M, Zghebi SS, Ashcroft DM, Buchan I, Chew-Graham C, Holt T, et al. The comorbidity burden of type 2 diabetes mellitus: patterns, clusters and predictions from a large English primary care cohort. BMC Medicine. 2019;17(1):145.)

Viewing the Impact of Diabetes Holistically

As those with DM are living longer than in previous decades, an increasing proportion of them live in poor health from an increasingly diverse set of conditions. The impact of DM on patients' lives has evolved our view of not only how we manage their holistic health throughout the duration of their condition but also how we measure this impact. Mortality risk has long been the metric of choice for assessing impacts of interventions, whether therapeutics or care pathways, but as patterns of health and illness have changed, other measures become as important to patient groups such as functionality or life lived in good health. Health-care resource utilization is a broad measure that captures the holistic impact on patients and health systems, although it is not without its limitations such as coding incentives that may distort trends. This could, however, provide clues for initial efforts to alleviate multimorbidity in those with DM. Not only would this improve the lived experience for those with DM, but given the large and diverse impacts on the health and care system along with the wider economy,[58–61] this approach would benefit health systems too. Although the patterns and sequence of multimorbidity will be unique to those with DM, the structural challenges are not. Multimorbidity is increasing as populations age, and these patients account for a disproportionately high share of increased primary and secondary care visits and hospital admissions,[35,48,62] particularly in those with a mental health comorbidity.[63]

Initial evidence suggests that older patients with moderate to long DM duration (>5 years), with depression, dementia, and end-organ complications, tend to have the most total inpatient admissions, whereas younger women with short to moderate T2DM duration and a high psychiatric burden had the most Accident & Emergency (A&E) and outpatient clinic visits.[35] As with the comorbidity burden, health-care utilization is also influenced by ethnicity and deprivation.[41,64] Uncertainty remains with regard to the leading drivers of ill health and health care usage in those with DM and related comorbidities.[65] Along with most health-care structures and training, specialties often sit in silos, which is increasingly divergent from the multimorbid patients treated by health systems.

Improvements in treatment and prevention over past decades have led to substantial gains in longevity for those with DM; to compress morbidity over coming decades, a shift of approach from single disease to multimorbidity is required. Health surveillance systems along with administrative data sets hold a plethora of untapped opportunities to provide insight to guide meaningful changes to those living with DM. These are substantial challenges to researchers, clinicians, and policymakers alike, but if tackled effectively, it could put life back into years lived for those with DM and provide a lifeline to health systems struggling under aging populations to do more with less.

Substantial improvements in longevity for those with DM over recent decades have been accompanied by a diversification in mortality, complications, and comorbidities throughout the life course. In parallel to this, the heterogeneity of trajectories in those with diabetes based on risk factors and yet-unknown factors appears to be increasing too. Rather than disease- and organ-focused approaches, holistic patient-centered approaches will be required across preventative and clinical pathways to compress morbidity in those with DM to improve the trajectories for DM patients and health systems alike. Unfortunately, however, population-level estimates of these trends are generally limited to high-income countries, with no comparable data in LMICs, severely limiting our understanding of trends in outcomes in DM populations in the majority of the world. Future efforts should promote stronger surveillance in LMICs in order to address these evidence gaps.

CLINICS CARE POINTS

- The prevalence of diabetes has increased substantially globally, but all-cause death rates have declined in several diabetes populations, driven in part by large declines in vascular disease mortality.
- There has been a diversification in cause of death, whereby a larger share of deaths in those with diabetes being attributable to nonvascular conditions, whereas the share of cancer deaths has remained stable or even increased in some countries.
- A similar pattern has emerged in complications but with large differences across age-groups so that around 90% of all acute complication events are in those younger than 65 years, whereas this is true for half of all events of microvascular complications and 40% of all events of macrovascular disease.
- Alongside this diversification, the health trajectory among those with diabetes appears to become more heterogenous based on both known and yet-unknown risk factors.
- Prevention and management approaches to those with diabetes should take a more holistic approach to encompass the breadth of condition-specific excess risk that these patients face.

DISCLOSURE

J. Pearson-Stuttard is supported by the Wellcome Trust 4i Programme at Imperial College London (203928/Z/16/Z). The authors also acknowledge the National Institute for Health Research (NIHR) Biomedical Research Center based at Imperial College Healthcare NHS Trust and Imperial College London. The views expressed are those of the author(s) and not necessarily those of the NHS, the NIHR or the Department of Health. J. Pearson-Stuttard is vice chairman of the Royal Society for Public Health, Partner at Lane Clark & Peacock LLP and reports personal fees from Novo Nordisk A/S all outside of the submitted work. All other authors declare no competing interests.

REFERENCES

1. (NCD-RisC) NRFC. Worldwide trends in diabetes since 1980: a pooled analysis of 751 population-based studies with 4.4 million participants. Lancet 2016; 387(10027):1513–30.
2. Muschik D, Tetzlaff J, Lange K, et al. Change in life expectancy with type 2 diabetes: a study using claims data from lower Saxony, Germany. Popul Health Metrics 2017;15(1):5.
3. Singh GM, Danaei G, Farzadfar F, et al. The age-specific quantitative effects of metabolic risk factors on cardiovascular diseases and diabetes: a pooled analysis. PLoS One 2013;8(7):e65174.
4. Genuth S, Eastman R, Kahn R, et al. Implications of the United kingdom prospective diabetes study. Diabetes Care 2003;26(Suppl 1):S28–32.
5. Fox CS, Matsushita K, Woodward M, et al. Associations of kidney disease measures with mortality and end-stage renal disease in individuals with and without diabetes: a meta-analysis. Lancet 2012;380(9854):1662–73.
6. Gregg EW, Li Y, Wang J, et al. Changes in diabetes-related complications in the United States, 1990–2010. N Engl J Med 2014;370(16):1514–23.
7. NICE. NICE Clinical Guidelines (NG28) - Type 2 diabetes in adults. Available at: https://www.nice.org.uk/guidance/ng28.
8. Gregg EW, Cheng YJ, Srinivasan M, et al. Trends in cause-specific mortality among adults with and without diagnosed diabetes in the USA: an

epidemiological analysis of linked national survey and vital statistics data. Lancet 2018;391(10138):2430–40.

9. Harding JL, Shaw JE, Peeters A, et al. Age-specific trends from 2000-2011 in all-cause and cause-specific mortality in type 1 and type 2 diabetes: a cohort study of more than one million people. Diabetes Care 2016;39(6):1018–26.

10. Lind M, Garcia-Rodriguez LA, Booth GL, et al. Mortality trends in patients with and without diabetes in Ontario, Canada and the UK from 1996 to 2009: a population-based study. Diabetologia 2013;56(12):2601–8.

11. Pearson-Stuttard J, Bennett J, Cheng YJ, et al. Trends in predominant causes of death in individuals with and without diabetes in England from 2001 to 2018: an epidemiological analysis of linked primary care records. Lancet Diabetes Endocrinol 2021;9(3):165–73.

12. Haffner SM, Lehto S, Rönnemaa T, et al. Mortality from coronary heart disease in subjects with type 2 diabetes and in nondiabetic subjects with and without prior myocardial infarction. N Engl J Med 1998;339(4):229–34.

13. (NIH) NIoH. Diabetes in America. 3rd ed. Bethesda, MD: NIH Pub; 2018.

14. CDC. Diabetes. 2020. Available at: www.cdc.gov/diabetes.

15. Harding JL, Pavkov ME, Magliano DJ, et al. Global trends in diabetes complications: a review of current evidence. Diabetologia 2019;62(1):3–16.

16. Gregg EW, Hora I, Benoit SR. Resurgence in diabetes-related complications. JAMA 2019;321(19):1867–8.

17. Harding JL, Benoit SR, Gregg EW, et al. Trends in rates of infections requiring hospitalization among adults with versus without diabetes in the U.S., 2000–2015. Diabetes Care 2020;43(1):106.

18. Benoit SR, Hora I, Albright AL, et al. New directions in incidence and prevalence of diagnosed diabetes in the USA. BMJ Open Diabetes Res Care 2019;7(1):e000657.

19. Geiss LS, Li Y, Hora I, et al. Resurgence of diabetes-related nontraumatic lower-extremity amputation in the young and middle-aged adult U.S. population. Diabetes Care 2019;42(1):50–4.

20. Nowakowska M, Zghebi SS, Ashcroft DM, et al. The comorbidity burden of type 2 diabetes mellitus: patterns, clusters and predictions from a large English primary care cohort. BMC Med 2019;17(1):145.

21. Marengoni A, Angleman S, Melis R, et al. Aging with multimorbidity: a systematic review of the literature. Ageing Res Rev 2011;10(4):430–9.

22. Kingston A, Robinson L, Booth H, et al. Projections of multi-morbidity in the older population in England to 2035: estimates from the population ageing and care simulation (PACSim) model. Age Ageing 2018;47(3):374–80.

23. Afshar S, Roderick PJ, Kowal P, et al. Multimorbidity and the inequalities of global ageing: a cross-sectional study of 28 countries using the World Health Surveys. BMC Public Health 2015;15:776.

24. Zhong VW, Juhaeri J, Cole SR, et al. Incidence and trends in hypoglycemia hospitalization in adults with type 1 and type 2 diabetes in England, 1998-2013: a retrospective cohort study. Diabetes Care 2017;40(12):1651–60.

25. Egede LE, Hull BJ, Williams JS. Infections associated with diabetes. Diabetes in America. 3rd edition. National Institutes of Health; 2017. NIH Pub No. 17-1468, pp. 30-31-30-25.

26. Pearson-Stuttard J, Blundell S, Harris T, et al. Diabetes and infection: assessing the association with glycaemic control in population-based studies. Lancet Diabetes Endocrinol 2016;4(2):148–58.

27. Tolman KG, Fonseca V, Dalpiaz A, et al. Spectrum of liver disease in type 2 diabetes and management of patients with diabetes and liver disease. Diabetes Care 2007;30(3):734.

28. Chatterjee S, Peters SA, Woodward M, et al. Type 2 diabetes as a risk factor for dementia in women compared with men: a pooled analysis of 2.3 million people comprising more than 100,000 cases of dementia. Diabetes Care 2016;39(2):300–7.

29. Tsilidis KK, Kasimis JC, Lopez DS, et al. Type 2 diabetes and cancer: umbrella review of meta-analyses of observational studies. BMJ 2015;350:g7607.

30. Pearson-Stuttard J, Zhou B, Kontis V, et al. Worldwide burden of cancer attributable to diabetes and high body-mass index: a comparative risk assessment. Lancet Diabetes Endocrinol 2018;6(6):e6–15.

31. Gläser S, Krüger S, Merkel M, et al. Chronic obstructive pulmonary disease and diabetes mellitus: a systematic review of the literature. Respiration 2015;89(3):253–64.

32. Ehrlich SF, Quesenberry CP Jr, Van Den Eeden SK, et al. Patients diagnosed with diabetes are at increased risk for asthma, chronic obstructive pulmonary disease, pulmonary fibrosis, and pneumonia but not lung cancer. Diabetes Care 2010;33(1):55–60.

33. Aga F, Dunbar SB, Kebede T, et al. The role of concordant and discordant comorbidities on performance of self-care behaviors in adults with type 2 diabetes: a systematic review. Diabetes Metab Syndr Obes 2019;12:333–56.

34. Holt RI, de Groot M, Golden SH. Diabetes and depression. Curr Diab Rep 2014; 14(6):491.

35. Seng JJB, Kwan YH, Lee VSY, et al. Differential health care use, diabetes-related complications, and mortality among five unique classes of patients with type 2 diabetes in Singapore: a latent class analysis of 71,125 patients. Diabetes Care 2020;43(5):1048–56.

36. Bădescu SV, Tătaru C, Kobylinska L, et al. The association between diabetes mellitus and depression. J Med Life 2016;9(2):120–5.

37. Hermanns N, Caputo S, Dzida G, et al. Screening, evaluation and management of depression in people with diabetes in primary care. Prim Care Diabetes 2013;7(1):1–10.

38. Roy T, Lloyd CE, Pouwer F, et al. Screening tools used for measuring depression among people with type 1 and type 2 diabetes: a systematic review. Diabet Med 2012;29(2):164–75.

39. Chen H, Zhang YY, Wu D, et al. Comorbidity in adult patients hospitalized with type 2 diabetes in northeast china: an analysis of hospital discharge data from 2002 to 2013. Biomed Res Int 2016;2016:9.

40. Hinton W, McGovern AP, Calderara S, et al. Ethnic and socioeconomic disparities in type 2 diabetes care: a trend analysis. Diabetologia 2017;60(1 Supplement 1):S344.

41. Whyte MB, Hinton W, McGovern A, et al. Disparities in glycaemic control, monitoring, and treatment of type 2 diabetes in England: A retrospective cohort analysis. PLoS Med 2019;16(10):e1002942.

42. Lynch CP, Gebregziabher M, Axon RN, et al. Geographic and racial/ethnic variations in patterns of multimorbidity burden in patients with type 2 diabetes. J Gen Intern Med 2015;30(1):25–32.

43. Gebregziabher M, Ward RC, Taber DJ, et al. Ethnic and geographic variations in multimorbidty: evidence from three large cohorts. Soc Sci Med 2018;211:198–206.

44. Lynch CP, Gebregziabher M, Zhao Y, et al. Impact of medical and psychiatric multimorbidity on mortality in diabetes: emerging evidence. BMC Endocr Disord 2014; 14(1):68.

45. Pearson-Stuttard J, Ezzati M, Gregg EW. Multimorbidity; a defining challenge for health systems. Lancet Public Health 2019;4(12):e599–600.

46. Whitty CJM. Triumphs and challenges in a world shaped by medicine. Royal College of Physicians; 2017.

47. Gruneir A, Markle-Reid M, Fisher K, et al. Comorbidity burden and health services use in community-living older adults with diabetes mellitus: a retrospective cohort study. Can J Diabetes 2016;40(1):35–42.

48. Lin PJ, Kent DM, Winn A, et al. Multiple chronic conditions in type 2 diabetes mellitus: prevalence and consequences. Am J Manag Care 2015;21(1):e23–34.

49. Luijks H, Schermer T, Bor H, et al. Prevalence and incidence density rates of chronic comorbidity in type 2 diabetes patients: an exploratory cohort study. BMC Med 2012;10:128.

50. Solomon TK, Rwebangira MR, Kurban G, et al, editors. Identifying subgroups of type II diabetes patients using cluster analysis. International Conference on Computational Science and Computational Intelligence (CSCI). Nevada, USA: IEEE; 2017.

51. Gao F, Chen J, Liu X, et al. Latent class analysis suggests four classes of persons with type 2 diabetes mellitus based on complications and comorbidities in Tianjin, China: a cross-sectional analysis. Endocr J 2017;64(10):1007–16.

52. Alonso-Moran E, Orueta JF, Esteban JIF, et al. Multimorbidity in people with type 2 diabetes in the Basque Country (Spain): Prevalence, comorbidity clusters and comparison with other chronic patients. Eur J Intern Med 2015;26(3):197–202.

53. Aguado A, Moratalla-Navarro F, López-Simarro F, et al. MorbiNet: multimorbidity networks in adult general population. Analysis of type 2 diabetes mellitus comorbidity. Sci Rep 2020;10(1):2416.

54. Khan A, Uddin S, Srinivasan U. Chronic disease prediction using administrative data and graph theory: The case of type 2 diabetes. Expert Syst Appl 2019; 136:230–41.

55. Khan A, Uddin S, Srinivasan U. Comorbidity network for chronic disease: a novel approach to understand type 2 diabetes progression. Int J Med Inform 2018; 115:1–9.

56. Li J, Shao YH, Gong YP, et al. Diabetes mellitus and dementia - a systematic review and meta-analysis. Eur Rev Med Pharmacol Sci 2014;18(12):1778–89.

57. Association AD. Introduction: standards of medical care in diabetes. Diabetes Care 2019;42(Supplement 1):S1–2.

58. McPhail SM. Multimorbidity in chronic disease: impact on health care resources and costs. Risk Manag Healthc Policy 2016;9:143–56.

59. Sum G, Hone T, Atun R, et al. Multimorbidity and out-of-pocket expenditure on medicines: a systematic review. BMJ Glob Health 2018;3(1):e000505.

60. Cannon A, Handelsman Y, Heile M, et al. Burden of illness in type 2 diabetes mellitus. J Manag Care Spec Pharm 2018;24(9-a Suppl):S5–13.

61. Hajat C, Stein E. The global burden of multiple chronic conditions: a narrative review. Prev Med Rep 2018;12:284–93.

62. Laiteerapong N, Gao Y, Cooper J, et al. Longitudinal A1C patterns and their associations with outcomes in type 2 diabetes. Diabetes 2015;64(SUPPL. 1):A415.

63. Calderon-Larranaga A, Abad-Diez JM, Gimeno-Feliu LA, et al. Global health care use by patients with type-2 diabetes: does the type of comorbidity matter? Eur J Intern Med 2015;26(3):203–10.

64. Mathur R, Palla L, Farmer RE, et al. Ethnic differences in the severity and clinical management of type 2 diabetes at time of diagnosis: a cohort study in the UK clinical practice research datalink. Diabetes Res Clin Pract 2020;160:108006.

65. Whitty CJM, MacEwen C, Goddard A, et al. Rising to the challenge of multimorbidity. BMJ 2020;368:l6964.

Screening for Diabetes and Prediabetes

Daisy Duan, MD[a], Andre P. Kengne, MD, PhD[b],
Justin B. Echouffo-Tcheugui, MD, PhD[a,c],*

KEYWORDS

- Screening • Prediabetes • Diabetes • Effectiveness • Cost-effectiveness

KEY POINTS

- Clinic-based opportunistic screening for prediabetes and diabetes among high-risk individuals is feasible using fasting plasma glucose and/or glycated hemoglobin.
- The management of screen-detected diabetes can be optimized using a multifactorial intervention that targets cardiovascular risk factors beyond glycemia.
- Prediabetes is primarily managed by lifestyle modification, but a select group of prediabetic individuals are eligible for initial metformin therapy.
- Screening for prediabetes and diabetes conducted at a 3-year interval is potentially cost-effective.

INTRODUCTION

Despite significant progress, screening for type 2 diabetes mellitus (T2DM) remains controversial, with a lack of uniform recommendation across professional organizations.[1–3]

There is a critical need for guidance on how to best use the available evidence, and thus implement an effective screening approach. Screening for prediabetes (ie, impaired glucose tolerance [IGT] and/or impaired fasting glucose [IFG]) and T2DM are inseparable, because they are part of a pathophysiologic continuum, are detected by the same tests, and have similar initial therapies (ie, lifestyle intervention and/or metformin). Trials conducted in various settings and populations have consistently shown the effectiveness of lifestyle modification and/or pharmacotherapy in preventing diabetes after identification of prediabetes.[4] However, most individuals with

[a] Division of Endocrinology, Diabetes and Metabolism, Department of Medicine, Johns Hopkins University School of Medicine, 5501 Hopkins Bayview Circle, Baltimore, MD 21224, USA; [b] Non-Communicable Diseases Research Unit, South African Medical Research Council, Francie van Zijl Drive Parowvallei, PO Box 19070, Tygerberg, Cape Town 7505, South Africa; [c] Welch Prevention Center for Prevention, Epidemiology and Clinical Research, Johns Hopkins University, Baltimore, MD, USA
* Corresponding author. 5501 Hopkins Bayview Circle, Baltimore, MD 21224.
E-mail address: jechouf1@jhmi.edu

Endocrinol Metab Clin N Am 50 (2021) 369–385
https://doi.org/10.1016/j.ecl.2021.05.002
endo.theclinics.com

prediabetes remain asymptomatic, and thus do not receive appropriate care.[5] More than 85% of US individuals with prediabetes are unaware of their diagnosis.[6] Consequently, screening for T2DM is a key first step for effective translation of diabetes prevention into practice.

This article presents a summary of the evidence to enhance clinician compliance with guideline-based diabetes preventive care.

RATIONALE FOR SCREENING
Extent of the Problem: Burden of Hyperglycemia

T2DM is highly prevalent in the United States. In 2018, 13% (34.1 million) of US adults had diabetes.[6] Strikingly, 21.4% of US adults with diabetes, or 2.8% of all US adults, had undiagnosed diabetes.[6] On a global scale, ~9.3% of the population (463 million people) had diabetes in 2019, and the prevalence is projected to increase to 10.9% by 2045.[7]

The risk of death among people with diabetes is twice that of those without diabetes.[8] Diabetes is the seventh leading cause of death in the United States.[6] Globally, diabetes contributed to 11.3% of deaths in 2019 (46.2% of deaths occurred in those younger than 60 years).[9] Among US adults, ~15% to 81% of those with T2DM have at least 1 cardiovascular complication.[10] The prevalence of chronic kidney disease in patients with T2DM is 43.5%,[11] and diabetes is the most common primary cause of end-stage renal disease (46.7% of cases).[12] Diabetic retinopathy is the leading cause of new cases of blindness among adults aged 20 to 74 years in developed countries.[13] Peripheral arterial disease, foot ulceration, and amputations are more prevalent among people with diabetes than those without it.[14]

The burden of diabetes is likely to increase over time, given the high prevalence of prediabetes. In 2018, 34.5% of US adults (88 million) had prediabetes.[6] Globally, there are 374 million adults with prediabetes, and nearly 540 million adults will have prediabetes by 2045.[7] Compared with normoglycemia, there is an increased risk of cardiovascular disease (CVD) in those with prediabetes.[15] Microvascular disease may also complicate prediabetes.[4]

The financial burden of diabetes is astoundingly high in the United States. Diabetes-related costs totaled $327 billion in 2017, which was a 25% increase from 2012.[16] The diabetes-related US medical expenditures in 2017 reached nearly $404 billion, representing a monetary burden averaging $1240 for each American.[17] Diabetes is associated with a substantially high lifetime medical expenditures, with ~ $124,600 excess lifetime spending when diagnosed at age 40 years.[18] Globally, diabetes imposes an enormous economic burden with an estimated global cost of US$1.31 trillion, accounting for 1.8% of the world gross domestic product.[19]

Identifiable Preclinical Phase

The natural history of dysglycemia is well understood, and includes an asymptomatic phase comprising 2 states: (1) prediabetes with an estimated duration of 8.5 to 10.3 years,[20] and (2) preclinical latent diabetes (after biological onset of the disease) that lasts at least 4 to 7 years.[21] Prediabetes includes the intermediate states of abnormal glucose regulation (IFG and/or IGT) preceding overt biological diabetes, and is associated with a high risk of progression to diabetes.[4] Latent diabetes refers to the time frame between the biological onset of diabetes and the clinical diagnosis of the disease. The public health burden of latent diabetes is reflected in the substantial proportion of undiagnosed diabetes (21.4% of all diabetes cases in the US population[6]).

The rationale for prediabetes screening includes the significant progression rate to T2DM, effectiveness of interventions for diabetes prevention, and the macrovascular and microvascular complications associated with prediabetes. Prediabetes (IFG and/ or IGT) is associated with a high risk of progression to overt T2DM. A meta-analysis found relative risks for diabetes of 4.32 for IFG defined using the American Diabetes Association (ADA) criteria, 5.47 for IFG defined using the World Health Organization (WHO) criteria, 3.61 for IGT, 6.90 for IFG and IGT, 5.55 for glycated hemoglobin (HbA$_{1C}$) level greater than 5.7%, and 10.10 for HbA$_{1C}$ level greater than 6.0%.[22] Moreover, there have been landmark studies showing the effectiveness of intensive lifestyle modification and drugs for preventing T2DM.[4] In addition, prediabetes increases the risks of macrovascular and microvascular diseases.[4]

Screening for preclinical diabetes is critical given the complications and morbidities already present at the time of the clinical diagnosis of diabetes. Hyperglycemia-related tissue damage is often already present during the asymptomatic T2DM stage. Approximately 50% of people with screen-detected diabetes already have macrovascular (coronary artery disease [CAD])[23] or microvascular complications (retinopathy, nephropathy, and neuropathy)[24] at diagnosis. In the Hoorn Screening Study, myocardial infarction (13.3% vs 3.4%), CAD (39.5% vs 24.1%), and retinopathy (7.6% vs 1.9%) were more frequent in screen-detected patients than in newly conventionally diagnosed patients.[23–25] In the Anglo-Danish-Dutch Study of Intensive Treatment In People with Screen Detected Diabetes in Primary Care (ADDITION)-Denmark, approximately 6.8% of screen-detected people with diabetes had retinopathy at diagnosis.[26]

TESTING FOR HYPERGLYCEMIA

The approaches to screen for prediabetes or diabetes include risk scoring tools and biochemical tests.

Risk Scores

Various risk models, consisting of a combination of known risk factors, have been developed to identify people at high risk of T2DM,[27] who account for most of the people with T2DM. These models involve the use of self-reported questionnaires, health service data, or newly collected data (anthropometric, lifestyle, or biochemical). Scores based on routinely collected clinical information may be more appropriate for clinical use. Using questionnaires or existing health service data may be more convenient because it allows population stratification before blood glucose testing, thus limiting those who undergo blood glucose testing to 20% to 25% of the overall population. However, such an approach relies on the availability of data on key variables. Clinic-derived risk scores may be convenient and widely available, and they have the best discriminatory accuracy in the populations in which they were developed. The external validation of these risk scores in other populations tends to be moderate to poor.[27] The extant risk assessment tools for prediabetes are limited by poor methodology and lack of data on calibration and external validation, and thus are not yet ready for clinical practice.[28]

In the United States, the most widely validated and simple-to-use risk screening tool is the ADA's diabetes risk test (https://www.diabetes.org/risk-test),[29] intended to identify asymptomatic adults who need glycemic assessment. However, the US Preventive Services Task Force (USPSTF) does not endorse the use of any specific risk tool.[2] The implementation of risk assessment tools in clinical practice is limited.[30] In a report, only 10 of the 65 available noninvasive diabetes risk assessment tools developed worldwide had been implemented in clinical practice.[30] Barriers to the implementation of these tools include factors related to health care providers (perceived lack of accuracy, lack of time and reimbursement support, and interference with physician-patient interaction) and patients (lack of perceived severity of T2DM; fear of complexity of the test; cultural and/or language barriers; uncertainties about next steps after identification of high risk of diabetes; and subsequent fear of the disease, treatment, and cost of care).[30] Strategies are needed to enhance the implementation of diabetes risk scores in daily clinical practice.

Biochemical Tests

The advantages and limitations of diabetes screening tests are summarized in **Table 1**.

The 75-g oral glucose tolerance test

The 75-g oral glucose tolerance test (OGTT) is accepted as the gold standard diagnostic test for diabetes and prediabetes. Both the ADA and WHO endorse the 2-hour postprandial glucose (2hPG) cutoff of 140 to 199 mg/dL for diagnosing prediabetes and greater than or equal to 200 mg/dL for diagnosing diabetes.[1,31] OGTT distinguishes between IFG and IGT, which represent distinct phenotypes, with their co-occurrence conferring a greater risk for diabetes than either alone.[32] IGT may be a better predictor of outcomes than fasting plasma glucose (FPG) or HbA$_{1C}$. Indeed, 2hPG is an independent predictor of diabetes, CVD, and mortality, beyond FPG and

Table 1
Practical advantages and limitations of biochemical screening tests for diabetes

Test	Advantages	Limitations
Random blood glucose	Easy to obtain; no fasting required; inexpensive	Prompt processing (<2 h) needed, thus the high risk of errors; measurement can be affected by numerous factors (eg, short-term lifestyle changes, time since prior meal)
Fasting plasma glucose	Cheap and simple; single plasma glucose level measured; highly correlated with presence of complications	Patient needs to fast overnight (at least 8 h); potential for processing error; measurement can be affected by short-term lifestyle changes; risks of phlebotomy
75-g Oral glucose tolerance test	Gold standard for the diagnosis of diabetes; most sensitive test for impaired glucose tolerance	Requires 8-h fast, lengthy, and requires commitment of nurse staff; overall test-retest reproducibility lower than with other tests
HbA$_{1C}$	Stable long-term glycemic marker; no fasting required; not affected by short-term lifestyle changes; requires venous blood or a point-of-care testing capillary sample; lower intraindividual variability (<2%) than fasting plasma glucose	Value may vary with assay method used; potential errors related to nonglycemic factors such as hemoglobinopathies and anemia; insensitive for detection of IGT; costly compared with glucose testing; limited availability in some areas of the world

HbA_{1C}, and thus could provide enhanced assessment of risk outcomes.[33] OGTT can detect additional cases not captured by other tests; for example, in a study, OGTT uncovered 5.6% and 20.7% of diabetes and prediabetes, not meeting diagnostic criteria based on HbA_{1C}.[34]

The routine use of OGTT is limited by the need for an overnight fast, a lengthy testing time, higher cost, intraindividual variability, differences in glucose absorption rates, and low reproducibility.[35] OGTT is almost never performed as the initial screening test for nonpregnant adults.

Random plasma glucose

The use of random plasma glucose (RPG) is limited by its low performance. An expert panel has recommended that RPG level 130 to 199 mg/dL (sensitivity of 63% and specificity of 87%) be considered a positive screening test for diabetes, based on validation against OGTT.[36] RPG may be helpful for patients who have a routine chemistry panel drawn for reasons other than diabetes, termed serendipitous screening. Individuals with glucose levels suggestive of diabetes would then undergo confirmatory tests. RPG would rarely ever serve as the initial screening test in ambulatory patients.

Fasting plasma glucose

FPG has modest sensitivity for hyperglycemia screening. The current cutoff of 7.0 mmol/L (126 mg/dL) for diabetes diagnosis has a sensitivity of 56% and specificity of 97.7%, when validated against 75-g OGTT.[37] IFG, defined as 100 to 125 mg/dL (5.6–6.9 mmol/L) by the ADA, was reduced from 110 to 125 mg/dL (6.1–6.9 mmol/L) in 2003 in order to optimize the sensitivity and specificity of predicting future diabetes.[38] Even with this lower threshold, FPG alone may detect 27.4% of individuals with prediabetes, compared with 87.1% of cases detected using a complete OGTT.[39]

Glycated hemoglobin

The ADA and WHO endorse HbA_{1C} for diabetes diagnosis.[1,40] As a screening tool, the current cutoff value of 6.5% has a sensitivity of 68.4% and specificity of 95.9% for the diagnosis of diabetes as validated with OGTT data.[37] The convenience of HbA_{1C} compared with FPG and OGTT should be balanced against its pitfalls,[41] including the genetic, hematologic, and illness-related factors that affect test accuracy, as well as age-related and ethnicity-related variations. The use of HbA_{1C} for defining prediabetes is complicated by varying definitions. ADA defines prediabetes with an HbA_{1C} level of 5.7% to 6.4%,[1] whereas the International Expert Committee uses HbA_{1C} of 6.0% to 6.4% to define high risk of developing diabetes.[42] The WHO has not endorsed the use of HbA_{1C} for prediabetes diagnosis.[40] A meta-analysis found HbA_{1C} to be neither sensitive nor specific for detecting prediabetes, with a mean sensitivity of 49% and specificity of 79% for prediabetes identification.[43]

Combining FPG and HbA_{1C} testing may be an optimal and accurate approach to identifying diabetes and prediabetes, but is not always the case in clinical practice. A community-based study showed that single-sample confirmatory testing for diagnosing diabetes has a high positive predictive value, and thus supports the use of a combination of increased FPG and HbA_{1C} levels from a single blood sample to identify undiagnosed diabetes.[44]

BENEFITS OF SCREENING FOR HYPERGLYCEMIA
Effectiveness of Screening

Randomized trials comparing people offered and not offered screening provide the highest level of evidence on the effect of screening for diabetes on morbidity and mortality. The ADDITION-Cambridge trial (with concurrent screening and no-screening groups) found that 1-time diabetes screening did not reduce mortality (all-cause, cardiovascular, or other causes) over 9.6 years.[45] A 7-year follow-up study on a subsample of the ADDITION-Cambridge (15% from the screening group and 40% from the no-screening group) reported no significant differences in self-reported cardiovascular morbidity.[46] A parallel-group population-based cohort UK (Ely) study found that diabetes screening (vs no screening) did not reduce all-cause mortality[47] or microvascular and macrovascular complications over 12 years of follow-up.[48] In contrast, the nonrandomized ADDITION-Denmark study found that the risk of CVD and mortality were lower in the screening group compared with a retrospectively constructed no-screening control group.[49] In a Swedish population-based cohort study, compared with clinically detected diabetes, patients with screen-detected diabetes had lower rates of all-cause mortality, CVD, renal disease, and retinopathy.[50] However, the aforementioned results may not be directly applicable to the US environment, because several contextual factors need consideration. The ADDITION-Cambridge study and the Ely studies were conducted in the United Kingdom, which has a good primary care infrastructure, and found only 3% with undiagnosed diabetes.[45,47] The United States has a less well-organized primary care system, which contributes to more cases of undiagnosed diabetes, as reflected in the high US prevalence of undiagnosed T2DM (21.4%).[6] Most participants in ADDITION were white, limiting the translation of findings to other racial/ethnic groups, more present in the United States.

Tight control of glucose, blood pressure, and lipid levels in screen-detected individuals can reduce diabetes-related cardiovascular and microvascular complications, as described in the UK Prospective Diabetes Study (UKPDS) and Steno-2 trials.[51,52] In the ADDITION-Europe (United Kingdom, Denmark, and Netherlands) trial, intensive treatment of multiple risk factors after diabetes screening led to small but significant improvements in HbA_{1C} level, blood pressure, and cholesterol level, with a nonsignificant reduction in CVD events compared with routine care group,[53] a tendency that persisted at 10-year follow-up.[54] Microvascular outcomes were also not significantly different between the routine care and the intensive management groups in the ADDITION-Europe study.[55] A simulation study using data from ADDITION-Europe estimated the absolute risk reduction of cardiovascular outcomes associated with screening and routine treatment to be 3.3% and 4.9% in the scenarios of a 3-year and 6-year delay in the diagnosis and treatment of diabetes, with relative risk reductions of 29% and 38% respectively.[56]

There are no clinical trials that directly evaluate the benefits of screening for prediabetes. However, landmark clinical trials have shown that diabetes can be prevented among individuals with prediabetes.[4] In these trials, over a 3-year to 6-year period, lifestyle interventions (dietary changes plus increased physical activity) reduced the incidence of diabetes by 28% to 58% compared with the placebo or minimal intervention groups.[4] In the US Diabetes Prevention Program (DPP) trial, metformin reduced the incidence of diabetes by 31% among people with prediabetes.[57] There was also a long-term reduction in diabetes incidence at 15-year posttrial follow-up caused by lifestyle modification.[58] In the Chinese Da Qing Study, diabetes prevention was associated with a reduction in diabetes incidence during the 6-year trial period[59] and after 30 years in the posttrial period.[60] The lifestyle modification was also associated with significantly decreased risks of CVD, cardiovascular deaths, microvascular disease (including a 40% reduction in severe retinopathy), and all-cause mortality after 30 years.[60]

Psychosocial Impact of Screening for Hyperglycemia

Studies have found limited or no psychological effect of screening on people with newly detected T2DM. The ADDITION-Cambridge trial showed no adverse psychosocial effect of diabetes screening. In the short and long term, the anxiety level, illness perception, and self-rated health of participants invited to screening (with or without diabetes at screening) do not differ from those of patients not invited, whether immediately after the test, at 6 weeks, at 3 to 6 months, or at 12 to 15 months.[61,62] In those who were tested, the screening outcome (positive or negative for diabetes) was not associated with anxiety or depression at 12 months.[63] Negative screening test results do not promote false reassurance (expressed as lower perceived risk, lower intentions for health-related behavioral change, or higher self-rated health)[64] or negatively affect health behaviors (smoking, alcohol consumption, dietary intake, or physical activity).[46]

The psychological effect of receiving a diagnosis of prediabetes remains unclear. Studies suggest that participation in a DPP is not associated with higher levels of anxiety, depression, or overall psychological distress than that of the general population,[65,66] but it is possibly associated with a better health-related quality of life,[67] and with lower levels of depression.[68]

Cost-Effectiveness of Screening for Hyperglycemia

A limited number of real-life studies have assessed the cost-effectiveness of prediabetes or diabetes screening. A simulation study postulated that diabetes prevention may avoid $124,600 and $91,200 in lifetime medical spending if a new case of diabetes can be prevented at age 40 years and age 50 years respectively.[18] Simulations have shown that diabetes prevention using lifestyle modification and metformin is cost-effective among patients with prediabetes (with longer duration of evaluation enhancing cost-effectiveness);[69] which is corroborated by actual cost data from DPP.[70] Furthermore, the nonrandomized ADDITION-Denmark showed that the modest cost of a diabetes screening program was offset within 2 years by savings in the health care system.[71] Overall, the economic studies of diabetes screening indicate that (1) screening for both IGT and diabetes would be cost-effective, (2) universal screening would be less cost-effective than targeted screening of high-risk groups, and (3) the single most important determinant of cost-effectiveness is treatment.[69,72]

Screening Intervals

The exact frequency of screening for diabetes is not known. There are no robust real-world data to rely on for the determination of an optimal screening frequency. A US-based simulation including individuals aged 45 to 74 years found that screening every 3 years yielded a good balance between true-positives and false-positives.[73] A more recent US-based simulation suggested that targeted screening for undiagnosed T2DM would be most cost-effective if started in the age range 30 to 45 years and repeated every 3 to 5 years.[74] In a UK cohort of diabetes-free individuals aged 40 to 65 years, a 5-year screening interval identified diabetes an average of 3.3 years earlier.[48] In a Japanese cohort of healthy adults, rescreening at intervals shorter than 3 years led to identification of less than or equal to 1% of incident diabetes.[75] Based on economic modeling studies and expert opinions, professional organizations have generally favored a 3-year interval.[1,2]

TREATMENT OF SCREEN-DETECTED DIABETES OR PREDIABETES

Therapies shown to be effective in preventing complications in people with clinically diagnosed diabetes, particularly macrovascular complications, can reasonably be applied to those with screen-detected disease. These therapies include optimal glycemic control,[52] lipid level–lowering therapy for CVD prevention,[76] antihypertensive treatment,[77] and aspirin therapy for CVD prevention when indicated.[78]

Multifactorial interventions have been studied in screen-detected individuals with diabetes. The ADDITION-Europe trial compared routine care of newly screen-detected T2DM with intensive multifactorial treatment to reduce cardiovascular outcomes[53] using an intervention modeled after the regimen used in the Steno-2 trial. The Steno-2study showed that intensified multifactorial intervention (lifestyle modification and multidrug therapy) to control cardiovascular risk factors was more cost-effective (in reducing macrovascular and microvascular complications and all-cause mortality) than standard therapy among people with long-standing T2DM and microalbuminuria.[51,79] In ADDITION Europe, intensive multifactorial treatment (targeting several cardiovascular risk factors) of screen-detected individuals with T2DM over 5 years provided a nonsignificant 17% reduction in a composite cardiovascular primary end point favoring intensive treatment compared with routine care, as well as in all individual components (12% reduction in cardiovascular deaths, 30% reduction in nonfatal myocardial infarction, and 21% reduction in revascularization).[53] There were also significant improvements in CVD risk factors (systolic and diastolic blood pressure, and total and low-density lipoprotein cholesterol),[53] and the frequency of microvascular complications (retinopathy and neuropathy) was lower for the intensive treatment group, but was not significant.[55] Both the macrovascular and microvascular results may partly be explained by improvements in the quality of diabetes care during the trial period, a phenomenon that can happen in any screening trial. The 10-year follow-up analysis of ADDITION-Europe showed that reductions in cardiovascular risk factors (weight, HbA_{1C}, blood pressure, and cholesterol) were sustained in both groups, but there was a nonsignificant 13% reduction in the composite cardiovascular primary end point, as well as nonsignificant reductions in individual CVD outcomes, including myocardial infarction (28% reduction), stroke (26% reduction) and revascularization (13% reduction), and in all-cause mortality (10% reduction).[54]

In recent years, the landscape of T2DM therapies has changed with the advent of glucagon-like peptide 1 (GLP-1) receptor agonists and sodium-glucose cotransporter 2 (SGLT2) inhibitors.[80] It is reasonable to think that although the current cardiovascular trials have been conducted in patients with established CVD or at very high risk for CVD, the cardiovascular benefits would translate to those with screen-detected diabetes.

As a result of diabetes detection programs, individuals with prediabetes are also identified. At present, less than one-third of prediabetic patients identified in clinical practice in the United States currently receive any therapy.[5] Prediabetic individuals can be effectively managed with lifestyle intervention and/or pharmacotherapy, with a stronger evidence for lifestyle intervention.[4] Trials showed that, over a 3-year to 6-year period, lifestyle interventions (dietary changes plus increased physical activity) reduced the incidence of diabetes by 28% to 58% compared with the placebo or minimal intervention (standard of care) groups.[4] The lifestyle interventions can be translated into real-life practice with the same level of beneficial effect as in the original trials.[81]

In the trials, the effects of lifestyle modification on the reduction of diabetes incidence persisted for 10 to 30 years after discontinuation of the active intervention, depending on the study.[4] In the Da Qing study, compared with the control group, the lifestyle modification group experienced significant reductions in the risks of CVD events, cardiovascular death, microvascular disease, and overall mortality over a 30-year period.[60]

Although multiple drugs (metformin, pioglitazone, troglitazone, rosiglitazone, acarbose, orlistat, voglibose, and liraglutide) have been tested for diabetes prevention,[4] most agents carry concerns regarding their costs, side effects, and lack of persistence of effect. Metformin has the best long-term safety profile, tolerability, and efficacy, and is therefore recommended by the ADA for preventing diabetes.[82] Metformin is most effective compared with lifestyle in patients with body mass index (BMI) of at least 35 kg/m^2, in younger patients (<60 years of age), and in women with prior gestational diabetes mellitus.[82]

CURRENT SCREENING RECOMMENDATIONS IN THE UNITED STATES

The available evidence does not support universal diabetes screening. Consequently, most professional organizations advocate a selective and opportunistic approach in high-risk populations (**Table 2**), including the ADA,[1] the US Preventive Services Task Force (USPSTF),[1,2] and the Endocrine Society,[3] which recommend diabetes screening at a 3-year interval but yearly among patients with prediabetes.[1,23]

The ADA recommends that patients detected with prediabetes be referred to an effective ongoing support program modeled on the DPP intervention. For patients with BMI greater than or equal to 35 kg/m^2, aged less than 60 years, and women with a history of gestational diabetes, metformin should be considered.[1,2]

The USPSTF and ADA recommendations were developed after a rigorous process of systematic review of the available evidence, and thus have a more reliable basis for clinical practice. However, the USPSTF guidelines include a more targeted population, with studies indicating that implementation of the USPSTF screening recommendations may miss close to half of those with undiagnosed diabetes.[83–85] A modeling study showed that the ADA guidelines would detect 38.9% more cases of prediabetes and 24.3% more cases of T2DM than the USPSTF guidelines. Because the most updated USPSTF guidelines have a set of limited criteria and a set of expanded criteria, a cross-sectional analysis found that using the limited criteria resulted in a sensitivity of 47.3% and specificity of 71.4%, whereas the expanded criteria yielded a higher sensitivity of 76.8% with a lower specificity of 33.8%.[86] In comparison, ADA recommendations would capture more individuals with undiagnosed diabetes with a sensitivity of 88.8% to 97.7% but with less specificity, ranging from 13.5% to 39.7%.[87]

Overall, targeted screening in individuals aged 45 years and older with additional risk factors as recommended by the ADA and USPSTF has been shown to be cost-effective.[88]

A special consideration is needed for ethnic/racial minorities, in whom the prevalence of diabetes and its related complications is higher than among white people. In 2017 to 2018, diabetes frequency was highest among American Indian/Alaska Natives (14.7%), followed by people of Hispanic origin (12.5%), non-Hispanic black people (11.7%), and non-Hispanic Asian people (9.2%), and lowest in non-Hispanic white people (7.5%).[6] Non-Hispanic black people have the highest rates of diabetes-related end-stage renal disease, and hospitalizations for lower extremity amputations and stroke.[6] The 2015 USPSTF recommendations included expanded criteria, recommending that the following racial/ethnic groups be considered for screening at a younger age or at a lower BMI than the traditional target population: African Americans, American Indians or Alaskan Natives, Asian Americans, Hispanic or Latino

Table 2
Diabetes and prediabetes screening recommendations from major professional organizations in the United States

Organization	ADA	USPSTF	Endocrine Society
Screening Criteria	1. Overweight or obese adults (BMI greater than or equal to 25 kg/m² or greater than or equal to 23 kg/m² in Asian Americans) with greater than or equal to 1 risk factor: • First degree relative with diabetes • High-risk race/ethnicity (eg, African American, Latino, Native American, Asian American, Pacific Islander) • History of CVD • Hypertension • HDL-cholesterol <35 mg/dL and/or triglyceride >250 mg/dL • PCOS • Physical inactivity • Other clinical conditions associated with insulin resistance (eg, severe obesity, acanthosis nigricans) 2. Patients with prediabetes 3. Women with prior diagnosis of GDM 4. For all other patients, testing should begin at age 45 years	1. Adults aged 40–70 years who are overweight or obese 2. Consider screening earlier in persons with greater than or equal to 1 risk factor: • Family history of diabetes •History of GDM or PCOS •Racial/ethnic groups (African American, American Indian or Alaskan Native, Asian American, Hispanic or Latino, or Native Hawaiian or Pacific Islander)	1. Adults aged 40–75 years, screen for all 5 components of metabolic risk: • Increased blood pressure • Increased waist circumference • Increased fasting triglyceride level • Low HDL-cholesterol level • Increased glycemia
Screening Tests	1. FPG 2. 75-g OGTT 3. HbA$_{1c}$	1. FPG 2. 75-g OGTT 3. HbA$_{1c}$	1. FPG 2. 75-g OGTT 3. HbA1c
Rescreening Intervals	1. Patients with prediabetes should be tested annually 2. Women with prior diagnosis of GDM should have lifelong testing at least every 3 y 3. For all other patients, rescreen at a minimum of 3-y intervals, with consideration of more frequent testing depending on initial results and risk status	Every 3 y	1. Patients with prediabetes should be tested at least annually 2. If do not yet have atherosclerotic CVD or T2DM and already have greater than or equal to 1 risk factor, screen every 3 y

Abbreviations: CVD, cardiovascular disease; FPG, fasting plasma glucose; GDM, gestational diabetes mellitus; HbA1c, glycosylated hemoglobin; HDL, high density lipoprotein; OGTT, oral glucose tolerance test; PCOS, polycystic ovary syndrome.

people, and Native Hawaiians or Pacific Islanders.[2] A study of the 2015 USPSTF criteria showed that the use of the limited screening criteria (without consideration of race/ethnicity as a separate risk factor) has a limited sensitivity for detecting dysglycemia in all minority groups.[86] This finding was more evident among Asian people, who are known to have an increased risk for developing diabetes at a lower BMI cutoff.[89] In another study, racial/ethnic minorities detected with dysglycemia using USPSTF screening criteria were younger and/or had a more normal weight compared with white people.[90] Lastly, the 2015 USPSTF systematic review of the evidence identified a significant research gap in evaluating the risks and benefits of screening on racial/ethnic minorities.[91]

SUMMARY

Screening for diabetes or prediabetes is dictated by the burden of the conditions; the recognizable prediabetic and prolonged latent diabetic phases; and the availability of reliable, high-performance, and widely acceptable detection tests. Screening for diabetes or prediabetes does not seem to have adverse psychosocial consequences. There are accepted and cost-effective treatments (lifestyle modification and metformin) for diabetes prevention, but the effect of these therapies on cardiovascular outcomes remains to be unequivocally proved. There is an incremental benefit of intensive multifactorial therapy compared with current standards in people with screen-detected diabetes. Economic models support targeted screening for both prediabetes and diabetes. Overall, there is adequate evidence to justify the implementation of opportunistic screening for undiagnosed diabetes and prediabetes among asymptomatic high-risk individuals, preferably using the ADA or USPSTF criteria, with a rescreening interval of 3 years.

CLINICS CARE POINTS

- Undiagnosed type 2 diabetes and prediabetes are frequent and generally asymptomatic disorders, and thus can be detected early.
- Opportunistic screening for undiagnosed type 2 diabetes or prediabetes in the clinical setting can be done among high-risk individuals at a 3-year frequency and using FPG and/or glycosylated hemoglobin.
- Screen-detected type 2 diabetes is treated using a multifactorial approach (lifestyle modification and drugs) targeting glycemia and other cardiovascular risk factors.
- Prediabetes is best addressed using lifestyle modification and metformin in a select number of cases.

DISCLOSURE

The authors have no conflict of interest related to this article. Dr J.B. Echouffo-Tcheugui was supported by NIH/NHLBI grant K23 HL153774. Dr D. Duan was supported by NIH/NHLBI grant 5T32HL110952.

REFERENCES

1. American Diabetes Association. 2. Classification and Diagnosis of Diabetes: Standards of Medical Care in Diabetes-2021. Diabetes Care 2021;43(Suppl 1): S15–33.

2. Siu AL. Screening for abnormal blood glucose and type 2 diabetes mellitus: U.S. preventive services task force recommendation statement. Ann Intern Med 2015; 163(11):861–8.

3. Rosenzweig JL, Bakris GL, Berglund LF, et al. Primary Prevention of ASCVD and T2DM in Patients at Metabolic Risk: An Endocrine Society* Clinical Practice Guideline. J Clin Endocrinol Metab 2019. https://doi.org/10.1210/jc.2019-01338.

4. Echouffo-Tcheugui JB, Selvin E. Pre-Diabetes and What It Means: The Epidemiological Evidence. Annu Rev Public Health 2021;42:59–77.

5. Karve A, Hayward RA. Prevalence, diagnosis, and treatment of impaired fasting glucose and impaired glucose tolerance in nondiabetic U.S. adults. Diabetes Care 2010;33(11):2355–9.

6. Centers for Disease Control and Prevention. National Diabetes Statistics Report, 2020. Estimates of Diabetes and Its Burden in the United State. 2020. Available at: https://www.cdc.gov/diabetes/pdfs/data/statistics/national-diabetes-statistics-report.pdf. Accessed February 18, 2021.

7. Saeedi P, Petersohn I, Salpea P, et al. Global and regional diabetes prevalence estimates for 2019 and projections for 2030 and 2045: Results from the International Diabetes Federation Diabetes Atlas, 9th edition. Diabetes Res Clin Pract 2019;157:107843.

8. Gu K, Cowie CC, Harris MI. Mortality in adults with and without diabetes in a National cohort of the U.S. Population, 1971-1993. Diabetes Care 1998;21(7): 1138–45.

9. Gregg EW, Cheng YJ, Srinivasan M, et al. Trends in cause-specific mortality among adults with and without diagnosed diabetes in the USA: an epidemiological analysis of linked national survey and vital statistics data. Lancet 2018; 391(10138):2430–40.

10. Vaidya V, Gangan N, Sheehan J. Impact of cardiovascular complications among patients with Type 2 diabetes mellitus: A systematic review. Expert Rev Pharmacoeconomics Outcomes Res 2015;15(3):487–97.

11. Bailey RA, Wang Y, Zhu V, et al. Chronic kidney disease in US adults with type 2 diabetes: An updated national estimate of prevalence based on Kidney Disease: Improving Global Outcomes (KDIGO) staging. BMC Res Notes 2014;7:415.

12. US Renal Data System. 2018 UKRDS Annual Data Report | Volume 2: ESRD in the United States - Chapter 1: Incidence, Prevalence, Patient Characteristics, and Treatment Modalities. Am J Kidney Dis 2019;73(3):S291–332.

13. Yau JWY, Rogers SL, Kawasaki R, et al. Global prevalence and major risk factors of diabetic retinopathy. Diabetes Care 2012;35(3):556–64.

14. Gregg EW, Gu Q, Williams D, et al. Prevalence of lower extremity diseases associated with normal glucose levels, impaired fasting glucose, and diabetes among U.S. adults aged 40 or older. Diabetes Res Clin Pract 2007;77(3):485–8.

15. Cai X, Zhang Y, Li M, et al. Association between prediabetes and risk of all cause mortality and cardiovascular disease: updated meta-analysis. BMJ 2020;370: m2297.

16. Yang W, Dall TM, Beronjia K, et al. Economic costs of diabetes in the U.S. in 2017. Diabetes Care 2018;41(5):917–28.

17. Dall TM, Yang W, Gillespie K, et al. The economic burden of elevated blood glucose levels in 2017: Diagnosed and undiagnosed diabetes, gestational diabetes mellitus, and prediabetes. Diabetes Care 2019;42(9):1661–8.

18. Zhuo X, Zhang P, Barker L, et al. The lifetime cost of diabetes and its implications for diabetes prevention. Diabetes Care 2014;37(9):2557–64.

19. Bommer C, Heesemann E, Sagalova V, et al. The global economic burden of diabetes in adults aged 20–79 years: a cost-of-illness study. Lancet Diabetes Endocrinol 2017;5(6):423–30.

20. Bertram MY, Vos T. Quantifying the duration of pre-diabetes. Aust N Z J Public Health 2010;34(3):311–4.

21. Harris MI, Klein R, Welborn TA, et al. Onset of NIDDM occurs at least 4-7 yr before clinical diagnosis. Diabetes Care 1992;15(7):815–9.

22. Richter B, Hemmingsen B, Metzendorf MI, et al. Development of type 2 diabetes mellitus in people with intermediate hyperglycaemia. Cochrane Database Syst Rev 2018;10(10):CD012661.

23. Spijkerman AMW, Henry RMA, Dekker JM, et al. Prevalence of macrovascular disease amongst type 2 diabetic patients detected by targeted screening and patients newly diagnosed in general practice: The Hoorn Screening Study. J Intern Med 2004;256(5):429–36.

24. Spijkerman AMW, Dekker JM, Nijpels G, et al. Microvascular complications at time of diagnosis of type 2 diabetes are similar among diabetic patients detected by targeted screening and patients newly diagnosed in general practice: The Hoorn Screening Study. Diabetes Care 2003;26(9):2604–8.

25. Spijkerman AMW, Adriaanse MC, Dekker JM, et al. Diabetic patients detected by population-based stepwise screening already have a diabetic cardiovascular risk profile. Diabetes Care 2002;25(10):1784–9.

26. Bek T, Lund-Andersen H, Hansen AB, et al. The prevalence of diabetic retinopathy in patients with screen-detected type 2 diabetes in Denmark: the ADDITION study. Acta Ophthalmol 2009;87(3):270–4.

27. Abbasi A, Peelen LM, Corpeleijn E, et al. Prediction models for risk of developing type 2 diabetes: Systematic literature search and independent external validation study. BMJ 2012;345:e5900.

28. Barber SR, Davies MJ, Khunti K, et al. Risk assessment tools for detecting those with pre-diabetes: A systematic review. Diabetes Res Clin Pract 2014;105(1):1–13.

29. Herman WH, Smith PJ, Thompson TJ, et al. A new and simple questionnaire to identify people at increased risk for undiagnosed diabetes. Diabetes Care 1995;18(3):382–7.

30. Dhippayom T, Chaiyakunapruk N, Krass I. How diabetes risk assessment tools are implemented in practice: A systematic review. Diabetes Res Clin Pract 2014;104(3):329–42.

31. World Health Organization. Definition and Diagnosis of Diabetes Mellitus and Intermediate. Geneva (Switzerland): World Health Organization; 2006.

32. Meigs JB, Muller DC, Nathan DM, et al. Baltimore Longitudinal Study of Aging. The natural history of progression from normal glucose tolerance to type 2 diabetes in the Baltimore Longitudinal Study of Aging. Diabetes 2003;52(6):1475–84.

33. Lu J, He J, Li M, et al. Predictive value of fasting glucose, postload glucose, and hemoglobin A1c on risk of diabetes and complications in Chinese adults. Diabetes Care 2019;42(8):1539–48.

34. Meijnikman AS, De Block CEM, Dirinck E, et al. Not performing an OGTT results in significant underdiagnosis of (pre)diabetes in a high risk adult Caucasian population. Int J Obes 2017;41(11):1615–20.

35. Bartoli E, Fra GP, Schianca GPC. The oral glucose tolerance test (OGTT) revisited. Eur J Intern Med 2011;22(1):8–12.

36. Saudek CD, Herman WH, Sacks DB, et al. A new look at screening and diagnosing diabetes mellitus. J Clin Endocrinol Metab 2008;93(7):2447–53.

37. Hoyer A, Rathmann W, Kuss O. Utility of HbA1c and fasting plasma glucose for screening of Type 2 diabetes: a meta-analysis of full ROC curves. Diabet Med 2018;35(3):317–22.

38. Genuth S, Alberti KGMM, Bennett P, et al. Follow-up Report on the Diagnosis of Diabetes Mellitus. Diabetes Care 2003;26(11):3160–7, 39.

39. Cheng C, Kushner H, Falkner BE. The utility of fasting glucose for detection of prediabetes. Metabolism 2006;55(4):434–8.

40. World Health Organization. Report of a world health organization Consultation: use of glycated haemoglobin (HbA1c) in the diagnosis of diabetes mellitus :Abbreviated report of a WHO Consultation. Geneva (Switzerland): World Health Organization; 2011.

41. Bergman M, Abdul-Ghani M, DeFronzo RA, et al. Review of methods for detecting glycemic disorders. Diabetes Res Clin Pract 2020;165:108233.

42. Nathan DM, Balkau B, Bonora E, et al. International Expert Committee report on the role of the A1C assay in the diagnosis of diabetes. Diabetes Care 2009; 32(7):1–8.

43. Barry E, Barry E, Roberts S, et al. Efficacy and effectiveness of screen and treat policies in prevention of type 2 diabetes: systematic review and meta-analysis of screening tests and interventions. BMJ 2017;356:i6538.

44. Selvin E, Wang D, Matsushita K, et al. Prognostic implications of single-sample confirmatory testing for undiagnosed diabetes: a prospective cohort study. Ann Intern Med 2018;169(3):156–64.

45. Simmons RK, Echouffo-Tcheugui JB, Sharp SJ, et al. Screening for type 2 diabetes and population mortality over 10 years (ADDITION-Cambridge): A cluster-randomised controlled trial. Lancet 2012;380(9855):1741–8.

46. Echouffo-Tcheugui JB, Simmons RKRK, Prevost ATT, et al. Long-Term effect of population screening for diabetes on cardiovascular morbidity, self-rated health, and health behavior. Ann Fam Med 2015;13(2):149–57.

47. Simmons RK, Rahman M, Jakes RW, et al. Effect of population screening for type 2 diabetes on mortality: Long-term follow-up of the Ely cohort. Diabetologia 2011; 54(2):312–9.

48. Rahman M, Simmons RK, Hennings SH, et al. How much does screening bring forward the diagnosis of type 2 diabetes and reduce complications? Twelve year follow-up of the Ely cohort. Diabetologia 2012;55(6):1651–9.

49. Simmons RK, Griffin SJ, Lauritzen T, et al. Effect of screening for type 2 diabetes on risk of cardiovascular disease and mortality: a controlled trial among 139,075 individuals diagnosed with diabetes in Denmark between 2001 and 2009. Diabetologia 2017;60(11):2192–9.

50. Feldman AL, Griffin SJ, Fhärm E, et al. Screening for type 2 diabetes: do screen-detected cases fare better? Diabetologia 2017;60(11):2200–9.

51. Gæde P, Lund-Andersen H, Parving H-H, et al. Effect of a Multifactorial Intervention on Mortality in Type 2 Diabetes. N Engl J Med 2008;358(6):580–91.

52. Holman RR, Paul SK, Bethel MA, et al. 10-year follow-up of intensive glucose control in type 2 diabetes. N Engl J Med 2008;359(15):1577–89.

53. Griffin SJ, Borch-Johnsen K, Davies MJ, et al. Effect of early intensive multifactorial therapy on 5-year cardiovascular outcomes in individuals with type 2 diabetes detected by screening (ADDITION-Europe): A cluster-randomised trial. Lancet 2011;378(9786):156–67.

54. Griffin SJ, Rutten GEHM, Khunti K, et al. Long-term effects of intensive multifactorial therapy in individuals with screen-detected type 2 diabetes in primary care: 10-year follow-up of the ADDITION-Europe cluster-randomised trial. Lancet Diabetes Endocrinol 2019;7(12):925–37.

55. Sandbæk A, Griffin SJ, Sharp SJ, et al. Effect of early multifactorial therapy compared with routine care on microvascular outcomes at 5 years in people with screen-detected diabetes: A randomized controlled trial. The ADDITION-Europe study. Diabetes Care 2014;37(7):2015–23.

56. Herman WH, Ye W, Griffin SJ, et al. Early detection and treatment of type 2 diabetes reduce cardiovascular morbidity and mortality: A simulation of the results of the Anglo-Danish-Dutch study of intensive treatment in people with screen-detected diabetes in primary care (ADDITION-Europe). Diabetes Care 2015; 38(8):1449–55.

57. Knowler WC, Barrett-Connor E, Fowler SE, et al. Reduction in the incidence of type 2 diabetes with lifestyle intervention or metformin. N Engl J Med 2002; 346(6):393–403.

58. Diabetes Prevention Program Research Group, Nathan DM, Barrett-Connor E, et al. Long-term effects of lifestyle intervention or metformin on diabetes development and microvascular complications over 15-year follow-up: The Diabetes Prevention Program Outcomes Study. Lancet Diabetes Endocrinol 2015;3(11): 866–75.

59. Pan XR, Li GW, Hu YH, et al. Effects of diet and exercise in preventing NIDDM in people with impaired glucose tolerance: The Da Qing IGT and diabetes study. Diabetes Care 1997;20(4):537–44.

60. Gong Q, Zhang P, Wang J, et al. Morbidity and mortality after lifestyle intervention for people with impaired glucose tolerance: 30-year results of the Da Qing Diabetes Prevention Outcome Study. Lancet Diabetes Endocrinol 2019;7(6):452–61.

61. Park P, Simmons RK, Prevost AT, et al. Screening for type 2 diabetes is feasible, acceptable, but associated with increased short-term anxiety: A randomised controlled trial in British general practice. BMC Public Health 2008;8:350.

62. Eborall HC, Griffin SJ, Prevost AT, et al. Psychological impact of screening for type 2 diabetes: Controlled trial and comparative study embedded in the ADDITION (Cambridge) randomised controlled trial. BMJ 2007;335(7618):486–9.

63. Paddison CAM, Eborall HC, French DP, et al. Predictors of anxiety and depression among people attending diabetes screening: A prospective cohort study embedded in the ADDITION (Cambridge) randomized control trial. Br J Health Psychol 2011;16(1):213–26.

64. Paddison CAM, Eborall HC, Sutton S, et al. Are people with negative diabetes screening tests falsely reassured? Parallel group cohort study embedded in the ADDITION (Cambridge) randomised controlled trial. BMJ 2010;340(7737):84.

65. Giel KE, Enck P, Zipfel S, et al. Psychological effects of prevention: Do participants of a type 2 diabetes prevention program experience increased mental distress? Diabetes Metab Res Rev 2009;25(1):83–8.

66. Rubin RR, Knowler WC, Ma Y, et al. Depression symptoms and antidepressant medicine use in diabetes prevention program participants. Diabetes Care 2005;28(4):830–7.

67. Florez H, Pan Q, Ackermann RT, et al. Impact of lifestyle intervention and metformin on health-related quality of life: the diabetes prevention program randomized trial. J Gen Intern Med 2012;27(12):1594–601.

68. Ruusunen A, Voutilainen S, Karhunen L, et al. How does lifestyle intervention affect depressive symptoms? Results from the Finnish Diabetes Prevention Study. Diabet Med 2012;29(7):e126–32.

69. Roberts S, Barry E, Craig D, et al. Preventing type 2 diabetes: Systematic review of studies of cost-effectiveness of lifestyle programmes and metformin, with and without screening, for pre-diabetes. BMJ Open 2017;7(11):e017184.

70. Diabetes Prevention Program Research Group. The 10-Year Cost-Effectiveness of Lifestyle Intervention or Metformin for Diabetes Prevention. Diabetes Care 2012;35(4):723–30.

71. Sortsø C, Komkova A, Sandbæk A, et al. Effect of screening for type 2 diabetes on healthcare costs: a register-based study among 139,075 individuals diagnosed with diabetes in Denmark between 2001 and 2009. Diabetologia 2018; 61(6):1306–14.

72. Waugh NR, Shyangdan D, Taylor-Phillips S, et al. Screening for type 2 diabetes: A short report for the National Screening Committee. Health Technol Assess (Rockv) 2013;17(35):1–89.

73. Johnson SL, Tabaei BP, Herman WH. The efficacy and cost of alternative strategies for systematic screening for type 2 diabetes in the U.S. population 45-74 years of age. Diabetes Care 2005;28(2):307–11.

74. Kahn R, Alperin P, Eddy D, et al. Age at initiation and frequency of screening to detect type 2 diabetes: a cost-effectiveness analysis. Lancet 2010;375(9723): 1365–74.

75. Takahashi O, Farmer AJ, Shimbo T, et al. A1C to detect diabetes in healthy adults: When should we recheck? Diabetes Care 2010;33(9):2016–7.

76. Costa J, Borges M, David C, et al. Efficacy of lipid lowering drug treatment for diabetic and non-diabetic patients: Meta-analysis of randomised controlled trials. BMJ 2006;332(7550):1115–8.

77. Turner R, Holman R, Stratton I, et al. Tight blood pressure control and risk of macrovascular and microvascular complications in type 2 diabetes: UKPDS 38. BMJ 1998;317(7160):703–13.

78. De Berardis G, Sacco M, Strippoli GFM, et al. Aspirin for primary prevention of cardiovascular events in people with diabetes: Meta-analysis of randomised controlled trials. BMJ 2009;339(7732):1238.

79. Gæde P, Vedel P, Larsen N, et al. Multifactorial Intervention and Cardiovascular Disease in Patients with Type 2 Diabetes. N Engl J Med 2003;348(5):383–93.

80. Das SR, Everett BM, Birtcher KK, et al. 2020 Expert Consensus Decision Pathway on Novel Therapies for Cardiovascular Risk Reduction in Patients With Type 2 Diabetes: A Report of the American College of Cardiology Solution Set Oversight Committee. J Am Coll Cardiol 2020;76(9):1117–45.

81. Ali MK, Echouffo-Tcheugui J, Williamson DF. How effective were lifestyle interventions in real-world settings that were modeled on the diabetes prevention program? Health Aff 2012;31(1):67–75.

82. American Diabetes Association. 3. Prevention or Delay of Type 2 Diabetes: Standards of Medical Care in Diabetes-2020. Diabetes Care 2021;44(Suppl 1):S34–9.

83. Sheehy AM, Flood GE, Tuan W-JJ, et al. Analysis of guidelines for screening diabetes mellitus in an ambulatory population. Mayo Clin Proc 2010;85(1):27–35.

84. Casagrande SS, Cowie CC, Fradkin JE. Utility of the U.S. Preventive Services Task Force criteria for diabetes screening. Am J Prev Med 2013;45(2):167–74.

85. Chung S, Azar KMJ, Baek M, et al. Reconsidering the age thresholds for type II diabetes screening in the U.S. Am J Prev Med 2014;47(4):375.

86. O'Brien MJ, Bullard KMK, Zhang Y, et al. Performance of the 2015 US Preventive Services Task Force Screening Criteria for Prediabetes and Undiagnosed Diabetes. J Gen Intern Med 2018;33(7):1100–8.

87. Bullard KMK, Ali MK, Imperatore G, et al. Receipt of glucose testing and performance of two us diabetes screening guidelines, 2007-2012. PLoS One 2015; 10(4):e0125249.

88. Li R, Zhang P, Barker LE, et al. Cost-effectiveness of interventions to prevent and control diabetes mellitus: A systematic review. Diabetes Care 2010;33(8): 1872–94.

89. Hsu WC, Araneta MRG, Kanaya AM, et al. BMI cut points to identify at-Risk asian americans for type 2 diabetes screening. Diabetes Care 2015;38(1):150–8.

90. O'Brien MJ, Lee JY, Carnethon MR, et al. Detecting Dysglycemia Using the 2015 United States Preventive Services Task Force Screening Criteria: A Cohort Analysis of Community Health Center Patients. Plos Med 2016;13(7):e1002074.

91. Selph S, Dana T, Blazina I, et al. Screening for type 2 diabetes mellitus: A systematic review for the U.S. preventive services task force. Ann Intern Med 2015; 162(11):765–76.

Prevention of Type 2 Diabetes

Mary Beth Weber, MPH, PhD[a],*, Saria Hassan, MD[a,b], Rakale Quarells, PhD[c],
Megha Shah, MD, MSc[d]

KEYWORDS

- Type 2 diabetes • Implementation and dissemination research • Prevention
- Prediabetes • Global health

KEY POINTS

- There is strong evidence for the efficacy and effectiveness of lifestyle interventions for diabetes prevention.
- Lifestyle interventions are not equally effective for all types of prediabetes, with the strongest evidence of effectiveness among those with impaired glucose tolerance or impaired glucose tolerance + impaired fasting glucose. Further research is needed to identify if and/or which lifestyle interventions are effective for reducing risk among individuals with isolated impaired fasting glucose.
- Implementation of proven programs faces unique challenges in the United States and globally.
- Well-designed implementation studies that consider the needs and realities of different communities, populations, and settings and clearly describe program adaptations are needed to increase successful scaling and dissemination of diabetes prevention interventions at the community level.

INTRODUCTION

Worldwide, a staggering number, an estimated 463 million people, have diabetes,[1] 90% to 95% of which is type 2 diabetes. This amount of people with diabetes has resulted in a significant burden, financially and in terms of population health and well-being.[1–3] In addition, a large population is at increased risk of developing type 2 diabetes; globally approximately 374 million people have impaired glucose tolerance

[a] Hubert Department of Global Health, Rollins School of Public Health, Emory University, 1518 Clifton Road, NE, Atlanta, GA 30322, USA; [b] Department of Medicine, Emory University School of Medicine, 100 Woodruff Circle, Atlanta, GA 30322, USA; [c] Cardiovascular Research Institute, Morehouse School of Medicine, 720 Westview Drive, SW NCPC-318, Atlanta, GA 30310, USA; [d] Department of Family and Preventive Medicine, Emory University School of Medicine, 100 Woodruff Circle, Atlanta, GA 30322, USA
* Corresponding author.
E-mail address: mbweber@emory.edu

Endocrinol Metab Clin N Am 50 (2021) 387–400
https://doi.org/10.1016/j.ecl.2021.05.003
0889-8529/21/© 2021 Elsevier Inc. All rights reserved.

(IGT; a type of prediabetes),[1] an underestimate of the true prediabetes burden, as impaired fasting glucose (IFG), another type of prediabetes, occurs more frequently in some race/ethnic groups.[4,5]

A reduction in the global burden of diabetes requires improved identification and treatment of diabetes and its complications but also an increased focus on implementing proven diabetes prevention programs in communities and clinics. Herein, the authors summarize the current evidence for type 2 diabetes prevention in the United States and globally. They consider lifestyle interventions, programs promoting diabetes risk reduction through diet improvement, increased physical activity, and/or weight loss, including efficacy trials and downstream implementation studies. They also discuss the challenges to effective implementation of proven programs and potential solutions. Finally, the authors present some possible future directions for diabetes prevention research.

CURRENT EVIDENCE
Efficacy of Lifestyle Interventions for Diabetes Prevention or Delay

Data from randomized controlled trials of individuals with IGT unequivocally show that lifestyle modification reduces diabetes incidence, improves glycemic control, and has beneficial effects on diabetes risk factors and its complications.[6–12] In the largest diabetes prevention study (n = 3234), the US Diabetes Prevention Program (DPP), trained lifestyle coaches delivered one-on-one, individualized education and guidance to help participants improve health behaviors, overcome barriers, and reach study goals (≥7% weight loss and ≥150 minutes of weekly, moderate-level physical activity).[13] The DPP reported a 58% reduction in diabetes incidence in intervention participants compared with controls.[9] A meta-analysis of randomized controlled trials of diabetes prevention studies reported that lifestyle interventions were associated with a 39% reduction in diabetes risk compared with controls (relative risk = 0.61, 95% confidence interval [CI] 0.54–0.68).[14]

Lifestyle programs have proven effectiveness in a variety of settings and populations, with positive results reported in studies in the United States, India, Europe, and China[9,10,15,16] and within the DPP, across age, sex, body mass index group, and race-ethnic identity.[9] Studies have shown reductions in diabetes risk even among those at highest risk for conversion to diabetes, including older adults and participants with a history of gestational diabetes, the highest levels of insulin sensitivity, and increased genetic risk for diabetes.[9,17,18]

Implementation of proven diabetes prevention programs could have wide-reaching impacts on public health. Efficacy trials have shown that effects of lifestyle intervention are long lasting. After 23 years of follow-up, Da Qing Diabetes Prevention Study participants had a 45% reduction in cumulative diabetes incidence (hazard ratio [HR]: 0.55, 95% CI, 0.40–0.76) and reductions in both cardiovascular and all-cause mortality (HR: 0.59, 95% CI, 0.36–0.96 and HR: 0.71, 95% CI, 0.51–0.99, respectively).[19] Participants in the DPP and the Da Qing Study whose glycemic levels returned to normal, even transiently, were less likely to develop diabetes[20] and lower incidence of cardiovascular and microvascular diseases[21,22] than participants who did not reach normoglycemia. In addition, the DPP, the Finnish Diabetes Prevention Study, and the Indian Diabetes Prevention Programme (IDPP) all reported that the lifestyle intervention in each program was cost-effective.[23–25]

Lifestyle interventions have resulted in diabetes prevention in some, but not all people with prediabetes. Studies in individuals with isolated impaired fasting glucose (iIFG) have not shown the same outcomes. A lifestyle intervention program in Japan was highly effective among individuals with IFG + IGT (HR: 0.41, 95% CI, 0.24–0.69) but did not reduce diabetes risk among individuals with iIFG (HR: 1.17, 95% CI, 0.50–2.74).[26] Similarly, the Diabetes Community Lifestyle Improvement Program (D-CLIP) study in India reported only a 12% relative risk reduction for diabetes in the iIFG group compared with 31% and 39% relative risk reductions in the iIGT and IFG + IGT groups, respectively.[27] Effective interventions for diabetes prevention among individuals with iIFG are needed.

Even so, based on the strong data from randomized controlled trials supporting lifestyle intervention for diabetes prevention, expert organizations, including the American, European, and Canadian Diabetes Associations, recommend lifestyle programs for diabetes prevention in high-risk groups.[28–30] In the United States and globally, there is a growing body of implementation and translation research describing the successes and challenges of delivering these proven programs at the clinic and community levels. Although these implementation studies show lower impact than efficacy studies, they do show that implementation of proven diabetes prevention programs in real-world settings can lead to improvements in participants' weight, glucose, and physical activity and reductions in diabetes risk.[31–33]

Implementation/Dissemination in the United States

The Centers for Disease Control and Prevention (CDC) created the National Diabetes Prevention Program (NDPP) to disseminate the DPP broadly in the United States.[33] The evidence-based curriculum materials, developed in collaboration with partners, are available to the public in multiple languages free of charge. The NDPP focuses on the 4 following key components to reach large-scale implementation: (1) training to increase the delivery workforce; (2) a recognition program to for quality assurances (Diabetes Prevention Recognition Program); (3) health marketing to improve uptake of the program; and (4) intervention sites and payment models to support sustainability, including the United States' largest private health insurer, United Health Group, and the YMCA.[34]

Participant-level analysis of the first 4 years of NDPP implementation through CDC-recognized sites demonstrated clinically meaningful findings. Participants attended a median of 14 sessions, and 35.5% achieved the 5% weight loss goal (average weight loss 4.2%, median 3.1%). Participants reported a weekly average of 152 minutes of physical activity with more than 40% meeting the physical activity goal (≥150 minutes per week).[33]

Even with these efforts, NDPP dissemination remains low. National survey data analyses show very low referral rates to CDC-recognized DPPs (<5%) and general weight loss programs (~20%) among at-risk individuals, and of those referred to programs, less than 40% report engaging.[35] In the NDPP, retention was low with less than half of participants continuing the program for more than 6 months.[33] Other studies have reported similar results, with low and dropping rates of participant engagement during the intervention period.[36,37] Given that participants who remain in the DPP for 6 months or more are more likely to achieve weight loss and activity goals,[33] there is an imperative need to better understand and address challenges to participant engagement.

Community-based and virtual adaptations

Although scaling proven interventions to real-world settings with diverse populations has been challenging with inconsistent outcomes, there are several examples of successful implementation of such programs. For example, participants in the DEPLOY Pilot Study at YMCAs showed significant reductions in weight, cholesterol, and blood pressure compared with baseline,[38] whereas the PREDICT Study, a church-based DPP program for African Americans, demonstrated feasibility yet no difference in weight loss between groups that did and did not receive the intervention.[39]

Cultural and linguistic adaptations have greatly improved the reach of the DPP,[40] and several studies have taken a community-based participatory research approach and/or sought stakeholder or community feedback to inform DPP adaptations in hopes of improving outcomes.[41] Resulting adaptations have included curriculum changes (eg, incorporation of faith-based content,[42] reducing session number,[40] incorporating additional hands-on exercise or cooking/food education[43]), group/family-based approaches,[44,45] or use of community health workers (CHW)/peer coaches.[40] Not all adaptations have been successful. For example, curriculum updates to reflect the psychosocial stressor of historical trauma did not increase success in a DPP translation for American Indian and Alaska Natives.[46]

Format adaptations to include peer support, lay health educators, and community leaders have demonstrated feasibility and acceptability in minority communities, without significant differences in outcomes.[31,47] The PREVENT-DM trial, which compared a CHW-led DPP translation for Hispanic women with metformin-only or control reported the greatest weight loss in the CHW-led group.[48] Other implementation studies have sought to optimize limited community resources by reducing DPP session number with some studies showing similar weight loss and HbA1c outcomes in shorter programs[49] and other studies reporting higher weight loss in programs with fewer modifications.[50]

DPP implementation trials are often of shorter duration and lack data on diabetes outcomes, instead relying on intermediate outcomes like weight. Among these, weight loss is low, potentially due in part to lower retention and engagement of participants in community-based programs.[51–53] Retention is markedly low in younger participants and racial/ethnic minorities.[41,51] Among African Americans in DPP translation studies, attendance ranges from 33% to 72%, and weight loss is markedly less.[54] Similarly, an NDPP study from Colorado found that Latinx, blacks, young adults, and uninsured individuals were less likely to achieve the 5% weight loss goal.[55] These findings support the need for continued cultural adaptation of diabetes prevention interventions but also the importance of implementation process evaluation to understand the factors contributing to reduced effectiveness in these populations.

As efforts to adapt and implement the DPP have grown, so too have the exploration and the need to incorporate novel technology and formats to meet the needs of various populations at risk for diabetes. One of the earliest adaptions was the use of telehealth to deliver the DPP curriculum. In partnership with local health systems, Montana's Department of Public Health implemented a version of the DPP using video conferencing. The completed study of 894 participants, comparing participation in the video conference format to in-person delivery of the NDPP, reported no significant differences between study arms in the number of sessions attended or percentage of participants reaching weight loss goals of 5% or 7%.[56]

With the growth of mobile technology, the use of smartphone applications, online programs, and wearable devices has been a growing area of research to address the challenges related to participant adherence in the DPP. *Prevent*, developed by Omada Health, is a DPP-based group lifestyle intervention integrating a private online social network, weekly lessons, health coaching, and a wireless scale and pedometer. This model has shown meaningful weight loss and HbA1c change among participants after 1 year.[57] Later iterations have also shown feasibility of online platforms to reach underserved communities, including Latinx, elderly, and rural populations.[56,58] Another study comparing an app-based DPP with virtual coaching to a group receiving a paper-based DPP curriculum with regular medical care with no formal intervention reported significantly better improvement in weight among the group receiving the mobile app-based program (−2.64 kg [standard error, 0.71; *P*<.001]).[59]

The creation and implementation of the NDPP have led to successful uptake and adaptations of the DPP, including in-person, community, Web-based, mobile delivery, and mixed interventions reporting weight loss of 3% or more.[31,40,60,61] Although various methods have been shown to be feasible, barriers at the participant level (eg, digital access, health literacy, behavior log burden, transportation, and activation), program level (eg, location, platform, class format), and system level (eg, payment model and marketing) must be addressed to achieve successful implementation and clinically meaningful outcomes.

Implementation/Dissemination Globally

The recent Global Burden of Disease Study estimates that the prevalence of diabetes will increase by almost 20% from 2019 to 2030 with most of the increase occurring in low- and middle-income countries (LMICs). With more than 80% of people with diabetes living in LMICs and 1 million deaths a year owing to diabetes alone, lower-income countries do not have the capacity to manage this rising burden of disease.[62] Diabetes prevention in LMICs is imperative. Most of the evidence for the effectiveness of diabetes prevention interventions comes from high-income countries. LMICs present a very different context, with differences at the provider, participant, and community level as well as limited availability of both human and material resources that impact translation of interventions. In the last several years, there has been a growing realization of the importance of considering context in implementation of interventions and the translation of evidence generated in high-income countries to LMICs. Effective translation must consider adaptation, implementation outcomes, innovative and appropriate implementation strategies, and sustainability for the LMIC context.[63,64]

Table 1 summarizes key studies of implementation and effectiveness of diabetes prevention initiatives in LMICs with a focus on studies in China (the highest number of people with diabetes), India (the second highest number of people with diabetes and the largest population with prediabetes), and Sub-Saharan Africa (largest projected growth in number of people with diabetes).[1] Understanding how and why components of the original evidence-based intervention were adapted is important for informing diabetes prevention in other settings. D-CLIP,[27] Lifestyle Africa,[65] and the Kerala Diabetes Prevention Program (K-DPP)[66] detail adaptations to the original diabetes prevention programs for the Indian and South African cultural context. These studies highlight the importance of engaging key stakeholders and people living with chronic disease in the process to understand barriers and facilitators to partaking in healthy lifestyle.

Implementation research engages key stakeholders to understand critical implementation outcomes, such as reach, adoption, acceptability, fidelity, and sustainability.[64] Understanding these outcomes facilitates the process of taking the intervention to scale. The K-DPP study and Lifestyle Africa provide important information on these implementation outcomes that can inform larger nationwide efforts. The K-DPP uses well-known implementation frameworks to report on reach/penetration adoption, acceptability, and fidelity.[67] Similarly, in Lifestyle Africa, investigators report on reach, acceptability, adoption, fidelity, and sustainability.[65]

Understanding the cost, cost-effectiveness, and cost utility of diabetes prevention interventions is important for policymakers in LMICs who have limited budgets, human resources, and many competing health-related priorities. Cost-effectiveness analysis of the IDPP showed it to be less cost-effective than K-DPP.[25,68] Cost in the D-CLIP[69]

Table 1
Implementation of diabetes prevention interventions globally: key examples from China, India, and Sub-Saharan Africa

Study Name	Study Population	Intervention Components	Mode of Delivery of the Intervention	Adaptation Reported; Implementation Outcomes Reported	Intervention Cost (INR to Prevent One Case of Diabetes)
Da Qing Diabetes Prevention Study[15]	China	Diet, exercise, or combined	In-person counseling sessions	N/A (original study)	Not reported
IDPP-1[16]	India	Lifestyle modification only Metformin only Lifestyle + Metformin	Lifestyle modification delivered via in-person and telephone counseling sessions	N/A (original study)	LSM $1052 Metformin $1095 LSM + Metformin $1,359[25]
IDPP mobile[70]	India (men only)	Diet and physical activity recommendations	Mobile phone messages tailored to transtheoretical model stage (based on IDPP)	Not reported	Not reported
LIMIT[71]	India	Lifestyle modification recommendations	Phone messages and e-mails	Not reported	$137.29 to prevent 1 case of overweight/obesity
D-CLIP[27]	India	Lifestyle modification modeled on DPP Metformin escalation	In-person group sessions Phone call follow-up	Documented DPP curriculum adaptations	$2604.1469
K-DPP[66,79]	India	Lifestyle modification modeled on DPP	In-person group sessions delivered by peers	Documented DPP curriculum adaptations Implementation outcomes assessed: reach, adoption, fidelity	$295.168
YOGA-DP[80]	India	Yoga-based exercises Program booklet	In-person; home video	Not reported	N/A

Lifestyle Africa[65]	South Africa	Lifestyle modification modeled on DPP	Video-based sessions modeled on DPP Sessions facilitated by CHWs	Documented adaptations on content, literacy/numeracy Implementation outcomes assessed: reach, fidelity, participant satisfaction	N/A
SA-DPP[81,82]	South Africa	Lifestyle modification modeled on the Finnish Diabetes Prevention Study	In-person sessions plus informational booklet	Documented adaptations	N/A

INR, international normalized ratio; LIMIT, lifestyle modification in information technology; LSM, lifestyle modification; N/A, not applicable; SA-DPP, South African Diabetes Prevention Program; YOGA-DP, Yoga Programme for Type 2 Diabetes Mellitus Prevention.

study was slightly higher than the IDPP or K-DPP. K-DPP showed a cost per diabetes case prevented of $295, whereas D-CLIP had a higher cost per diabetes case prevented at $2604.

These studies also provide great examples of innovative implementation strategies that can increase the reach of interventions. The use of mobile technology and text messaging in India is 1 example of a program component that lessens the requirement for more costly and time-intensive in-person sessions. Virtual tools also overcome transportation barriers often cited for missing sessions. Phone-based messaging was successfully used in 2 studies in India.[70,71] In Lifestyle Africa, the US-DPP was modified to include video-assisted sessions, which required less training and experience for individuals delivering the intervention.[65] Although encouraging, the use of innovative delivery methodologies to facilitate scale-up of interventions in LMICs still requires comparative studies to understand the effectiveness and cost-effectiveness of these approaches compared with more traditional, in-person delivery.

The increased reporting of implementation outcomes, adaptation, and cost analysis for diabetes prevention interventions in LMICs is encouraging. However, as the evidence base for implementation of diabetes prevention interventions in different LMIC contexts increases, there is a need to ensure that there is a parallel effort to translate these findings into effective and sustainable scale-up (implementing programs at the subnational/national level) and scale-out (implementing programs in similar contexts) initiatives, for example, the statewide scale-up of the K-DPP[67] or scale-out of Lifestyle Africa to in other sub-Saharan Africa countries with high diabetes and prediabetes burdens, such as Nigeria. Studies must also consider longer-term follow-up to understand the factors that impact sustainability of and adherence to interventions.

DISCUSSION

Despite strong evidence for lifestyle interventions for diabetes prevention, implementation of these programs at the community level, particularly in LMIC settings, is lagging, and there are significant gaps in the available literature to guide these efforts. There is need for research to identify successful methods to overcome challenges seen within diabetes prevention studies, including loss of program gains over time (eg, weight gain, decreases in physical activity) and identification of successful interventions for individuals with non-IGT prediabetes or normal weight individuals with prediabetes. Novel intervention methods for diabetes prevention, for example, a Health at Every Size approach[72] or high-intensity interval training exercise,[73] should be tested within the context of diabetes prevention studies to determine their efficacy within different populations. Behavioral nudges, small changes in the environment that nudge an individual to make certain choices,[74] and financial incentives should be tested more widely in the context of improving health behaviors and participant outcomes in diabetes prevention research.[75,76]

There is a need for more detailed reporting and evaluation of implementation processes to guide further implementation, scale-up, and dissemination. Few diabetes prevention implementation studies describe what adaptations were made or document the reasons for these changes. Providing these pieces of granular data would be highly beneficial to guide additional tailoring of proven diabetes prevention programs across settings. There is a need for data from implementation trials assessing longer-term outcomes, including diabetes incidence, a deeper understanding of barriers to participant engagement and retention paired with methods to improve these metrics, and additional work testing novel methods for cultural adaptation. A greater number of implementation studies should be designed to assess fidelity, cost and cost-effectiveness, acceptability, and sustainability.

Future diabetes prevention efforts within communities should focus on delivering programs to overcome barriers to attendance; for example, worksite-based interventions can ease participation barriers to reaching at-risk individuals at a location where they already spend much of their time.[77] Similarly, mobile or online programs can be delivered anywhere and may be more appealing to some populations; however, barriers to digital access or digital literacy may prevent the reach and uptake of such models. Additional research is needed to understand how to best leverage and use digital tools (eg, wearable fitness trackers, continuous glucose monitoring) and platforms to support diabetes prevention.[78] This attention to digital DPP delivery is particularly appropriate currently, as the COVID-19 pandemic necessitated that on-going DPP programming adapt to comply with social distancing measures. Studies are needed to understand how existing programs responded to the global COVID-19 crisis and use this knowledge to create more nimble diabetes prevention programming that can quickly respond to similar breaks in delivery in the future (eg, during a natural disaster).

SUMMARY

Randomized controlled trials provide strong evidence for the efficacy of lifestyle interventions focused on increasing physical activity, improving diet quality and quantity, and/or weight loss for reducing diabetes incidence and improving cardiometabolic health among individuals at elevated risk for type 2 diabetes. Implementation studies, in the United States and globally, have successfully applied these models at the community level. However, additional research is needed to better guide community implementation and dissemination, understand diabetes prevention across different prediabetes groups, and improve participant engagement and retention in diabetes prevention programs.

CLINICS CARE POINTS

- There is strong evidence that diabetes can be prevented or delayed in high-risk adults by increasing physical activity, reducing weight, and improving diet quality and quantity.

- Clinicians should consider the cultural appropriateness of lifestyle advice and work with patients to find solutions to barriers, both personal and cultural, to achieve the needed behavior change.

- Clinicians should regularly screen individuals at risk for prediabetes to identify patients who could benefit from proven diabetes prevention programs.

- Patients with prediabetes should be referred to existing diabetes prevention programs (community or payer-based programs), and clinicians should provide support and encouragement to help patients find programs that work for them; these include virtual or other remote applications that may improve acceptability for some patients. Resources for health professionals are available through the Centers for Disease Control and Prevention at https://www.cdc.gov/diabetes/prevention/info-hcp.html.

- Clinicians should be prepared to escalate therapy for patients with prediabetes struggling with weight loss or lifestyle behavior changes. This includes following up with patients regarding their prediabetes diagnosis and diabetes prevention program referral and helping them overcome resistance to joining and remaining engaged in these programs.

DISCLOSURES

The authors have no conflicts of interest to declare.

The authors declare the following grant support: M.B.W. NIH/NIDDK P30DK111024, S.H. NIH/NHLBI K23 HL152368, and M.S. NIH/NIMHD K23MD015088.

REFERENCES

1. International Diabetes Federation. IDF diabetes atlas. 9th Edition. Brussels, Belgium: International Diabetes Federation; 2019.
2. Seuring T, Archangelidi O, Suhrcke M. The economic costs of type 2 diabetes: a global systematic review. Pharmacoeconomics 2015;33(8):811–31.
3. Liu J, Ren ZH, Qiang H, et al. Trends in the incidence of diabetes mellitus: results from the Global Burden of Disease Study 2017 and implications for diabetes mellitus prevention. BMC Public Health 2020;20(1):1415.
4. Anjana RM, Pradeepa R, Deepa M, et al. Prevalence of diabetes and prediabetes (impaired fasting glucose and/or impaired glucose tolerance) in urban and rural India: phase I results of the Indian Council of Medical Research-INdia DIABetes (ICMR-INDIAB) study. Diabetologia 2011;54:3022–7.
5. Sentell TL, He G, Gregg EW, et al. Racial/ethnic variation in prevalence estimates for United States prediabetes under alternative 2010 American Diabetes Association criteria: 1988-2008. Ethn Dis 2012;22(4):451–8.
6. Crandall JP, Knowler WC, Kahn SE, et al. The prevention of type 2 diabetes. Nat Clin Pract Endocrinol Metab 2008;4(7):382–93.
7. Lindstrom J, Ilanne-Parikka P, Peltonen M, et al. Sustained reduction in the incidence of type 2 diabetes by lifestyle intervention: follow-up of the Finnish Diabetes Prevention Study. Lancet 2006;368(9548):1673–9.
8. Li G, Zhang P, Wang J, et al. The long-term effect of lifestyle interventions to prevent diabetes in the China Da Qing Diabetes Prevention Study: a 20-year follow-up study. Lancet 2008;371(9626):1783–9.
9. Knowler WC, Barrett-Connor E, Fowler SE, et al. Reduction in the incidence of type 2 diabetes with lifestyle intervention or metformin. N Engl J Med 2002; 346(6):393–403.
10. Lindstrom J, Louheranta A, Mannelin M, et al. The Finnish Diabetes Prevention Study (DPS): lifestyle intervention and 3-year results on diet and physical activity. Diabetes Care 2003;26(12):3230–6.
11. Ratner R, Goldberg R, Haffner S, et al. Impact of intensive lifestyle and metformin therapy on cardiovascular disease risk factors in the diabetes prevention program. Diabetes Care 2005;28(4):888–94.
12. Wing RR. Long-term effects of a lifestyle intervention on weight and cardiovascular risk factors in individuals with type 2 diabetes mellitus: four-year results of the look AHEAD trial. Arch Intern Med 2010;170(17):1566–75.
13. Diabetes Prevention Program Research Group. The Diabetes Prevention Program. Design and methods for a clinical trial in the prevention of type 2 diabetes. Diabetes Care 1999;22(4):623–34.
14. Haw JS, Galaviz KI, Straus AN, et al. Long-term sustainability of diabetes prevention approaches: a systematic review and meta-analysis of randomized clinical trials. JAMA Intern Med 2017;177(12):1808–17.
15. Pan XR, Li GW, Hu YH, et al. Effects of diet and exercise in preventing NIDDM in people with impaired glucose tolerance. The Da Qing IGT and Diabetes Study. Diabetes Care 1997;20(4):537–44.

16. Ramachandran A, Snehalatha C, Mary S, et al. The Indian Diabetes Prevention Programme shows that lifestyle modification and metformin prevent type 2 diabetes in Asian Indian subjects with impaired glucose tolerance (IDPP-1). Diabetologia 2006;49(2):289–97.

17. Ratner RE, Christophi CA, Metzger BE, et al. Prevention of diabetes in women with a history of gestational diabetes: effects of metformin and lifestyle interventions. J Clin Endocrinol Metab 2008;93(12):4774–9.

18. Li G, Hu Y, Yang W, et al. Effects of insulin resistance and insulin secretion on the efficacy of interventions to retard development of type 2 diabetes mellitus: the DA Qing IGT and Diabetes Study. Diabetes Res Clin Pract 2002;58(3):193–200.

19. Li G, Zhang P, Wang J, et al. Cardiovascular mortality, all-cause mortality, and diabetes incidence after lifestyle intervention for people with impaired glucose tolerance in the Da Qing Diabetes Prevention Study: a 23-year follow-up study. Lancet Diabetes Endocrinol 2014;2(6):474–80.

20. Perreault L, Pan Q, Mather KJ, et al. Effect of regression from prediabetes to normal glucose regulation on long-term reduction in diabetes risk: results from the Diabetes Prevention Program Outcomes Study. Lancet 2012;379(9833):2243–51.

21. Chen Y, Zhang P, Wang J, et al. Associations of progression to diabetes and regression to normal glucose tolerance with development of cardiovascular and microvascular disease among people with impaired glucose tolerance: a secondary analysis of the 30 year Da Qing Diabetes Prevention Outcome Study. Diabetologia 2021;64(6):1279–87.

22. Perreault L, Pan Q, Schroeder EB, et al. Regression from prediabetes to normal glucose regulation and prevalence of microvascular disease in the Diabetes Prevention Program Outcomes Study (DPPOS). Diabetes Care 2019;42(9):1809–15.

23. Lindgren P, Lindstrom J, Tuomilehto J, et al. Lifestyle intervention to prevent diabetes in men and women with impaired glucose tolerance is cost-effective. Int J Technol Assess Health Care 2007;23(2):177–83.

24. Diabetes Prevention Program Research Group. Within-trial cost-effectiveness of lifestyle intervention or metformin for the primary prevention of type 2 diabetes. Diabetes Care 2003;26(9):2518–23.

25. Ramachandran A, Snehalatha C, Yamuna A, et al. Cost-effectiveness of the interventions in the primary prevention of diabetes among Asian Indians: within-trial results of the Indian Diabetes Prevention Programme (IDPP). Diabetes Care 2007;30(10):2548–52.

26. Saito T, Watanabe M, Nishida J, et al. Lifestyle modification and prevention of type 2 diabetes in overweight Japanese with impaired fasting glucose levels: a randomized controlled trial. Arch Intern Med 2011;171(15):1352–60.

27. Weber MB, Ranjani H, Staimez LR, et al. The stepwise approach to diabetes prevention: results from the D-CLIP randomized controlled trial. Diabetes Care 2016;39(10):1760–7.

28. American Diabetes Association. 3. Prevention or delay of type 2 diabetes: standards of medical care in diabetes-2020. Diabetes Care 2020;43(Suppl 1):S32–6.

29. Diabetes Canada Clinical Practice Guidelines Expert C, Prebtani APH, Bajaj HS, Goldenberg R, et al. Reducing the risk of developing diabetes. Can J Diabetes 2018;42(Suppl 1):S20–6.

30. Cosentino F, Grant PJ, Aboyans V, et al. 2019 ESC guidelines on diabetes, prediabetes, and cardiovascular diseases developed in collaboration with the EASD: the Task Force for diabetes, pre-diabetes, and cardiovascular diseases of the European Society of Cardiology (ESC) and the European Association for the Study of Diabetes (EASD). Eur Heart J 2020;41(2):255–323.

31. Ali MK, Echouffo-Tcheugui J, Williamson DF. How effective were lifestyle interventions in real-world settings that were modeled on the diabetes prevention program? Health Aff (Millwood) 2012;31(1):67–75.

32. Galaviz KI, Weber MB, Straus A, et al. Global diabetes prevention interventions: a systematic review and network meta-analysis of the real-world impact on incidence, weight, and glucose. Diabetes Care 2018;41(7):1526–34.

33. Ely EK, Gruss SM, Luman ET, et al. A national effort to prevent type 2 diabetes: participant-level evaluation of CDC's National Diabetes Prevention Program. Diabetes Care 2017;40(10):1331–41.

34. Albright AL, Gregg EW. Preventing type 2 diabetes in communities across the U.S.: the National Diabetes Prevention Program. Am J Prev Med 2013;44(4 Suppl 4):S346–51.

35. Ali MK, McKeever Bullard K, Imperatore G, et al. Reach and use of diabetes prevention services in the United States, 2016-2017. JAMA Netw Open 2019;2(5): e193160.

36. Ackermann RT, Kang R, Cooper AJ, et al. Effect on health care expenditures during nationwide implementation of the diabetes prevention program as a health insurance benefit. Diabetes Care 2019;42(9):1776–83.

37. Ali MK, Wharam F, Kenrik Duru O, et al. Advancing health policy and program research in diabetes: findings from the Natural Experiments for Translation in Diabetes (NEXT-D) Network. Curr Diab Rep 2018;18(12):146.

38. Ackermann RT, Finch EA, Caffrey HM, et al. Long-term effects of a community-based lifestyle intervention to prevent type 2 diabetes: the DEPLOY extension pilot study. Chronic Illn 2011;7(4):279–90.

39. Faridi Z, Shuval K, Njike VY, et al. Partners reducing effects of diabetes (PREDICT): a diabetes prevention physical activity and dietary intervention through African-American churches. Health Educ Res 2010;25(2):306–15.

40. Tabak RG, Sinclair KA, Baumann AA, et al. A review of diabetes prevention program translations: use of cultural adaptation and implementation research. Transl Behav Med 2015;5(4):401–14.

41. AuYoung M, Moin T, Richardson CR, et al. The diabetes prevention program for underserved populations: a brief review of strategies in the real world. Diabetes Spectr 2019;32(4):312–7.

42. Berkley-Patton J, Bowe Thompson C, Bauer AG, et al. A multilevel diabetes and CVD risk reduction intervention in African American churches: Project Faith Influencing Transformation (FIT) feasibility and outcomes. J Racial Ethn Health Disparities 2020;7(6):1160–71.

43. Weber MB, Hennink MM, Narayan KMV. Tailoring lifestyle programmes for diabetes prevention for US South Asians. Fam Med Community Health 2020;8(2):e000295.

44. Azar KMJ, Nasrallah C, Szwerinski NK, et al. Implementation of a group-based diabetes prevention program within a healthcare delivery system. BMC Health Serv Res 2019;19(1):694.

45. Palmer KNB, Garr Barry VE, Marrero DG, et al. Intervention delivery matters: what mothers at high risk for type 2 diabetes want in a diabetes prevention program-results from a comparative effectiveness trial. Diabetes Ther 2020;11(10):2411–8.

46. Rosas LG, Vasquez JJ, Hedlin HK, et al. Comparing enhanced versus standard diabetes prevention program among indigenous adults in an urban setting: a randomized controlled trial. BMC Public Health 2020;20(1):139.

47. Shah M, Kaselitz E, Heisler M. The role of community health workers in diabetes: update on current literature. Curr Diab Rep 2013;13(2):163–71.

48. O'Brien MJ, Perez A, Scanlan AB, et al. PREVENT-DM comparative effectiveness trial of lifestyle intervention and metformin. Am J Prev Med 2017;52(6):788–97.

49. Johnson M, Jones R, Freeman C, et al. Can diabetes prevention programmes be translated effectively into real-world settings and still deliver improved outcomes? A synthesis of evidence. Diabet Med 2013;30(1):3–15.

50. Neamah HH, Sebert Kuhlmann AK, Tabak RG. Effectiveness of program modification strategies of the diabetes prevention program: a systematic review. Diabetes Educ 2016;42(2):153–65.

51. Cannon MJ, Masalovich S, Ng BP, et al. Retention among participants in the national diabetes prevention program lifestyle change program, 2012-2017. Diabetes Care 2020;43(9):2042–9.

52. Nhim K, Gruss SM, Porterfield DS, et al. Using a RE-AIM framework to identify promising practices in national diabetes prevention program implementation. Implement Sci 2019;14(1):81.

53. Ritchie ND, Baucom KJW, Sauder KA. Current perspectives on the impact of the National Diabetes Prevention Program: building on successes and overcoming challenges. Diabetes Metab Syndr Obes 2020;13:2949–57.

54. Samuel-Hodge CD, Johnson CM, Braxton DF, et al. Effectiveness of diabetes prevention program translations among African Americans. Obes Rev 2014; 15(Suppl 4):107–24.

55. Clennin MN, Maytag A, Ellis J, et al. Weight loss disparities among Hispanic and underserved participants, Colorado, 2015-2018. Prev Chronic Dis 2020;17:E162.

56. Vadheim LM, Patch K, Brokaw SM, et al. Telehealth delivery of the diabetes prevention program to rural communities. Transl Behav Med 2017;7(2):286–91.

57. Sepah SC, Jiang L, Peters AL. Translating the diabetes prevention program into an online social network: validation against CDC standards. Diabetes Educ 2014;40(4):435–43.

58. Fontil V, McDermott K, Tieu L, et al. Adaptation and feasibility study of a digital health program to prevent diabetes among low-income patients: results from a partnership between a digital health company and an academic research team. J Diabetes Res 2016;2016:8472391.

59. Toro-Ramos T, Michaelides A, Anton M, et al. Mobile delivery of the diabetes prevention program in people with prediabetes: randomized controlled trial. JMIR Mhealth Uhealth 2020;8(7):e17842.

60. Aziz Z, Absetz P, Oldroyd J, et al. A systematic review of real-world diabetes prevention programs: learnings from the last 15 years. Implement Sci 2015;10:172.

61. Joiner KL, Nam S, Whittemore R. Lifestyle interventions based on the diabetes prevention program delivered via eHealth: a systematic review and meta-analysis. Prev Med 2017;100:194–207.

62. Saeedi P, Petersohn I, Salpea P, et al. Global and regional diabetes prevalence estimates for 2019 and projections for 2030 and 2045: results from the International Diabetes Federation Diabetes Atlas, 9th edition. Diabetes Res Clin Pract 2019;157:107843.

63. Karachaliou F, Simatos G, Simatou A. The challenges in the development of diabetes prevention and care models in low-income settings. Front Endocrinol (Lausanne) 2020;11:518.

64. Haregu TN, Mahat K, Miller SM, et al. Improving diabetes prevention and management amidst varied resources: from local implementation to global learnings. Transl Behav Med 2020;10(1):1–4.

65. Catley D, Puoane T, Goggin K, et al. Adapting the diabetes prevention program for low- and middle-income countries: preliminary implementation findings from Lifestyle Africa. Transl Behav Med 2020;10(1):46–54.

66. Thankappan KR, Sathish T, Tapp RJ, et al. A peer-support lifestyle intervention for preventing type 2 diabetes in India: a cluster-randomized controlled trial of the Kerala Diabetes Prevention Program. Plos Med 2018;15(6):e1002575.

67. Ravindranath R, Oldenburg B, Balachandran S, et al. Scale-up of the Kerala Diabetes Prevention Program (K-DPP) in Kerala, India: implementation evaluation findings. Transl Behav Med 2020;10(1):5–12.

68. Sathish T, Oldenburg B, Thankappan KR, et al. Cost-effectiveness of a lifestyle intervention in high-risk individuals for diabetes in a low- and middle-income setting: trial-based analysis of the Kerala Diabetes Prevention Program. BMC Med 2020;18(1):251.

69. Islek D, Weber MB, Ranjit Mohan A, et al. Cost-effectiveness of a stepwise approach vs standard care for diabetes prevention in India. JAMA Netw Open 2020;3(7):e207539.

70. Ramachandran A, Snehalatha C, Ram J, et al. Effectiveness of mobile phone messaging in prevention of type 2 diabetes by lifestyle modification in men in India: a prospective, parallel-group, randomised controlled trial. Lancet Diabetes Endocrinol 2013;1(3):191–8.

71. Limaye T, Kumaran K, Joglekar C, et al. Efficacy of a virtual assistance-based lifestyle intervention in reducing risk factors for type 2 diabetes in young employees in the information technology industry in India: LIMIT, a randomized controlled trial. Diabet Med 2017;34(4):563–8.

72. Ritchie ND. Solving the puzzle to lasting impact of the National Diabetes Prevention Program. Diabetes Care 2020;43(9):1994–6.

73. Jelleyman C, Yates T, O'Donovan G, et al. The effects of high-intensity interval training on glucose regulation and insulin resistance: a meta-analysis. Obes Rev 2015;16(11):942–61.

74. Thaler RH, Sunstein CR. Nudge: improving decisions about health, wealth, and happiness. New Haven: Yale University Press; 2008.

75. VanEpps EM, Volpp KG, Halpern SD. A nudge toward participation: improving clinical trial enrollment with behavioral economics. Sci Transl Med 2016;8(348): 348fs313.

76. Desai JR, Vazquez-Benitez G, Taylor G, et al. The effects of financial incentives on diabetes prevention program attendance and weight loss among low-income patients: the We Can Prevent Diabetes cluster-randomized controlled trial. BMC Public Health 2020;20(1):1587.

77. Conn VS, Hafdahl AR, Cooper PS, et al. Meta-analysis of workplace physical activity interventions. Am J Prev Med 2009;37(4):330–9.

78. Fagherazzi G, Ravaud P. Digital diabetes: perspectives for diabetes prevention, management and research. Diabetes Metab 2019;45(4):322–9.

79. Aziz Z, Mathews E, Absetz P, et al. A group-based lifestyle intervention for diabetes prevention in low- and middle-income country: implementation evaluation of the Kerala Diabetes Prevention Program. Implement Sci 2018;13(1):97.

80. Chattopadhyay K, Mishra P, Singh K, et al. Yoga programme for type-2 diabetes prevention (YOGA-DP) among high risk people in India: a multicentre feasibility randomised controlled trial protocol. BMJ Open 2020;10(9):e036277.

81. Hill J, Lavigne Delville C, Auorousseau AM, et al. Development of a tool to increase physical activity among people at risk for diabetes in low-resourced communities in Cape Town. Int J Environ Res Public Health 2020;17(3):865.

82. Hill J, Peer N, Jonathan D, et al. Findings from community-based screenings for type 2 diabetes mellitus in at risk communities in Cape Town, South Africa: a pilot study. Int J Environ Res Public Health 2020;17(8):2876.

Population-Level Approaches to Preventing Type 2 Diabetes Globally

Karen R. Siegel, PhD, MPH[a,b,*], Ann L. Albright, PhD, RD[a]

KEYWORDS

- Type 2 diabetes • Prevention • Population-level • Nutrition • Physical activity
- Built environment

KEY POINTS

- Effective interventions at both the individual and population levels can help address type 2 diabetes (T2DM) prevention worldwide.
- Individual-level risk factors for T2DM are rooted in society; population-level approaches aim to address the upstream societal drivers of unhealthy food consumption, physical inactivity levels, and obesity.
- Population-level approaches to preventing T2DM include modifications to the food environment (pricing strategies, improvement of the food supply/availability, and educational and information strategies); modifications to the built environment for physical activity (strategies that combine 1 or more interventions to improve pedestrian or bicycle transportation systems with 1 or more land use and environmental design interventions); and programs and policies to address social and economic factors.
- There is evidence that some population-based approaches for T2DM prevention are cost-saving or cost-effective.
- Rigorous natural experiments can help fill knowledge gaps by evaluating the real-world effectiveness of major policies and their impact on disease outcomes, particularly in diverse populations, and help prioritize and implement such approaches.

INTRODUCTION

In 2019, 463 million people had diabetes worldwide, with 80% from low-income and middle-income countries. As previous articles in this special issue of *Endocrinology & Metabolism Clinics* have described (CITE), diabetes is associated with increased mortality, including excess deaths from cardiovascular disease, renal disease, and some cancers, as well as morbidity from macrovascular and microvascular complications.

[a] Division of Diabetes Translation, Centers for Disease Control and Prevention, 4770 Buford Highway Northeast, Atlanta, GA 30341, USA; [b] Hubert Department of Global Health, Rollins School of Public Health, Emory University, Atlanta, GA, USA
* Corresponding author. Division of Diabetes Translation, Centers for Disease Control and Prevention, 4770 Buford Highway Northeast, Atlanta, GA 30341.
E-mail address: Yuo0@cdc.gov

Endocrinol Metab Clin N Am 50 (2021) 401–414
https://doi.org/10.1016/j.ecl.2021.05.010
0889-8529/21/Published by Elsevier Inc.

On average, diabetes reduces life expectancy in people aged 40 to 60 years by 4 to 10 years and independently increases the risk of death from cardiovascular disease, renal disease, and cancer by 1.3 to 3 times, and is among the leading causes of non-traumatic lower-extremity amputation and blindness, especially in people of working age.[1]

The majority (approximately 95%) of the global diabetes burden is type 2 diabetes (T2DM), and individuals with prediabetes are at elevated risk for developing T2DM. In the United States (US), more than 88 million adults—1 in 3—have prediabetes. Although the complexities of prediabetes identification (COLAGIURI / TCHEUGUI) make global estimates challenging, the prevalence of impaired glucose tolerance (IGT) among individuals aged 20 to 79 years is often used. In 2017, global IGT prevalence was estimated at 7.3% of the adult population (352.1 million individuals) and projected to increase to 587 million individuals by 2045 (8.3% of the adult population).[2]

Importantly, T2DM can be prevented or delayed in high-risk adults through structured lifestyle programs focused on improved nutrition, physical activity, and weight loss (WEBER). Stress reduction and coping skills are often a crucial part of lifestyle programs because the psychosocial and emotional components of behavior change are so important.[3] Large randomized controlled trials (RCTs) conducted in the US,[4] China,[5] Finland,[6] and India[7] have shown 30% to 60% reductions in T2DM incidence in high-risk adults, and follow-up studies show that the benefits of these interventions, including a greater likelihood of regression to normoglycemia,[8] sustained reductions in T2DM incidence, and fewer long-term eye complications[9] and cardiovascular deaths,[10] can be sustained long after the intervention has ended. Findings from trials form the evidence base for current programs, such as the National Diabetes Prevention Program in the US, and are critical for identifying people of high risk and allowing preventive services to be reserved for and directed to people most likely to benefit.[11,12]

Although the most robust scientific evidence for preventing T2DM comes from research conducted in high-risk individuals, T2DM is increasingly thought of as an epidemic rooted in modern society as much as in individual behavior.[1,13] We know that at the individual level, the risk of developing T2DM is increased by higher consumption of overall calories,[14] red and processed meats,[15] refined grains,[16] and sugar-sweetened beverages (SSBs)[17]; lower consumption of fruits and vegetables,[18] whole grains,[16] and nuts[14]; lower physical activity and high physical inactivity[19]; and being overweight or having obesity.[20] Globalization, urbanization, and the nutrition transition have changed how people live and eat, and increased mass media (marketing) has led to greater exposure to and concentration of individual risk factors. In low-income and middle-income countries—and poorer communities in high-income countries—food insecurity and the unaffordability of fruits, vegetables, and whole grains further preclude healthy diets.[21,22] As a result, global diets are increasingly high in sugar, fat, and salt and low in whole grains, fruits, and vegetables,[23] and global obesity prevalence[24] and physical inactivity[25] levels are increasing.

Addressing the T2DM burden thus involves a dual approach, simultaneously addressing high-risk individuals and whole populations. Although prevention efforts for high-risk individuals (ie, those with prediabetes) focus on structured lifestyle programs to make and sustain behavior changes, efforts to reduce T2DM incidence may be optimized if population-wide changes in dietary risk factors and physical activity levels are also achieved.[11,12] Population-targeted approaches, including modifications to the food and built environments and social and economic factors underpinning T2DM risk, may also benefit people across the spectrum of T2DM—including high-risk individuals (**Fig. 1**). Within this context, this article summarizes the evidence for population-level approaches to prevent T2DM.

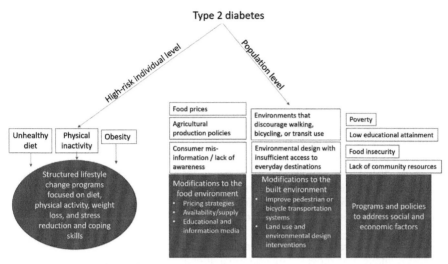

Fig. 1. High-risk individual-level and population-level approaches to type 2 diabetes prevention.

POPULATION-LEVEL APPROACHES TO PREVENTING TYPE 2 DIABETES

Population-level approaches aim to shift the distribution of a risk factor in a healthy direction, even if by a small degree, to significantly affect the proportion of individuals in a population who develop a disease.[26] In the case of T2DM, population approaches can address the upstream societal drivers of unhealthy food consumption, physical inactivity levels, and obesity. Such approaches can be categorized broadly as (1) modifications to the food environment, (2) modifications to the built environment and physical activity, and (3) programs and policies to address social and economic factors. This section summarizes the current evidence base for each of these strategies related to preventing T2DM and the knowledge gaps that still exist.

Food Environment

The bulk of the evidence for population-level approaches to prevent T2DM comes from modifications to the food environment. Such approaches include pricing strategies (taxes and subsidies), improvement of the food supply/availability (including food and agricultural policies), and educational and information strategies (food and menu labeling, mass media campaigns).

Pricing strategies

Food prices are important in determining dietary choices, and strategies to promote healthy diets can include taxes (or disincentives) on unhealthy foods, subsidies (or incentives) on healthy foods, and other price manipulations.[27] Overall, evidence from prospective observational and interventional studies of pricing strategies to improve diet suggests that a 10% price reduction or subsidy increases consumption of healthful foods/beverages by 14%, whereas a 10% price increase or tax reduces the consumption of unhealthful foods/beverages by 7%.[28] In many low-income and middle-income countries, fruits and vegetables in particular remain prohibitively expensive: the cost of purchasing the recommended servings of fruits and vegetables is almost one-fifth of the average household's income in these countries, and both fruit and vegetable consumption declines as their relative price per serving increases.[21] A systematic review found that consumer-level subsidies may have a positive impact on consumption: 4 studies in the review that modeled fruit and vegetable subsidies of around 10% showed increases in consumption of around 5%, with 1 study estimating a 1.5% increase in consumption in response to a 1.8% price decrease.[29]

Taxes and subsidies may have an impact not just on consumption patterns but also on health outcomes. Researchers used a comparative risk assessment to model the potential effects of 10% and 30% price subsidies on fruits, vegetables, whole grains, and nuts/seeds and 10% and 30% taxes on processed meat, unprocessed red meats, and SSBs on subsequent diabetes-related mortality in the US. They found that jointly altering the prices of these 7 dietary factors (10% each) could prevent 2274 diabetes deaths per year, whereas a larger price change (30%) in all 7 dietary factors could prevent 6287 diabetes deaths per year. Diabetes deaths would be most influenced by price changes in SSBs (1.5% reduction in deaths) and processed meats (0.7% reduction).[30] Modeling studies in South Africa[31] and India[32] have found similar results, where a 20% SSB tax was estimated to reduce diabetes prevalence by 4% over 20 years.

Over the past decade, the SSB tax, a potential policy lever for reducing population-level SSB intake, has received much global attention.[17,33] There are now 7 US cities and more than 30 countries worldwide that have implemented an SSB tax, and major evaluation efforts have been conducted in US cities (Berkeley, California,[34] and Philadelphia, Pennsylvania[35,36]) and Mexico.[37,38] In Berkeley, the first municipality in the US to implement a penny-per-ounce tax on SSBs (together with an information campaign), in March 2015, the tax was associated with decreased sales of SSBs (by 9.6%) and increased sales of untaxed beverages (by 3.5%), especially water (by 15.6%) after just 1 year.[39] Three years after the tax was implemented, people in Berkeley were drinking 52% fewer servings of SSBs than they did pretax and consuming 29% more water.[34] Similarly, Mexico's excise tax of 1 peso per liter (an approximately 10% tax) on SSBs, implemented in 2014, was associated with a 9.7% reduction in the consumption of these products in 2015, with steeper declines (17%) in lower-income households.[38] These evaluations provide important real-world understandings of the impact of population-level policies on consumer purchasing and consumption, although the impacts on more distal outcomes such as obesity and T2DM still must be estimated using simulation models.

In the US, researchers have studied the potential impact of pricing strategies implemented within low-income populations, which tend to be disproportionately affected by T2DM. There is evidence that changes (subsidizing fruits, vegetables, and other healthy foods, and restricting or disincentivizing unhealthy products) to the Supplemental Nutrition Assistance Program (SNAP), the largest federal nutrition program that provides $68 billion per year for food to 40 million low-income Americans, could improve diets among SNAP participants. In 2012, the Healthy Incentive Pilot (HIP) study randomized SNAP-participating households in 1 county in Massachusetts to receive either standard SNAP benefits (a monthly deposit of about $4 per person per day) or standard SNAP benefits plus an additional incentive for fruit and vegetable purchases (for every $1 of SNAP benefits spent on fruits and vegetables, participants received 30-cents additional benefit). The study found that those who received the additional benefit purchased 0.24 cup equivalents more produce per day—a 26% increase.[40]

Although these studies suggest the potential effectiveness of food pricing strategies on improving dietary factors to help prevent T2DM, there are limitations. First, most of these findings are from mathematical models rather than from real-world implementations and evaluations. Second, where the findings are from real-world evaluations (such as the SSB tax in Berkeley and Mexico), the outcomes assessed are mostly proximal (sales and consumption of SSBs). Longer follow-up times would be valuable to investigate the impact on health outcomes and the overall impact of these policies long-term.

Improvement of food availability and supply

Scientific evidence on what constitutes a healthy diet for preventing T2DM exists; however, many food and agricultural policies that determine the production and availability of food encourage the production of less healthy foods. For example, many countries provide producer-end subsidies for grain crops and meat/dairy, incentivizing farmers to grow these items while creating disincentives for fruit and vegetable production.[41] A partial result is that the global supply of fruits and vegetables is insufficient to meet population needs according to nutritional guidance (more than 5 servings of fruits and vegetables, or approximately 400 g, per day).[42] Moreover, despite a wealth of evidence of the health benefits of fruits and vegetables, their lack of affordability and accessibility present challenges, particularly in low-income and middle-income countries.[43]

Ecological analyses suggest that food supply matters: a country's availability (as determined by production, imports, exports, and accounting for food losses) of sugar,[44] animal fats,[45] and high-fructose corn syrup[46] is directly associated with that country's national diabetes prevalence, whereas the availability of fruits and vegetables[45] is inversely associated with national diabetes prevalence. In the US, higher consumption of calories from major subsidized food commodities—corn, soybeans, wheat, rice, dairy, and livestock—has been associated with a greater probability of obesity (overall and abdominal) and dysglycemia.[47,48]

More research would be beneficial to better understand what specific approaches could help better align food/agricultural policies with nutrition recommendations and promote healthier diets. As a start, encouraging the production of crops associated with lower T2DM prevalence (including fruits and vegetables, whole grains) over crops used in products associated with higher T2DM prevalence (meat and dairy) could transition the food supply toward healthier options. This research could be done in concert with farmers to understand facilitators and barriers—incentives and disincentives—to growing crops related to healthier foods. Importantly, 1 current barrier to fruit and vegetable availability is the large amount of food loss and waste at all parts of the food chain. Globally, 40% to 50% of root crops, fruits, and vegetables are wasted each year, perishing during harvest, storage, transport, packaging, and distribution,[49] and this is particularly true in warm climates where fruits and vegetables are prone to spoiling before reaching their market destinations. Investments in a sustainable solution to the lack of cold chains could potentially prevent up to 25% of food waste in developing countries.[50]

Educational and information strategies

Addressing food and menu labeling and mass media campaigns are 2 potential ways to encourage healthy diets through information.

Food labeling supports informed consumer choice and can effectively change consumer behavior and stimulate industry reformulation. A 2018 meta-analysis of the influence of food and beverage labeling on consumer behaviors and industry responses (in terms of reformulation) found that overall, food labeling reduced consumer intake of calories by 6.6%, total fat by 10.6%, and other generally unhealthy choices by 13% while increasing vegetable intake by 13.5%.[51] There was little evidence that food labels affected the intake of total carbohydrates, protein, saturated fat, or sodium, nor did they influence the consumption of fruits or whole grains. At the time of the meta-analysis, there were too few studies to assess the impact of food labels—such as the new and improved US nutrition facts label with "Added Sugars"—on intake of added sugars or the effects of labels on more distal health outcomes. It is also unknown which food labels, in terms of design, simplicity, and types of included nutrients or food components, have the greatest impact on consumer behavior.

In terms of industry responses and product reformulation, the same 2018 meta-analysis found that mandated food labels led to manufacturers reducing the amount of artificial trans fat in food by 64% and sodium by 8%, although there was little effect on total calories and the amounts of saturated fat, dietary fiber, or other healthy or unhealthy components (although relatively few studies included those endpoints). One example of product reformulation comes from Chile, where front-of-package labels with "black box" (black stop-sign-shaped) symbols to highlight excessive levels of calories, sugar, saturated fat, and sodium were adopted in 2018. Although the direct food consumption and health impacts have not yet been evaluated, the regulation led manufacturers to reformulate 25% of foods to avoid having to put "high in" labels on their products.[52] Another example comes from the experience with trans-fat labeling in the US, which was implemented in 2006. By 2011%, 58% of products containing trans fat had reduced their trans-fat content by at least 0.2 g per serving, and among all products with trans fat, the mean trans-fat content decreased by 44%.[53]

It is important to note that food labeling alone can exacerbate disparities across socioeconomic status. Evaluation studies of menu calorie labeling have highlighted that the strongest data evaluating purchases at typical fast-food restaurants (which might attract more low-income individuals) suggest menu labels do not alter consumer purchases, while there is evidence that labels do encourage lower-energy purchases in other settings such as coffee chains and full-service restaurants (which might attract higher-income patrons on average).[54] This has implications for label design—simple and straightforward labels that include graphics rather than words may be more impactful—and for implementing labeling approaches in combination with mass media campaigns and other strategies (education, environment/structural changes, price incentives), particularly in disadvantaged populations, to minimize potential widening of disparities.[28]

Studies suggest that a focused mass media campaign targeting a single dietary factor or related dietary factors can improve diet, although the effectiveness of mass media campaigns on dietary targets beyond fruits, vegetables, or salt is not established. A meta-analysis of the association of national mass media campaigns, including the US national 5 A Day campaign, indicated that a typical national campaign increases fruit and vegetable intake and reduces SSB intake by approximately 7% each.[55] However, further investigation would be valuable on the influence of varying intensity, penetration, and duration of mass media campaigns, as well as cost-effectiveness and effects on disparities relative to other strategies.[28]

Built Environment and Physical Activity

Effective population-based approaches implemented in communities can help to increase physical activity, and built-environment interventions that aim to create or modify community environmental characteristics to make physical activity easier or more accessible offer 1 such approach. The Community Preventive Services Task Force recommends built environment strategies that combine 1 or more interventions to improve pedestrian or bicycle transportation systems with 1 or more land use and environmental design interventions.[56,57] These recommendations can be applied at the macrolevel (overall community design related to walkability) or the microlevel (bicycle racks, street-crossing amenities) in urban, suburban, and rural environments, and increased collaboration within and across sectors, including health care, can help to amplify and extend existing efforts.

Specifically, improving transportation systems involves creating activity-friendly routes (ie, pedestrian, bicycle, or public transit access) that are a direct and convenient connection with common or everyday destinations, and components can include

- Street pattern design and connectivity
- Pedestrian infrastructure
- Bicycle infrastructure
- Public transit infrastructure and access.

Land use and environmental design involve creating and enhancing walking, bicycling, and public transit access to everyday destinations (eg, grocery stores, schools, worksites, libraries, parks, restaurants, and health care facilities).[57] Specific components can include

- Mixed land use (development with 2 or more major uses, such as residential, commercial, office, or institutional)
- Increased residential density
- Proximity to community or neighborhood destinations
- Parks and recreational facility access.

Related to this, the recent Lancet Commission on Diabetes proposed several actions that could influence physical activity.[1] These include, at the national or regional level, taxes on transport mode (eg, fuel duty) or subsidies to promote healthy travel (eg, bike-to-work schemes and subsidized public transport); at the regional level, social marketing and mass media campaigns; and at the local level, promotion of walking and cycling infrastructure; development of local space for physical activity (eg, parks, leisure centers, playing fields); use of local planning regulation to promote walkable neighborhoods; and use of local fiscal levers to promote healthy travel (eg, subsidized public transport, parking charges, and congestion charging).

There are evidence gaps that remain to be filled through longitudinal assessments of policy, systems, and environmental intervention approaches. Studies describing the implementation and evaluation of coordinated built-environment approaches, such as complete streets,[58] would strengthen the evidence base and provide direct guidance and support to help community planners. More studies would be beneficial to evaluate combinations of microscale interventions in different settings and populations. Additional research would be valuable to assess intervention effectiveness among different populations (eg, racial/ethnic minorities, people with lower socioeconomic status) and in different settings that may lack activity-supportive environments and services.

Social and Economic Factors

Efforts to address the underlying social determinants of health are important to consider as potential levers for changing population health behaviors and outcomes. For example, modifying the food or built environment may have little impact on populations that are primarily focused on ensuring shelter and safe housing.[59] Such approaches may not improve health behaviors or outcomes as the primary goal but nonetheless have implicit health-related impacts.

One such example is the 1994 to 1998 initiative by the Department of Housing and Urban Development (HUD)[60] in which women with children living in public housing in high-poverty urban census tracts (≥40% of residents with incomes below the federal poverty threshold, or FPL) were randomly assigned to 1 of 3 groups: (1) received housing vouchers that were redeemable only if they moved to a low-poverty census tract (<10% of residents below FPL), and counseling on moving; (2) received unrestricted, traditional vouchers with no counseling; and (3) offered neither of these opportunities. Although health was not the primary motivation for the initiative, results showed that the opportunity to move from a neighborhood with a high level of poverty to one with a lower level of poverty was associated with significant reductions in the prevalence of extreme obesity and diabetes.

Another example comes from the New Leaf project in Vancouver, Canada, which awards one-time cash transfers to individuals aged 19 years and older who have recently become homeless as a way to empower individuals to move beyond homelessness.[61] An initial evaluation of the program found that in addition to improving housing stability and savings, it decreased spending on goods such as alcohol, cigarettes, and drugs by 39% and increased food security; 67% of cash recipients were food secure after 1 month, an increase of 37% points from baseline (compared with a 2% point increase in the noncash group during the same period), and the cash recipients maintained greater food security over the entire 12 months of the evaluation.

COST-EFFECTIVENESS OF POPULATION-LEVEL APPROACHES TO PREVENTING TYPE 2 DIABETES

One of the most important considerations for policymakers is whether an intervention is cost-effective—that is, do the health and economic benefits of the intervention outweigh its cost? A recent systematic review of population-based approaches for T2DM prevention found evidence that these interventions are generally cost-saving or cost-effective. SSB taxes were found to be cost-saving from both health care system and government perspectives, with the potential to benefit a large population. However, the cost-effectiveness of many population-based interventions (including subsidies for fruits and vegetables, community-based education programs, and modifications to the built environment) were inconclusive, and further investigation with real-world data would be valuable.[62]

There is evidence that food package labeling has the potential to be cost-effective or cost-saving. In 2016, the US Food and Drug Administration mandated the labeling of added sugar content on all packaged foods and beverages. Researchers used a microsimulation model to estimate T2DM cases averted and cost-effectiveness of 2 policy scenarios: (1) implementation of the added sugar labeling policy and (2) further accounting for corresponding industry reformulation. Between 2018 and 2037, the sugar label is estimated to prevent 599,300 T2DM cases and save $31 billion in net health care costs of $61.9 billion societal costs; the sugar label + reformulation scenario resulted in an estimated 1.2 million T2DM cases averted and savings of $57.6 billion and $113.2 billion, respectively. Both scenarios were estimated to be cost-saving by 2023.

There is little cost information on the 1990s HUD study of women who received housing vouchers, although studies have found that while moving to a less impoverished neighborhood did not affect adult earnings or employment, moving to a less impoverished neighborhood in childhood (before age 13) increased future annual income by the midtwenties by approximately $3500 (31%).[63] However, whether this intervention could be cost-effective scaled to the larger population remains unknown.

One important consideration is the target population being studied. For example, although evidence of the cost-effectiveness of interventions to promote the consumption of fruits and vegetables was inconclusive for the general population, studies of fruit and vegetable subsidies implemented in the SNAP program suggest this approach may be cost-effective in SNAP participants.[64,65] Specifically, a modeled cost-effectiveness analysis of the HIP pilot program described above, expanded to SNAP participants nationally, estimated that such a subsidy could reduce T2DM incidence by 1.7% (95% CI 1.2, 2.2) and obesity by 0.2% (95% CI 0.1, 0.3), and be cost-saving from a societal perspective, largely attributable to long-term reductions in T2DM and cardiovascular diseases.

Another simulation model evaluated 3 potential interventions within SNAP, including (1) a 30% subsidy for purchases of fruits and vegetables (F + V), (2) a fruit and vegetable incentive with restriction of SSBs (FV + SSB), and (3) a broader incentive/disincentive program that preserves choice, combining a 30% subsidy for purchases of fruits and vegetables, nuts, whole grains, fish, and plant-based oils and a 30% disincentive for purchases of SSBs, junk food, and processed meats (SNAP+). The second and third interventions were estimated to prevent 171,000 and 147,000 cases of T2DM over a lifetime, and all interventions were cost-saving from a societal perspective.[66]

IMPORTANCE OF NATURAL EXPERIMENTS IN EVALUATING POPULATION-BASED APPROACHES

While evidence for individual-level approaches to diabetes prevention comes from real-world trials and programs, what we know about the impact of population-level approaches often comes from simulation modeling (that estimates cost and effectiveness using numerous assumptions), due to ethical and practical issues of performing RCTs of such approaches, as well as the large sample sizes needed. For example, in the US, nutrition assistance programs such as SNAP and the Special Supplemental Nutrition Program for Women, Infants, and Children account for a large proportion of federal nutrition program spending, but researchers have been unable to examine the effects of participation in these programs on T2DM-related health outcomes or costs, in large part due to the ethical and practical barriers of randomizing low-income populations to nutrition assistance or control. Natural experiments— wherein researchers formally evaluate the health impact of policies and programs as they are occurring in the real world—can also help to identify specific segments of the population that may be more likely to receive benefit from interventions (such as in the case of SSB taxes, low-income populations, or food/menu labeling on individuals with lower education or literacy levels).

Another aspect of population-targeted interventions is that they carry logistic and political challenges and sometimes the risk of unintended consequences. For example, what factors are needed to successfully implement these policies, and how does this vary across different communities and cultures? What is the impact of SSB tax revenues on health, equity, and community well-being?

SUMMARY

The strongest evidence for T2DM prevention comes from RCTs in which people at high risk for T2DM have participated in a structured lifestyle intervention that addresses nutrition, physical activity, weight loss, and stress reduction and coping skills, but a growing body of evidence suggests that population-level approaches implemented alongside approaches for those at high risk have the potential to reduce T2DM risk in the general population. Population-level approaches include modifications to the food environment (taxes and subsidies, changes to the food supply and availability, food and menu labeling, and mass media campaigns) and to the built environment (improving pedestrian or bicycle transportation systems and land use and environmental design interventions), as well as interventions that address underlying social and economic factors related to T2DM risk.

Efforts to address population-level risk factors and implement change in communities across the globe utilizing the current knowledge base would be valuable, while research to build upon the evidence can help to further understand how to improve nutrition and physical activity at the population level. Rigorous natural experiments can play a role here, helping to fill knowledge gaps by providing science-based evaluations of the real-world effectiveness of major policies and their impact on disease outcomes, particularly in diverse populations, and to guide the prioritization and implementation of such approaches.

DISCLAIMER

The findings and conclusions in this report are those of the authors and do not necessarily represent the official position of the Centers for Disease Control and Prevention.

DISCLOSURE

The authors have nothing to disclose.

REFERENCES

1. Chan JCN, Lim LL, Wareham NJ, et al. The Lancet Commission on diabetes: using data to transform diabetes care and patient lives. Lancet 2020;396(10267): 2019–82.
2. Hostalek U. Global epidemiology of prediabetes - present and future perspectives. Clin Diabetes Endocrinol 2019;5:5.
3. Mensa-Wilmot Y, Bowen SA, Rutledge S, et al. Early Results of States' Efforts to Support, Scale, and Sustain the National Diabetes Prevention Program. Prev Chronic Dis 2017;14:E130.
4. Knowler WC, Barrett-Connor E, Fowler SE, et al. Reduction in the incidence of type 2 diabetes with lifestyle intervention or metformin. N Engl J Med 2002; 346(6):393–403.
5. Pan XR, Li GW, Hu YH, et al. Effects of diet and exercise in preventing NIDDM in people with impaired glucose tolerance. The Da Qing IGT and Diabetes Study. Diabetes Care 1997;20(4):537–44.
6. Tuomilehto J, Lindstrom J, Eriksson JG, et al. Prevention of type 2 diabetes mellitus by changes in lifestyle among subjects with impaired glucose tolerance. N Engl J Med 2001;344(18):1343–50.
7. Ramachandran A, Snehalatha C, Mary S, et al. The Indian Diabetes Prevention Programme shows that lifestyle modification and metformin prevent type 2 diabetes in Asian Indian subjects with impaired glucose tolerance (IDPP-1). Diabetologia 2006;49(2):289–97.
8. Perreault L, Kahn SE, Christophi CA, et al. Regression from pre-diabetes to normal glucose regulation in the diabetes prevention program. Diabetes Care 2009;32(9):1583–8.
9. Diabetes Prevention Program Research Group. Long-term effects of lifestyle intervention or metformin on diabetes development and microvascular complications over 15-year follow-up: the Diabetes Prevention Program Outcomes Study. Lancet Diabetes Endocrinol 2015;3(11):866–75.
10. Li G, Zhang P, Wang J, et al. Cardiovascular mortality, all-cause mortality, and diabetes incidence after lifestyle intervention for people with impaired glucose

tolerance in the Da Qing Diabetes Prevention Study: a 23-year follow-up study. Lancet Diabetes Endocrinol 2014;2(6):474–80.

11. Albright A. Prevention of Type 2 Diabetes Requires BOTH Intensive Lifestyle Interventions and Population-Wide Approaches. Am J Manag Care 2015; 21(Suppl 7):S238–9.

12. Albright AL, Gregg EW. Preventing type 2 diabetes in communities across the U.S.: the National Diabetes Prevention Program. Am J Prev Med 2013;44(4 Suppl 4):S346–51.

13. Colagiuri R, Colagiuri S, Yach D, et al. The answer to diabetes prevention: science, surgery, service delivery, or social policy? Am J Public Health 2006; 96(9):1562–9.

14. Schwingshackl L, Hoffmann G, Lampousi AM, et al. Food groups and risk of type 2 diabetes mellitus: a systematic review and meta-analysis of prospective studies. Eur J Epidemiol 2017;32(5):363–75.

15. Micha R, Wallace SK, Mozaffarian D. Red and processed meat consumption and risk of incident coronary heart disease, stroke, and diabetes mellitus: a systematic review and meta-analysis. Circulation 2010;121(21):2271–83.

16. Aune D, Norat T, Romundstad P, et al. Whole grain and refined grain consumption and the risk of type 2 diabetes: a systematic review and dose-response meta-analysis of cohort studies. Eur J Epidemiol 2013;28(11):845–58.

17. Malik VS, Popkin BM, Bray GA, et al. Sugar-sweetened beverages, obesity, type 2 diabetes mellitus, and cardiovascular disease risk. Circulation 2010;121(11): 1356–64.

18. Lock K, Pomerleau J, Causer L, et al. Low fruit and vegetable consumption. In: WHO, editor. Comparative Quantification of health risks. Geneva (Switzerland): WHO; 2006.

19. Colberg SR, Sigal RJ, Yardley JE, et al. Physical Activity/Exercise and Diabetes: A Position Statement of the American Diabetes Association. Diabetes Care 2016; 39(11):2065–79.

20. American Diabetes A. 5. Prevention or Delay of Type 2 Diabetes: Standards of Medical Care in Diabetes-2018. Diabetes Care 2018;41(Suppl 1):S51–4.

21. Miller V, Yusuf S, Chow CK, et al. Availability, affordability, and consumption of fruits and vegetables in 18 countries across income levels: findings from the Prospective Urban Rural Epidemiology (PURE) study. Lancet Glob Health 2016; 4(10):e695–703.

22. Rose D, Oliveira V. Nutrient intakes of individuals from food-insufficient households in the United States. Am J Public Health 1997;87(12):1956–61.

23. Hu FB. Globalization of diabetes: the role of diet, lifestyle, and genes. Diabetes Care 2011;34(6):1249–57.

24. Collaboration NCDRF. Trends in adult body-mass index in 200 countries from 1975 to 2014: a pooled analysis of 1698 population-based measurement studies with 19.2 million participants. Lancet 2016;387(10026):1377–96.

25. Lavie CJ, Ozemek C, Carbone S, et al. Sedentary Behavior, Exercise, and Cardiovascular Health. Circ Res 2019;124(5):799–815.

26. Rose G. Sick individuals and sick populations. Int J Epidemiol 1985;14(1):32–8.

27. Powell LM, Chriqui JF, Khan T, et al. Assessing the potential effectiveness of food and beverage taxes and subsidies for improving public health: a systematic review of prices, demand and body weight outcomes. Obes Rev 2013;14(2): 110–28.

28. Afshin A, Penalvo J, Del Gobbo L, et al. CVD Prevention Through Policy: a Review of Mass Media, Food/Menu Labeling, Taxation/Subsidies, Built Environment,

School Procurement, Worksite Wellness, and Marketing Standards to Improve Diet. Curr Cardiol Rep 2015;17(11):98.

29. Thow AM, Downs S, Jan S. A systematic review of the effectiveness of food taxes and subsidies to improve diets: understanding the recent evidence. Nutr Rev 2014;72(9):551–65.

30. Penalvo JL, Cudhea F, Micha R, et al. The potential impact of food taxes and subsidies on cardiovascular disease and diabetes burden and disparities in the United States. BMC Med 2017;15(1):208.

31. Manyema M, Veerman JL, Chola L, et al. Decreasing the Burden of Type 2 Diabetes in South Africa: The Impact of Taxing Sugar-Sweetened Beverages. PLoS One 2015;10(11):e0143050.

32. Basu S, Vellakkal S, Agrawal S, et al. Averting obesity and type 2 diabetes in India through sugar-sweetened beverage taxation: an economic-epidemiologic modeling study. Plos Med 2014;11(1):e1001582.

33. Hu FB. Resolved: there is sufficient scientific evidence that decreasing sugar-sweetened beverage consumption will reduce the prevalence of obesity and obesity-related diseases. Obes Rev 2013;14(8):606–19.

34. Lee MM, Falbe J, Schillinger D, et al. Sugar-Sweetened Beverage Consumption 3 Years After the Berkeley, California, Sugar-Sweetened Beverage Tax. Am J Public Health 2019;109(4):637–9.

35. Zhong Y, Auchincloss AH, Lee BK, et al. The Short-Term Impacts of the Philadelphia Beverage Tax on Beverage Consumption. Am J Prev Med 2018;55(1):26–34.

36. Zhong Y, Auchincloss AH, Lee BK, et al. Sugar-Sweetened and Diet Beverage Consumption in Philadelphia One Year after the Beverage Tax. Int J Environ Res Public Health 2020;17(4):1336.

37. Colchero MA, Popkin BM, Rivera JA, et al. Beverage purchases from stores in Mexico under the excise tax on sugar sweetened beverages: observational study. BMJ 2016;352:h6704.

38. Colchero MA, Rivera-Dommarco J, Popkin BM, et al. In Mexico, Evidence Of Sustained Consumer Response Two Years After Implementing A Sugar-Sweetened Beverage Tax. Health Aff (Millwood) 2017;36(3):564–71.

39. Silver LD, Ng SW, Ryan-Ibarra S, et al. Changes in prices, sales, consumer spending, and beverage consumption one year after a tax on sugar-sweetened beverages in Berkeley, California, US: A before-and-after study. Plos Med 2017;14(4):e1002283.

40. Olsho LE, Klerman JA, Wilde PE, et al. Financial incentives increase fruit and vegetable intake among Supplemental Nutrition Assistance Program participants: a randomized controlled trial of the USDA Healthy Incentives Pilot. Am J Clin Nutr 2016;104(2):423–35.

41. Siegel KR. Insufficient Consumption of Fruits and Vegetables among Individuals 15 Years and Older in 28 Low- and Middle-Income Countries: What Can Be Done? J Nutr 2019;149(7):1105–6.

42. WHO/FAO. Diet, nutrition and the prevention of chronic diseases: report of a joint WHO/FAO expert consultation. Geneva (Switzerland): World Health Organization; 2003.

43. Frank SM, Webster J, McKenzie B, et al. Consumption of Fruits and Vegetables Among Individuals 15 Years and Older in 28 Low- and Middle-Income Countries. J Nutr 2019;149(7):1252–9.

44. Basu S, Yoffe P, Hills N, et al. The relationship of sugar to population-level diabetes prevalence: an econometric analysis of repeated cross-sectional data. PLoS One 2013;8(2):e57873.

45. Siegel KR, Echouffo-Tcheugui JB, Ali MK, et al. Societal correlates of diabetes prevalence: An analysis across 94 countries. Diabetes Res Clin Pract 2012; 96(1):76–83.

46. Goran MI, Ulijaszek SJ, Ventura EE. High fructose corn syrup and diabetes prevalence: a global perspective. Glob Public Health 2013;8(1):55–64.

47. Do WL, Bullard KM, Stein AD, et al. Consumption of Foods Derived from Subsidized Crops Remains Associated with Cardiometabolic Risk: An Update on the Evidence Using the National Health and Nutrition Examination Survey 2009-2014. Nutrients 2020;12(11):3244.

48. Siegel KR, McKeever Bullard K, Imperatore G, et al. Association of Higher Consumption of Foods Derived From Subsidized Commodities With Adverse Cardiometabolic Risk Among US Adults. JAMA Intern Med 2016;176(8):1124–32.

49. FAO. Global initiative on food loss and waste reduction. Rome: FAO; 2014.

50. A tank of cold: cleantech leapfrog to a more food secure world. London (UK): Institution of Mechanical Engineers; 2014.

51. Shangguan S, Afshin A, Shulkin M, et al. A Meta-Analysis of Food Labeling Effects on Consumer Diet Behaviors and Industry Practices. Am J Prev Med 2019;56(2):300–14.

52. Jacobson MF, Krieger J, Brownell KD. Potential Policy Approaches to Address Diet-Related Diseases. JAMA 2018;320(4):341–2.

53. Otite F, Jacobson MF, Dahmub A, et al. Trends in trans fatty acids reformulations of US supermarket and brand-name foods from 2007 through 2011. Prev Chronic Dis 2013;10:E85.

54. VanEpps EM, Roberto CA, Park S, et al. Restaurant Menu Labeling Policy: Review of Evidence and Controversies. Curr Obes Rep 2016;5(1):72–80.

55. Afshin A, ON A, AB N, et al. Abstract P087: effectiveness of mass media campaigns for improving dietary behaviors: a systematic review and meta-analysis. Circulation 2013;127(AP087).

56. CPSTF. Physical activity: built environment approaches combining transportation system interventions with land use and environmental design. The community guide. Atlanta (GA): Centers for Disease Control and Prevention; 2016.

57. Omura JD, Carlson SA, Brown DR, et al. Built Environment Approaches to Increase Physical Activity: A Science Advisory From the American Heart Association. Circulation 2020;142(11):e160–6.

58. Zaccaro HN, Atherton E. Bright spots, physical activity investments that work-Complete Streets: redesigning the built environment to promote health. Br J Sports Med 2018;52(18):1168–9.

59. Thompson T, Kreuter MW, Boyum S. Promoting Health by Addressing Basic Needs: Effect of Problem Resolution on Contacting Health Referrals. Health Educ Behav 2016;43(2):201–7.

60. Ludwig J, Sanbonmatsu L, Gennetian L, et al. Neighborhoods, obesity, and diabetes–a randomized social experiment. N Engl J Med 2011;365(16):1509–19.

61. Foundations for Social Change: The New Leaf Project. Taking Bold Action on Homelessness. 2020. Available at: https://static1.squarespace.com/static/5f07a92f21d34b403c788e05/t/5f751297fcfe7968a6a957a8/1601507995038/2020_09_30_FSC_Statement_of_Impact_w_Expansion.pdf. Accessed October 15, 2020.

62. Zhou X, Zhang P. Response to Comment on Zhou et al. Cost-effectiveness of Diabetes Prevention Interventions Targeting High-risk Individuals and Whole Populations: A Systematic Review. Diabetes Care 2020;43:1593–616. Diabetes Care. 2020;43(12):e206-e207.

63. Chetty R, Hendren N, Katz LF. The Effects of Exposure to Better Neighborhoods on Children: New Evidence from the Moving to Opportunity Experiment. Am Econ Rev 2016;106(4):855–902.
64. Basu S, Seligman H, Bhattacharya J. Nutritional policy changes in the supplemental nutrition assistance program: a microsimulation and cost-effectiveness analysis. Med Decis Making 2013;33(7):937–48.
65. Choi SE, Seligman H, Basu S. Cost Effectiveness of Subsidizing Fruit and Vegetable Purchases Through the Supplemental Nutrition Assistance Program. Am J Prev Med 2017;52(5):e147–55.
66. Mozaffarian D, Liu J, Sy S, et al. Cost-effectiveness of financial incentives and disincentives for improving food purchases and health through the US Supplemental Nutrition Assistance Program (SNAP): A microsimulation study. Plos Med 2018; 15(10):e1002661.

Prevention of Diabetes Macrovascular Complications and Heart Failure

Naveed Sattar, MD, PhD, FMedSci*

KEYWORDS

- Hypertension • LDL-cholesterol • Obesity • Countries • Ethnicity • Metformin
- SGLT2i • GLP-1RA

KEY POINTS

- Glucose reduction per se lowers atherosclerotic cardiovascular disease (ASCVD) risk modestly but multifactorial risk management, incorporating LDL-cholesterol and systolic blood pressure reductions and smoking cessation, in addition to glucose management, can lead to substantial reductions in risk for ASCVD.
- Priority in low- and middle-income countries should be given toward sustainable supplies of cheap metformin, statin, and blood pressure medications to lower cardiovascular (CV) risks for people with diabetes.
- Large-scale weight loss can lessen or reverse type 2 diabetes but may also meaningfully lower ASCVD and heart failure risks—ongoing trials will refute or confirm this notion in the next 5 years.
- The sodium/glucose cotransporter-2 inhibitors and glucagon-like peptide-1 receptor agonists class lower CV outcomes, with greater reductions in cardiorenal outcomes for the former and atherothrombotic outcomes (eg, stroke and peripheral artery disease) for the latter. Such benefits are independent of glycaemia and background metformin therapy. These findings have led to revisions of clinical guidelines.
- Further reductions in CV risk may stem from delaying diabetes in those at high risk, as well as from better messaging and adoption of sustainable lifestyle changes.

INTRODUCTION

As described previously, type 2 diabetes (T2D) is associated with accelerated vascular risk, which accounts for around half of the life years lost from diabetes.[1] However, in high-income countries, many factors inclusive of earlier diagnosis and better management of several risk factors have driven down cardiovascular risks. Declining risk for

University of Glasgow, Institute of Cardiovascular and Medical Sciences, BHF Glasgow Cardiovascular Research Centre, 126 University Place, Glasgow, G12 8TA, United Kingdom
* Corresponding author.
E-mail address: Naveed.Sattar@glasgow.ac.uk
Twitter: @MetaMedTeam (N.S.)

Endocrinol Metab Clin N Am 50 (2021) 415–430
https://doi.org/10.1016/j.ecl.2021.05.004
0889-8529/21/© 2021 Elsevier Inc. All rights reserved.

atherosclerotic cardiovascular disease has led, in turn, to increasing deaths from cancer in people with diabetes.[2] However, premature cardiovascular deaths from T2D in many low- and middle-income countries are increasing. At the same time, more people with diabetes in high-income countries, such as the United Kingdom, now develop peripheral arterial disease or heart failure (HF) as their first "vascular" presentation.[3] This chapter summarizes the major therapeutic modalities to lessen cardiovascular outcomes and HF in people with T2D. It will rely, wherever possible, on meta-analysis of outcome trials, supplemented by other outcome trials or best-quality observational data. The data will show that good glycemia control per se lowers risk modestly but that multifactorial risk factor management, also targeting lipids, smoking, and blood pressure, gives far greater protection against adverse vascular outcomes. In addition, it will describe recent gains from a series of landmark trials that have helped establish newer diabetes therapies—sodium-glucose cotransporter-2 inhibitors (SGLT2is) and glucagon-like peptide-1 receptor agonists (GLP-1RAs)—as important in further lowering of atherosclerotic cardiovascular disease (ASCVD) or cardiorenal risks in people with T2D.

Impact of Glucose Lowering Per Se

Although diabetes is diagnosed based on elevated glucose or HbA1c levels higher than specific diagnostic criteria, both the pathophysiology of T2D (excess weight/ectopic fat[4]) and patterns of risk factors in people with prediabetes (higher body mass index [BMI], systolic blood pressure [SBP], abnormal lipids) indicate that many risk factors linked to ASCVD are already worsened before frank diabetes develops.[5] Even so, once frank diabetes develops, further elevations in glucose levels independently add to adverse cardiovascular risk; keeping glucose level lower will therefore protect against ASCVD.

Although the impact of intensive glucose lowering has been questioned, a meta-analysis that combined data from 5 major glucose-lowering trials, using differing glucose-lowering regimens, showed that for each 0.9% lower HbA1c, there was a 17% reduction in events of nonfatal myocardial infarction (odds ratio 0.83, 95% confidence interval [CI] 0.75–0.93) (**Fig. 1**) and a 15% reduction in coronary heart disease (0.85, 0.77–0.93), although there was no impact on all-cause mortality (1.02, 0.87–1.19).[6] Those in the intensive glucose arm did not have lower HF risks, however, and were on average 2.5 kg heavier, linked to greater use of therapies known to increase weight (sulfonylureas and insulin and pioglitazone in the proactive trial). The same meta-analysis[6] also helped place these HbA1c findings into context by comparing how many events would be prevented should 200 people with diabetes have their glucose-lowered versus typical benefits from statins or blood pressure medications (**Fig. 2**). This figure helps reiterate the concept of multifactorial treatment, as it shows blood pressure and LDL-cholesterol (LDL-c) reductions can do more in the short term to lower cardiovascular risks than targeting glucose alone. Furthermore, although glucose lowering is important to protect against ASCVD, the benefits seem less than perhaps many first imagined and take some years to emerge. Of course, it must be remembered most of the aforementioned trials were done in predominantly white individuals, who on average develop T2D later than many other ethnicities. It is therefore entirely possible that due to earlier development of T2D in other ethnic groups, and often with more rapid glycemic deterioration, hyperglycemia has a greater weighting for ASCVD outcomes in many nonwhite groups. This speculation requires direct study.

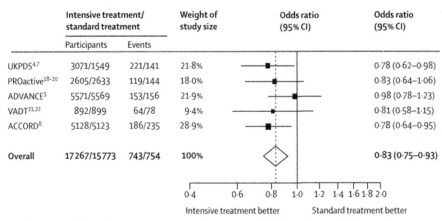

Intensive treatment/ standard treatment		Weight of study size	Odds ratio (95% CI)	Odds ratio (95% CI)
Participants	Events			
UKPDS[4,7] 3071/1549	221/141	21·8%		0·78 (0·62–0·98)
PROactive[18-20] 2605/2633	119/144	18·0%		0·83 (0·64–1·06)
ADVANCE[5] 5571/5569	153/156	21·9%		0·98 (0·78–1·23)
VADT[21,22] 892/899	64/78	9·4%		0·81 (0·58–1·15)
ACCORD[8] 5128/5123	186/235	28·9%		0·78 (0·64–0·95)
Overall 17267/15773	743/754	100%		0·83 (0·75–0·93)

0·4   0·6   0·8   1·0   1·2 1·4 1·6 1·8 2·0

Intensive treatment better   Standard treatment better

Fig. 1. Probability of events of nonfatal myocardial infarction with intensive glucose-lowering versus standard treatment. (*From* Ray KK, Seshasai SRK, Wijesuriya S, et al. Effect of intensive control of glucose on cardiovascular outcomes and death in patients with diabetes mellitus: a meta-analysis of randomised controlled trials. Lancet. 2009;373(9677):1765-1772; with permission of Elsevier, Inc.)

Lipids Lowering

LDL-c is causally related to adverse outcomes in all populations, and ample evidence supports statins lowering ASCVD outcomes in people with and without diabetes. In people with diabetes, the Cholesterol Treatment Trialists' Collaborators showed that a 1 mmol/L reduction in LDL-c led to a 21% reduction in major vascular events and a 13% reduction in vascular mortality.[7] For this reason, most guidelines around the

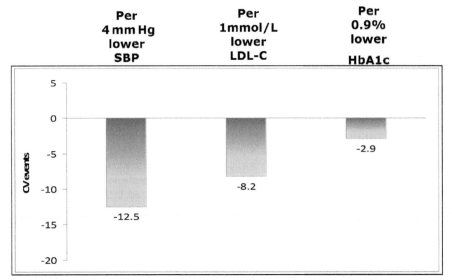

Fig. 2. Number of cardiovascular events prevented per every 200 individuals treated for 5 years with relevant agents in each class. (*Data from* Ray KK, Seshasai SRK, Wijesuriya S, et al. Effect of intensive control of glucose on cardiovascular outcomes and death in patients with diabetes mellitus: a meta-analysis of randomised controlled trials. *Lancet.* 2009;373(9677):1765–1772).

world recommend statin use in people with T2D, with lower targets for those with existing ASCVD; additional trial evidence shows that the lower the achieved LDL-c, the greater the reduction in ASCVD outcomes. Furthermore, genetic data now confirm elevated apolipoprotein B levels as the causal element in development of ASCVD.[8]

More recently, 2 other nonstatin agents that lower LDL-c have also shown to lower vascular risks in people with diabetes, as summarized in a recent article[9] (**Table 1**). This includes the once-daily oral agent, ezetimibe, which seems to have a particularly good effect in people with diabetes, and PCSK9 inhibitors, which are given as injections every 2 of 4 weeks. Ezetimibe lowers LDL-c by around 24%, whereas PCSK9i lowers LDL-c around 60%. Both agents are now licensed for use in diabetes, although PCSK9i remain expensive, so their use is restricted to those at greatest risks and in whom statins or ezetimibe do not allow patients to reach reasonable LDL-c levels. Ezetimibe is, however, available in generic forms, and lower cost makes it a good agent when maximally tolerated statin doses do not help patients achieve their LDL-c goals. The evidence for outcome benefit with other lipid lowering agents is either currently lacking (bempedoic acid) or controversial (high-dose fish oils and fibrates—more trials ongoing), although it seems more LDL-c–lowering agents will be licensed soon, increasing the lipid-lowering armoury to help prevent or delay ASCVD.

Blood Pressure Lowering

In a recent paper that looked at differences in cardiovascular (CV) risk factors between people with and without T2D by age of onset, SBP was higher by around 7 to 9 mm Hg across all ethnicities in those with diabetes diagnosed aged 20 to 39 years.[10] The link between diabetes and hypertension is highly robust, and it may be that the processes that lead to development of T2D—for example, ectopic fat gain, excess caloric intake, lower activity levels—also lead to increments in SBP. For this reason, and as higher SBP is causally related to ASCVD and key microvascular complications, lowering blood pressure is another cornerstone in the management of people with T2D. Blood pressure reduction lowers all major vascular outcomes in people with diabetes (a 10 mm Hg reduction in SBP lowering risk by 12%, 95% CI: 6%–28%), although the benefits seem to be somewhat less in people with diabetes compared with those without for incident coronary heart disease (12% risk reduction) but similar for stroke (26% risk reduction).[11] Blood pressure reduction also lowers HF and all-cause mortality in people with diabetes (**Fig. 3**).

Recent guidance on blood pressure reduction has advocated lower targets than previously, aiming for less than 130 mm Hg for most of the people with type 2 diabetes mellitus (T2DM), but less strict targets (typically to <150 mm Hg) for those who are older or frail.[12] Likely, most physicians will aim for an SBP somewhere between 130 to 140 mm Hg in their patients, although if they can tolerate levels less than 130 without side effects, then gains will be greater. Most favored blood pressure drugs are angiotensin-converting enzyme inhibitors or angiotensin-receptor blockers (due to their effects to lessen albuminuria risks), followed by calcium channel blockers and diuretics, and more recently spironolactone has come into favor. The emerging consensus for better SBP control is to use lower doses of 2 drugs than a larger dose of a single agent.

Lifestyle Measures and Atherosclerotic Cardiovascular Disease Outcomes

Weight loss
Surprisingly, although modest weight loss protects against development of diabetes in those at elevated risk, and larger weight loss can lead many people with T2DM to

Table 1
Lipid-lowering medications and their impacts in people with diabetes and brief relevant clinical implications

Classification of Drug	Key Trials	Findings	Clinical Implications
Statins	CTT	LDL-c reduction of 1 mmol/L results in approximately 21% reduction in CV event. Intensive statin regimes result in statistically significant 15% further reduction in major vascular events, without significant side effects.	Statins as first-line therapy in patients with diabetes. Nowadays, the most used are atorvastatin and rosuvastatin. Both have greater benefits on TG reduction than the older simvastatin and pravastatin.
Ezetimibe	IMPROVE-IT	Reduced CV mortality, major CV event, and stroke by 5.5% absolute RR (hazard ratio, 0.85; 95% confidence interval, 0.78–0.94). The largest relative reductions occurred in patients with DM were in MI (24%) and stroke (39%)	First add-on therapy if patients are not reaching targets for LDL-c or non-HDL-c despite maximally tolerated statin therapy
PCSK9 inhibitor	FOURIER	Evolocumab reduced cardiovascular outcomes in patients with diabetes: HR 0.83 (95% CI 0.75–0.93; $P = .0008$) for primary composite endpoint. Similar data for alirocumab	Currently reserved for patients at very high absolute risk for ASCVD, including patients with HF or existing ASCVD, with sustained elevations in LDL-c despite maximally tolerated statin therapy plus ezetimibe
Fibrates	ACCORD	Modest changes seen in the reduction of TG levels and increase in HDL-c levels	Add-on to statins for mixed hyperlipidemia, without robust evidence demonstrating improved outcomes in ASCVD risk. Further ongoing trials with newer fibrates
Icosapent ethyl; eicosapentaenoic acid (EPA) ethyl ester	REDUCE-IT	Primary endpoint event occurred in 17.2% of treated patients compared with 22.0% in placebo group (HR 0.75; 95% CI 0.68–0.83; $P < .001$)	Potential new therapy with modest lowering of TG levels. Outcome benefits may be largely independent of TG lowering. Other trials in same space were negative, lending some doubt on the REDUCE-IT trial result
Bempedoic acid; ATP citrate lyase inhibitor	CLEAR-Harmony	Treatment reduced the mean LDL-c level −16.5% from baseline (difference vs placebo in change from baseline, −18.1% points; 95% CI, −20.0 to −16.1; $P < .001$)	Potential new therapy for LDL-c lowering. Can be combined to ezetimibe to achieve LDL-c reduction equivalent to modest dose statin

Abbreviations: RR, relative risk; TG, triglyceride.
Adapted from Sillars A, Sattar N. Management of Lipid Abnormalities in Patients with Diabetes. *Curr Cardiol Rep.* 2019;21(11):147.

Subgroup	Studies	Baseline SBP	Events Intervention	Participants Intervention	Events Control	Participants Control	RR per 10 mm Hg lower SBP	RR (95% CI)
Major Cardiovascular Events								
Diabetes	23	145	3999	30796	4007	28977		0.88 [0.82; 0.94]
No Diabetes	18	153	3494	52616	4035	46427		0.75 [0.70; 0.80]
Fixed effect model								0.81 [0.77; 0.85]
Test for interaction: p=0.0006								
Coronary Heart Disease								
Diabetes	19	144	1404	26688	1487	25441		0.88 [0.80; 0.97]
No Diabetes	15	153	1143	41462	1389	35389		0.77 [0.70; 0.86]
Fixed effect model								0.83 [0.77; 0.89]
Test for interaction: p=0.0827								
Stroke								
Diabetes	21	144	1263	29643	1368	28421		0.74 [0.65; 0.84]
No Diabetes	19	153	1691	52920	1978	46852		0.74 [0.67; 0.81]
Fixed effect model								0.74 [0.68; 0.80]
Test for interaction: p=0.9533								
Heart Failure								
Diabetes	13	143	1028	21424	1094	20536		0.84 [0.72; 0.98]
No Diabetes	10	143	263	18578	373	18442		0.75 [0.65; 0.87]
Fixed effect model								0.79 [0.71; 0.88]
Test for interaction: p=0.277								
Renal Failure								
Diabetes	9	143	760	14549	774	13641		0.88 [0.75; 1.03]
No Diabetes	4	146	592	9921	638	9952		0.92 [0.79; 1.07]
Fixed effect model								0.90 [0.81; 1.01]
Test for interaction: p=0.7275								
All-cause Mortality								
Diabetes	20	144	2324	27562	2309	25782		0.87 [0.79; 0.97]
No Diabetes	17	153	1952	45588	2033	39414		0.83 [0.76; 0.90]
Fixed effect model								0.85 [0.79; 0.90]
Test for interaction: p=0.4544								

0.5   1   2   3

Fig. 3. Standardized effect of a 10 mm Hg reduction in systolic blood pressure (SBP) on the relative risk (RR) of major cardiovascular events, coronary heart disease, stroke, heart failure, renal failure, and all-cause mortality stratified by subgroups in which all (DM) or none (No DM) of the participants had diabetes mellitus at baseline. DM, diabetes mellitus. (*From* Ettehad D, Emdin CA, Kiran A, et al. Blood pressure lowering for prevention of cardiovascular disease and death: a systematic review and meta-analysis. Lancet. 2016;387(10022):957-967; with permission of Elsevier, Inc.)

undergo remission, trial evidence linking intentional weight loss to hard outcome benefits in T2DM is lacking. The Look AHEAD trial, a randomized trial of intensive lifestyle versus usual care in people with T2DM, did not establish outcome benefits of modest weight loss.[13] However, most considered this trial to have recruited too low a risk population to have sufficient power to see gains, and as noted, overall average weight loss was modest. A post hoc analysis from the same trial showed that those people who achieved a greater than 10% weight loss in the first year had a 21% (95% CI: 2% to 36%) lower risk of the primary outcome (composite of death from cardiovascular causes, nonfatal acute myocardial infarction, nonfatal stroke, or admission to hospital for angina[14]). This work allied to other trials, which show modest weight loss does not lead to ASCVD outcome benefits in the short term (eg, Lorcaserin in the CAMELLIA-TIMI 61 trial[15]), suggests larger weight loss may be needed to show outcome benefits.

In the DiRECT trial, which helped people with T2DM achieve around a 10 kg weight loss, the number of adverse events, albeit admittedly low, was significantly lower by second year of follow-up in the control group.[16] The authors were also able to show significant benefits in terms of lipids and blood pressure in the intervention group relative to controls. In unpublished data, they noted remarkable improvements in a protein pattern–associated incident cardiovascular outcomes by the end of the first year relative to control participants, in keeping with a significant reduction in future cardiovascular risk. Ongoing clinical outcome trials perhaps in particular SUR-PASS,[17] which is comparing the effects of tirzepatide (dual glucose-dependent insulinotropic polypeptide and GLP-1 receptor agonist) versus dulaglutide (GLP-1RA with proved ASCVD benefits[18]). As the former drug is associated with sustainably greater weight loss, this trial should help gauge the benefits of intentional weight loss in people with T2DM.

Outside of randomized trials, a series of studies using bariatric surgery suggests even greater weight loss may give important CV outcome benefits in people with diabetes. For example, using the Swedish Diabetes Registry, we reported that gastric bypass surgery (GBP) was associated with remarkably lower risks for major outcomes in people with T2DM who had on average a BMI greater than 40 at baseline. Risks for incident HF (hazard ratio [HR] 0.33 [95% CI 0.24, 0.46]) and CV mortality (HR 0.36 [95% CI 0.22, 0.58]) were substantially lowered by GBP as were renal outcomes.[19] In a linked study, we also showed GBP surgery to be associated with a lower risk for incident atrial fibrillation (AF) and to lower risk of mortality in people with T2DM who had prevalent HF.[20] Although such findings are of major interest, one must remember that these are not randomized trials and biases exist in people who choose to undergo bariatric surgery versus those who do not. Even so, the totality of findings suggest large weight loss may yield important cardiovascular outcome benefits in people with T2DM, extending beyond ASCVD to include AF, renal, and HF benefits. With the advent of stronger incretin-based drugs for weight loss, and ongoing clinical outcome trials, the impact of large-scale weight loss (ie, >10 kg) on cardiovascular outcomes in people with T2D should soon be confirmed or refuted.

Other lifestyle measures

There is no dubiety smoking is a strong risk factor for ASCVD, and people with diabetes have as much reason not to smoke as those without diabetes. There are now excellent ways to help people stop smoking, including nicotine patches and a range of medications.[21] Face-to-face support also seems more helpful than self-help materials. All people with T2DM who smoke should be encouraged to try to stop smoking and given the best possible help to achieve success.

In terms of activity, there are no randomized trials linked to CV outcomes, but clearly, greater activity levels help maintain muscle mass; keeps BMI, lipids, and blood pressure levels lower; and may have additional benefits across a range of pathways (liver fat, inflammation etc.). Perhaps the best recent data on activity and mortality come from the UK Biobank, a general population study that included people with T2DM. Using data from wearable devices, Strain and colleagues were able to show greater physical activity energy expenditure was associated with lower all-cause mortality.[22] More intense activity levels were also associated with lower risk for mortality, independent of amount of total activity volume. If we accept activity lessens CV outcomes, if people with T2DM can find sustainable ways to increase their activity levels, including even walking a little more, this could help offset CV disease. The manner in which health care professionals discuss activity with their patients can improve and perhaps needs to be more prescriptive. For example, as most people have iPhones, even simple targets of modest increase in steps (eg, extra 500 per day on average, increasingly gradually) may allow people to focus on achievable changes.

Antihyperglycemic agents

Aside from their glucose-lowering abilities that lower vascular risk, albeit modestly and slowly, it is important to assess whether antihyperglycemic agents (AHAs) lower cardiovascular risk beyond their glucose-lowering actions. A short summary of the quality of evidence for each agent is given in the following section for each major AHA used in clinical care.

Metformin. Metformin is an excellent glucose-lowering agent that does not cause weight gain or potentiate hypoglycemia. The UKPDS trial identified a cardiovascular benefit for metformin, but because this evidence stemmed from a subgroup analysis and involved low outcome numbers, many in the cardiovascular community remain skeptical. Subsequent meta-analyses have not added additional support for a metformin-associated CV benefit.

Sulfonylureas. There is no good evidence to suggest sulfonylureas lower cardiovascular risk, beyond their glucose-lowering benefits. In a recent large, randomized trial (CAROLINA[23]), there was no clear benefit of the dipeptidyl peptidase-4 (DPP-4) inhibitor, linagliptin, versus the sulfonylureas, glimepiride: primary outcome occurred in 356 of 3023 participants (11.8%) in the linagliptin group and 362 of 3010 (12.0%) in the glimepiride group (HR, 0.98 [95.47% CI, 0.84–1.14]). Because DPP-4 inhibitors have not been shown to lower ASCVD risk compared with placebo (see later discussion), by extension, glimepiride is unlikely to do so either.

Insulin. The ORIGIN trial (n = 12,537 people) did not show insulin lowers cardiovascular risk compared with standard when given in early diabetes or prediabetes. Incident cardiovascular outcomes rates were 2.94 and 2.85 per 100 person years in the insulin-glargine and standard-care groups, respectively, for the first coprimary outcome (HR, 1.02; 95% CI, 0.94–1.11; $P = 0.63$).

Dipeptidyl peptidase-4 inhibitors. Four DPP-4 inhibitor outcome trials testing alogliptin, saxagliptin, sitagliptin, and linagliptin[24–27] failed to demonstrate any superiority compared with placebo in patients with T2DM and high CV risk. In addition, there was an unexpected higher risk of hospitalization for HF reported with saxagliptin in SAVOR-TIMI-53.

Pioglitazone. In the PROACTIVE trial, pioglitazone reduced the secondary outcome composite of all-cause mortality, nonfatal myocardial infarction, and stroke in patients with T2D who had a high risk of cardiovascular events.[28] However, HF risk increased significantly. Pioglitazone also lowered stroke and myocardial infarction risks in patients with prediabetes and insulin resistance in the IRIS (Insulin Resistance Intervention after Stroke) trial.[29] However, because the drug causes weight gain, is linked to greater fracture risk, and increases HF risk in people with diabetes, it is less favored compared with available alternatives. This trial helped generate the idea that some drugs can have differential effects on ASCVD and HF, so that the pathophysiological processes can be differentially influenced depending on the drugs actions.

Sodium-glucose cotransporter-2 inhibitors. The most notable results from recent cardiovascular outcome trials come from the SGLT2i and GLP-1RA classes. As reported in a recent meta-analysis of 5 SGLT2i outcome trials, this class lowers major adverse cardiovascular events (MACE) risk modestly (around 10%), significant only in those with prior ASCVD (**Fig. 4A**[30]). However, more notable is a far greater reduction in the risk of incident HF hospitalization (HFH) in both those with (by 30%) and without (by 37%) prior ASCVD (see **Fig. 4B**). As noted in other papers, these drugs also lower

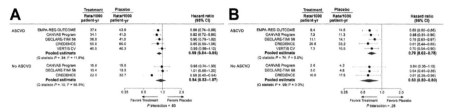

Fig. 4. The MACE (*A*) and HFH (*B*) benefits across people with diabetes with and without prevalent ASCVD in recent SGLT2i cardiovascular outcome trials. HFH, heart failure hospitalization. (*From* McGuire DK, Shih WJ, Cosentino F, et al. Association of SGLT2 Inhibitors With Cardiovascular and Kidney Outcomes in Patients With Type 2 Diabetes: A Meta-analysis. *JAMA Cardiol.* 2021;6(2):148–158; with permission).

incident renal outcomes and slow decline in estimated glomerular filtration rate. It has also been established that such benefits do not relate to glucose-lowering effects but to multiple other actions, chief among these likely to be hemodynamic effects leading to lessening of glomerular hyperfiltration and adverse cardiac remodeling.[31–33] However, cellular changes arising from SGLT2i actions on nutrient fluxes may also play a role.[34] Whatever the mechanism, multiple ongoing mechanistic trials are underway to add more insights, so called reverse translation (**Fig. 5**[35]). Finally, this class has also been shown to lessen HF or CV death in people with HF with reduced ejection fraction (HFrEF) in 2 recent seminal trials that have established SGLT2i as foundational in the treatment of such patients, whether they have diabetes or not.[36] The SGLT2i drugs with the best benefits to safety ratio seem to be empagliflozin and dapagliflozin, although canagliflozin is also licensed for some indications.

Glucagon-like peptide-1 receptor agonists. The GLP-1RA class, mostly injectable therapies, but a recent oral drug introduced, has also shown outcome benefits but these appear more consistently in the ASCVD domain. A recent meta-analysis that included all seven outcome trials to date showed the class lessens MACE and CV death by 12%, myocardial infarction risk by 9% and stroke risk by 16%[37] (**Fig. 6**). These HRs are likely modest underestimates as the meta-analysis included ELIXA (The Evaluation of Lixisenatide in Acute Coronary Syndrome), a universally null trial that tested the short-acting GLP-1RA, lixisenatide. The agents with the best evidence include liraglutide, dulaglutide, albiglutide, and semaglutide, although albiglutide has

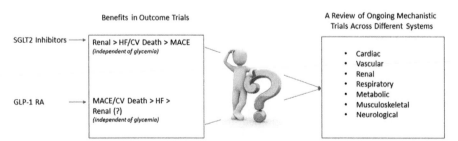

Fig. 5. Reverse translation of the outcome benefits seen with SGLT2i and GLP-1RAs. (*From* Lee MMY, Petrie MC, McMurray JJV, Sattar N. How Do SGLT2 (Sodium-Glucose Cotransporter 2) Inhibitors and GLP-1 (Glucagon-Like Peptide-1) Receptor Agonists Reduce Cardiovascular Outcomes? *Arterioscler Thromb Vasc Biol.* 2020;40(3):506–522; with permission).

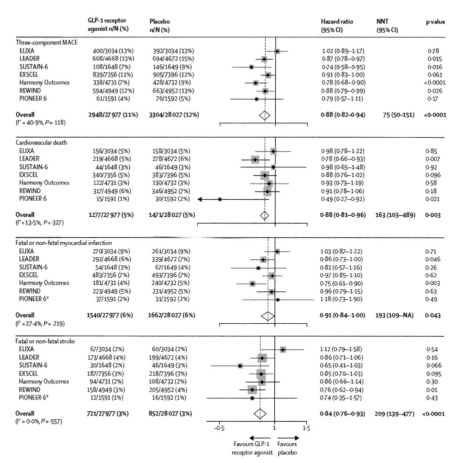

Fig. 6. Risk of MACE and each of its components. Three-component MACE consisted of cardiovascular death, myocardial infarction, and stroke. NNTs are calculated over an estimated median follow-up of 3·2 years. NNT = number needed to treat. (*From* Kristensen SL, Rørth R, Jhund PS, et al. Cardiovascular, mortality, and kidney outcomes with GLP-1 receptor agonists in patients with type 2 diabetes: a systematic review and meta-analysis of cardiovascular outcome trials. *Lancet Diabetes Endocrinol.* 2019;7(10):776–785; with permission).

not been licensed for use. There is some evidence that these drugs may lessen incident HFH but far more modestly (9% reduction) than seen with SGLT2is.

Side-effect profiles of SGLT2i and GLP-1RA classes

The advantage of both classes over some other AHA agents is that they help weight loss, do not increase hypoglycemia, and lower blood pressure. The SGLT2i class does increase risk for genital infections and diabetic ketoacidosis, but these can be minimized by patient education and better targeting of drugs to suitable patients. Genetical infections are also easily treated. The GLP-1RA class causes nausea and vomiting early on in treatment, an effect that can be minimized by starting low and escalating the doses slowly. Such effects tend to lessen with continued use.

Guideline implications of recent evidence

Because of their consistent results, the SGLT2i and GLP-1RA classes have been recommended in recent guidelines for treatment of patients with diabetes and existing

ASCVD.[38,39] The SGLT2i class is also recommended for patients with T2DM and HF and chronic kidney disease. These 2 classes have also been variably suggested for patients at elevated risk for ASCVD, but, as we recently reviewed,[40] cardiovascular- and diabetes-led guidelines recommend somewhat different categories of at-risk patients who would merit treatment. However, all groups now agree such classes can be used independently of glycaemia levels, and increasing evidence shows that both classes work independently of background metformin therapy, as recently reviewed,[41] so that there is no need to start with metformin in patients recommended for such therapies. This latter point remains somewhat debated in diabetes circles.

Greater outcome benefits in Asians

Finally, in a recent meta-analysis of outcome trials where primary endpoints data for Asian ethnicity were able to be extracted, the authors showed that the GLP-1RA class may lessen MACE in people with diabetes more greatly in Asians than in whites (**Fig. 7**).[42] The same pattern seemed true for the SGLT2i class in lessening incident HFH/CV death in those with HFrEF. If these observations hold true, they are clinically

Study		Hazard Ratio with 95% CI	Weight (%)
Asian			
LEADER		0.70 [0.46, 1.04]	4.59
SUSTAIN-6		0.58 [0.25, 1.34]	1.43
EXSCEL		0.81 [0.57, 1.14]	4.73
HARMONY OUTCOMES		0.73 [0.36, 1.48]	1.36
REWIND		0.71 [0.40, 1.24]	2.35
PIONEER 6		0.44 [0.20, 0.97]	2.76
Heterogeneity: $\tau^2 = 0.00$, $I^2 = 0.00\%$, $H^2 = 1.00$		0.68 [0.53, 0.84]	
Test of $\theta_i = \theta_j$: Q(5) = 2.49, P = .78			
White			
LEADER		0.90 [0.80, 1.02]	18.19
SUSTAIN-6		0.76 [0.58, 1.00]	7.86
EXSCEL		0.95 [0.85, 1.05]	19.91
HARMONY OUTCOMES		0.76 [0.64, 0.89]	15.89
REWIND		0.90 [0.79, 1.02]	17.39
PIONEER 6		0.83 [0.56, 1.23]	3.56
Heterogeneity: $\tau^2 = 0.00$, $I^2 = 28.58\%$, $H^2 = 1.40$		0.87 [0.81, 0.94]	
Test of $\theta_i = \theta_j$: Q(5) = 7.00, P = .22			
Overall		0.84 [0.77, 0.90]	
Heterogeneity: $\tau^2 = 0.00$, $I^2 = 26.68\%$, $H^2 = 1.36$			
Test of $\theta_i = \theta_j$: Q(11) = 15.00, P = .18			
Test of group differences: $Q_b(1) = 4.87$, P = .03			

0.00   0.50   1.00   1.50

Random-effects DerSimonian-Laird model

Fig. 7. GLP-1RA cardiovascular outcome trials reporting MACE outcome by race. (*From* Lee MMY, Ghouri N, McGuire DK, Rutter MK, Sattar N. Meta-analyses of Results From Randomized Outcome Trials Comparing Cardiovascular Effects of SGLT2is and GLP-1RAs in Asian vs White Patients With and Without Type 2 Diabetes. *Diabetes Care.* March 2021:dc203007; with permission).

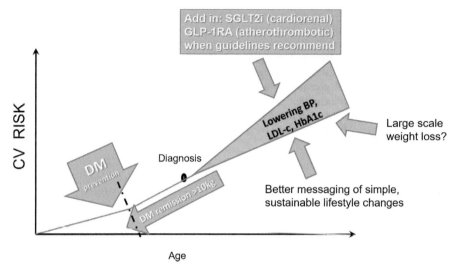

Fig. 8. Different factors that are either fully proved to help lessen CV risk in people with diabetes or may be shown to do so in future. If diabetes can be prevented or delayed in those at higher risk, this delay can offset CV risk. Earlier diagnosis can also lower overall glycemic exposure. Early after diagnosis, consideration of multifactorial risk factor management, targeting glucose, cholesterol, and blood pressure, as well as smoking cessation, will lead to considerable benefits. There are ongoing trials testing agents that yield substantial weight loss, and their CV outcomes are also eagerly awaited. Whether better messaging of lifestyle advice (or facilitating adoption of such changes) can lessen CV risks is not known but seems sensible. Finally, 2 newer classes of diabetes drugs have shown substantial CV benefits and, wherever possible (and affordable), should be initiated at some point in the diabetes life course, in line with national or local diabetes guidelines.

important as greater than 60% of the world's population is Asian, and it is here where diabetes rates are escalating most rapidly. However, more work is needed to validate these observations and, if validated, to test whether they apply to all Asians or only specific ethnicities within this large population.

SUMMARY

Cardiovascular risk in people with T2DM has substantially declined in high-income countries over the last 3 to 4 decades, with early gains achieved from a combination of glucose reductions, lipid lowering via statins, and blood pressure treatments, on the background of falling smoking rates. In low- and middle-income countries, CV risks remain high, and the goals are for earlier diagnosis of diabetes, and prediabetes, so that more can be prevented from developing diabetes or it can be meaningfully delayed. Thereafter, a reliable supply of cheap metformin, statin, and blood pressure medications would do much to lessen CV risks in these countries. It is insufficient to target only glucose reduction.

In high-income countries, cardiovascular improvements accrued over a few decades may have started to plateau in the last decade, perhaps due to a slowing or even reversal of risk factor improvements. That noted, the last 10 years have seen a remarkable number of outcome trials that convincingly showed reductions in ASCVD and incident HFH in people with diabetes using 2 newer classes of drugs. At the same time, there is growing interest in the benefits of large weight loss to further lessen risks of important CV outcomes in people with diabetes who are living with obesity or severe obesity. There is a parallel growing interest in helping recently diagnosed people with diabetes achieve remission, a process that should also lessen CV risks. Further strategies to test remission protocols in many countries are being widely tested or planned. Going forward, the toolbox to help lessen CV outcomes in people with diabetes across its life course has expanded significantly (**Fig. 8**), with gains at both ends of the diabetes life course.

Finally, despite all these medical advances, it is also important that health care professionals do not forget to help their patients with diabetes achieve small but sustainable improvements in their diets and activity levels, even if trials are lacking to show the hard outcome benefits of such changes. There is other ample evidence that lifestyle improvements can have profound benefits on future health, and the messaging of these needs to improve going forward. Such points are particularly pertinent in the post-COVID era, as better lifestyles are needed to help offset all the metabolic and vascular harms imposed by the pandemic, effects that disproportionately affect people living with diabetes.

CLINICS CARE POINTS

- To help prevent important CV complications, it is critical to adopt a multifactorial risk factor approach and not just focus on glucose reduction.

- Many people with diabetes will be recommended for statins. The risk for myopathy associated with statin has been proved to be exaggerated in recent n-of-1 trials. Patients who claim to suffer muscle side effects (unless severe or associated with measurable creatine kinase elevations) should be encouraged to stop and restart statin, initially at same dose and then at a lower dose, or type of statin switched. If statins cannot be tolerated, ezetimibe should be recommended.

- When starting blood pressure treatments, it is better to consider dual therapy, each drug given at low dose.

- Give simpler messaging for lifestyle advice so that patients can attempt achievable goals, which must also be sustainable. If such advice fails to make a difference, multiple other options to help aid weight loss could be signposted.

- Discuss diabetes drug options with patients, pointing out the benefits and side effects and explain that some drugs can give meaningful CV benefits without necessarily altering glucose concentrations.

- If local resources allow, consider discussing the potential option for diabetes remission clinics in people with recently diagnosed diabetes, as this can also lower CV risk.

DISCLOSURE

N.S. has received grant and personal fees from Boehringer Ingelheim, and personal fees from Amgen, AstraZeneca, Eli Lilly, Merck Sharp & Dohme, Novartis, Novo Nordisk, Pfizer, and Sanofi outside the submitted work.

ACKNOWLEDGMENTS

This work was supported by the British Heart Foundation Research Excellence Award (RE/18/6/34217). The author thanks Liz Coyle, University of Glasgow, for her assistance in the preparation of this article.

REFERENCES

1. Rao Kondapally Seshasai S, Kaptoge S, Thompson A, et al. Diabetes mellitus, fasting glucose, and risk of cause-specific death. N Engl J Med 2011;364(9): 829–41.
2. Bjornsdottir HH, Rawshani A, Rawshani A, et al. A national observation study of cancer incidence and mortality risks in type 2 diabetes compared to the background population over time. Sci Rep 2020;10(1):17376.
3. Shah AD, Langenberg C, Rapsomaniki E, et al. Type 2 diabetes and incidence of cardiovascular diseases: A cohort study in 1·9 million people. Lancet Diabetes Endocrinol 2015;3(2):105–13.
4. Taylor R, Al-Mrabeh A, Sattar N. Understanding the mechanisms of reversal of type 2 diabetes. Lancet Diabetes Endocrinol 2019;7(9):726–36.
5. Welsh C, Welsh P, Celis-Morales CA, et al. Glycated Hemoglobin, Prediabetes, and the Links to Cardiovascular Disease: Data From UK Biobank. Diabetes Care 2020;43(2):440–5.
6. Ray KK, Seshasai SRK, Wijesuriya S, et al. Effect of intensive control of glucose on cardiovascular outcomes and death in patients with diabetes mellitus: a meta-analysis of randomised controlled trials. Lancet 2009;373(9677):1765–72.
7. Cholesterol Treatment Trialists' (CTT) Collaborators. Efficacy of cholesterol-lowering therapy in 18 686 people with diabetes in 14 randomised trials of statins: a meta-analysis. Lancet 2008;371(9607):117–25.
8. Ference BA, Kastelein JJP, Catapano AL. Lipids and lipoproteins in 2020. JAMA 2020;324(6):595–6.
9. Sillars A, Sattar N. Management of lipid abnormalities in patients with diabetes. Curr Cardiol Rep 2019;21(11):147.
10. Wright AK, Welsh P, Gill JMR, et al. Age-, sex- and ethnicity-related differences in body weight, blood pressure, HbA1c and lipid levels at the diagnosis of type 2 diabetes relative to people without diabetes. Diabetologia 2020;63(8):1542–53.
11. Ettehad D, Emdin CA, Kiran A, et al. Blood pressure lowering for prevention of cardiovascular disease and death: a systematic review and meta-analysis. Lancet 2016;387(10022):957–67.
12. Williams B, Mancia G, Spiering W, et al. 2018 ESC/ESH Guidelines for the management of arterial hypertension: The Task Force for the management of arterial hypertension of the European Society of Cardiology and the European Society of Hypertension: The Task Force for the management of arterial hypertension of the European Society of Cardiology and the European Society of Hypertension. J Hypertens 2018;36(10):1953–2041.
13. Look AHEAD Research Group, Wing RR, Bolin P, Brancati FL, et al. Cardiovascular Effects of Intensive Lifestyle Intervention in Type 2 Diabetes. N Engl J Med 2013;369(2):145–54.
14. Gregg E, Jakicic J, Blackburn G, et al. Association of the magnitude of weight loss and changes in physical fitness with long-term cardiovascular disease outcomes in overweight or obese people with type 2 diabetes: a post-hoc analysis of the Look AHEAD randomised clinical trial. Lancet Diabetes Endocrinol 2016; 4(11):913–21.
15. Bohula EA, Wiviott SD, McGuire DK, et al. Cardiovascular safety of lorcaserin in overweight or obese patients. N Engl J Med 2018;379(12):1107–17.
16. Lean MEJ, Leslie WS, Barnes AC, et al. Durability of a primary care-led weight-management intervention for remission of type 2 diabetes: 2-year results of the

DiRECT open-label, cluster-randomised trial. Lancet Diabetes Endocrinol 2019; 7(5):344–55.

17. A Study of Tirzepatide (LY3298176) Compared With Dulaglutide on Major Cardiovascular Events in Participants With Type 2 Diabetes. Available at: https://clinicaltrials.gov/ct2/show/NCT04255433. Accessed March 26, 2021.

18. Gerstein HC, Colhoun HM, Dagenais GR, et al. Dulaglutide and cardiovascular outcomes in type 2 diabetes (REWIND): a double-blind, randomised placebo-controlled trial. Lancet 2019;394(10193):121–30.

19. Liakopoulos V, Franzén S, Svensson AM, et al. Renal and cardiovascular outcomes after weight loss from gastric bypass surgery in type 2 diabetes: cardiorenal risk reductions exceed atherosclerotic benefits. Diabetes Care 2020;43(6): 1276–84.

20. Höskuldsdóttir G, Sattar N, Miftaraj M, et al. Potential effects of bariatric surgery on the incidence of heart failure and atrial fibrillation in patients with type 2 diabetes mellitus and obesity and on mortality in patients with preexisting heart failure: a nationwide, matched, observational cohort. J Am Heart Assoc 2021; 69(Supplement 1):e019323.

21. Lindson N, Klemperer E, Hong B, et al. Smoking reduction interventions for smoking cessation. Cochrane Database Syst Rev 2019;9(9):CD013183.

22. Strain T, Wijndaele K, Dempsey PC, et al. Wearable-device-measured physical activity and future health risk. Nat Med 2020;26(9):1385–91.

23. Rosenstock J, Kahn SE, Johansen OE, et al. Effect of linagliptin vs glimepiride on major adverse cardiovascular outcomes in patients with type 2 diabetes: the CAROLINA randomized clinical trial. JAMA 2019;322(12):1155–66.

24. White WB, Cannon CP, Heller SR, et al. Alogliptin after acute coronary syndrome in patients with type 2 diabetes. N Engl J Med 2013;369(14):1327–35.

25. Scirica BM, Bhatt DL, Braunwald E, et al. Saxagliptin and cardiovascular outcomes in patients with type 2 diabetes mellitus. N Engl J Med 2013;369(14): 1317–26.

26. Green JB, Bethel MA, Armstrong PW, et al. Effect of sitagliptin on cardiovascular outcomes in type 2 diabetes. N Engl J Med 2015;373(3):232–42.

27. Rosenstock J, Perkovic V, Johansen OE, et al. Effect of linagliptin vs placebo on major cardiovascular events in adults with type 2 diabetes and high cardiovascular and renal risk. JAMA 2019;321(1):69–79.

28. Dormandy JA, Charbonnel B, Eckland DJA, et al. Secondary prevention of macrovascular events in patients with type 2 diabetes in the PROactive Study (PROspective pioglitAzone Clinical Trial in macroVascular Events): A randomised controlled trial. Lancet 2005;366(9493):1279–89.

29. Spence JD, Viscoli CM, Inzucchi SE, et al. Pioglitazone therapy in patients with stroke and prediabetes: a post hoc analysis of the iris randomized clinical trial. JAMA Neurol 2019;76(5):526–35.

30. McGuire DK, Shih WJ, Cosentino F, et al. Association of SGLT2 inhibitors with cardiovascular and kidney outcomes in patients with type 2 diabetes: a meta-analysis. JAMA Cardiol 2021;6(2):148–58.

31. Sattar N, McLaren J, Kristensen SL, et al. SGLT2 Inhibition and cardiovascular events: why did EMPA-REG outcomes surprise and what were the likely mechanisms? Diabetologia 2016;59(7):1333–9.

32. Lee MMY, Brooksbank KJM, Wetherall K, et al. Effect of empagliflozin on left ventricular volumes in patients with type 2 diabetes, or prediabetes, and heart failure with reduced ejection fraction (SUGAR-DM-HF). Circulation 2021;143(6):516–25.

33. Butler J, Hamo CE, Filippatos G, et al. The potential role and rationale for treatment of heart failure with sodium-glucose co-transporter 2 inhibitors. Eur J Heart Fail 2017;19(11):1390–400.

34. Packer M. Molecular, cellular, and clinical evidence that sodium-glucose cotransporter 2 inhibitors act as neurohormonal antagonists when used for the treatment of chronic heart failure. J Am Heart Assoc 2020;9(16):e016270.

35. Lee MMY, Petrie MC, McMurray JJV, et al. How do SGLT2 (sodium-glucose co-transporter 2) inhibitors and GLP-1 (glucagon-like peptide-1) receptor agonists reduce cardiovascular outcomes? Arterioscler Thromb Vasc Biol 2020;40(3):506–22.

36. McMurray JJV, Solomon SD, Inzucchi SE, et al. Dapagliflozin in patients with heart failure and reduced ejection fraction. N Engl J Med 2019;381(21):1995–2008.

37. Kristensen SL, Rørth R, Jhund PS, et al. Cardiovascular, mortality, and kidney outcomes with GLP-1 receptor agonists in patients with type 2 diabetes: a systematic review and meta-analysis of cardiovascular outcome trials. Lancet Diabetes Endocrinol 2019;7(10):776–85.

38. Cosentino F, Grant PJ, Aboyans V, et al. 2019 ESC Guidelines on diabetes, pre-diabetes, and cardiovascular diseases developed in collaboration with the EASD. Eur Heart J 2020;41(2):255–323.

39. Buse JB, Wexler DJ, Tsapas A, et al. 2019 Update to: Management of Hyperglycemia in Type 2 Diabetes, 2018. A Consensus Report by the American Diabetes Association (ADA) and the European Association for the Study of Diabetes (EASD). Diabetes Care 2020;43(2):487–93.

40. Sattar N, McMurray JJV, Cheng AYY. Cardiorenal risk reduction guidance in diabetes: can we reach consensus? Lancet Diabetes Endocrinol 2020;8(5):357–60.

41. Sattar N, McGuire DK. Prevention of CV outcomes in antihyperglycaemic drug-naïve patients with type 2 diabetes with, or at elevated risk of, ASCVD: to start or not to start with metformin. Eur Heart J 2020;ehaa879. https://doi.org/10.1093/eurheartj/ehaa879.

42. Lee MMY, Ghouri N, McGuire DK, et al. Meta-analyses of results from randomized outcome trials comparing cardiovascular effects of SGLT2is and GLP-1RAs in Asian versus white patients with and without type 2 diabetes. Diabetes Care 2021;44(5):1236–41.

Prevention of Microvascular Complications of Diabetes

Winston Crasto, MBBS, MRCP, MD[a,*],
Vinod Patel, MD, FRCP, DRCOG, MRCGP, FHEAA, RCPathME[a,b],
Melanie J. Davies, CBE, MBChB, MD, FRCP, FRCGP, FMedSci[c],
Kamlesh Khunti, FRCGP, FRCP, MD, PhD, FMedSci[c]

KEYWORDS

- Cardiovascular • Diabetes • Diabetic kidney disease • Diabetic retinopathy
- Diabetic neuropathy

KEY POINTS

- Microvascular complications of diabetes present with diverse clinical presentations, seem to be strongly intercorrelated, and are a cause of significant morbidity and cardiovascular mortality.
- Hyperglycemia mainly drives the development and progression of microvascular disease, whereas the synergistic effects of hypertension, dyslipidemia, smoking, and genetic and hereditary susceptibility also contribute.
- Preventative strategies should focus on tight control of modifiable cardiovascular risk factors including hypertension and dyslipidemia, with particular emphasis on individualized glycemic control.
- Increased awareness and education; pragmatic, low-cost screening; and affordable specialist care are important measures toward reducing the increasing global microvascular disease burden due to diabetes.

INTRODUCTION

Global prevalence estimates from 2019 suggest that the number of people diagnosed with diabetes was 463 million and is projected to increase to 700 million by the year 2045.[1] The growing prevalence and increase in life-years spent with diabetes has a significant impact on the development of macrovascular and microvascular complications and places a huge societal and financial burden on almost every health care system in the world.[2] Although, declining trends in cardiovascular complications, cardiovascular-related mortality and lower extremity amputation rates have been reported over the last 2 decades, particularly from high-income countries including

[a] Department of Diabetes and Endocrinology, George Eliot Hospitals NHS Trust, College street, Nuneaton CV10 7DJ, UK; [b] Warwick Medical School, University of Warwick, Coventry, UK; [c] Diabetes Research Centre, College of Life Sciences, University of Leicester, Leicester General Hospital, Leicester, LE5 4PW, UK
* Corresponding author.
E-mail address: winston.crasto@geh.nhs.uk

Endocrinol Metab Clin N Am 50 (2021) 431–455
https://doi.org/10.1016/j.ecl.2021.05.005 **endo.theclinics.com**

Europe and North America, the global burden of cardiovascular disease, blindness due to retinopathy, and end-stage kidney disease (ESKD) in people with diabetes compared with those without has increased alarmingly.[3] The "DISCOVER" observational study program from 2014 to 2019 reported that the global crude prevalence of microvascular complications in people with type 2 diabetes was 18.8%, being highest in Europe (23.5%) and lowest in Africa (14.5%).[4] Among individuals with a median duration of type 2 diabetes of 4.1 years, the prevalence of peripheral neuropathy was 7.7%, chronic kidney disease 5.0%, and albuminuria 4.3%.

Epidemiologic studies suggest a strong correlation between the vascular related complications of diabetes.[5,6] For example, diabetic retinopathy (DR) is strongly associated with the risk of developing diabetic kidney disease (DKD) and is a strong predictor of stroke and cardiovascular disease.[5] Furthermore, in people with type 2 diabetes, individual microvascular complications indicate cardiovascular risk better than classic risk factors such as blood pressure, HbA1c, and LDL-cholesterol, whereas multiple complications are associated with doubling of cardiovascular risk and cardiovascular mortality.[7] These findings suggest that screening for microvascular complications offers a convenient and inexpensive tool to improve risk prediction in people with diabetes and that early use of cardioprotective therapies can prevent or delay these debilitating events with minimal impact.[8]

Microvascular complications typically develop over several years but can manifest even at diagnosis, particularly in people with type 2 diabetes. Although, hyperglycemia is the "sine qua non" in the causation of microvascular disease, the mechanisms by which it disrupts normal microvessel structure or function are multiple and not clearly defined.[9] In addition, the synergistic effects of hypertension, dyslipidemia (low HDL and often elevated triglycerides), smoking, and duration of diabetes, play an important role in its causation, development, and progression. In recent years, the interaction between genetic and environmental modifications (diet, lifestyle) is a plausible mechanism in the development of microvascular complications of diabetes.[10] Indeed, retinopathy and microalbuminuria are often present both in prediabetes states and prehypertension.[11]

This review discusses the pathogenesis, risk factors, diagnosis, and prevention of microvascular complications of diabetes mainly affecting the target organs including the eye, kidneys, and peripheral and autonomic nervous systems. It also summarizes best practice clinical care recommendations that can guide health care professionals to better manage people with these conditions.

DIABETES RETINOPATHY

Global prevalence estimates from 2015 suggest that nearly 2.6 million people had moderate or severe vision impairment due to DR, and the numbers are expected to increase to 3.2 million by 2020, which is approximately 1% of the total population with diabetes.[12] In high-income countries such as the United Kingdom, there has been a significant decline in DR prevalence due to improved surveillance and effective specialist care and is no longer the commonest cause of blindness.[13] Furthermore, it is estimated that between 2010 and 2030, the number of adults with diabetes will increase by 69% in low-income and middle-income countries compared with only 20% in high-income countries.

Pathogenesis

Increased pericyte loss, endothelial cell apoptosis, leaky retinal capillary endothelial cells, accumulation of advanced glycation end products, and thickening of the basement membrane occur early in DR.[14] Leukocyte adherence to retinal vascular endothelium, vascular leakage, and capillary closure leads to the formation of micro-aneurysms, cotton wool spots, and hard exudates.[14] Occlusion of retinal capillaries and arterioles leads to retinal ischemia, which promotes increased intraocular production of vascular endothelial growth factor (VEGF). Subsequently, leakage of blood from fragile neoproliferative blood vessels, loss of retinal astrocytes and photoreceptors due to microglial fibrosis, leads on to loss of vision.[14]

RISK FACTORS FOR DIABETES RETINOPATHY

Poor glycemic control, longer duration of diabetes, hypertension, dyslipidemia (total cholesterol and low-density lipoprotein cholesterol), anemia, smoking, and microalbuminuria are recognized risk factors for DR.[15] Ethnicity is a complex, independent risk factor, and sight-threatening DR and diabetic macular oedema (DMO) are found to be higher in people of South Asian, African, Latin American, and indigenous tribal descent.[14] Genetic susceptibility has been linked to progression of DR, although validated genotype-phenotype associations have not yet been found. Interestingly, in people with type 2 diabetes and hypothyroidism, thyroid hormone replacement seems to have a protective effect on the development of DR.[16]

DIAGNOSIS AND CLASSIFICATION OF DIABETIC RETINOPATHY

Although grading systems vary across the world, the American Academy of Ophthalmology International Clinical Diabetic Retinopathy Disease Severity scale is a practical and valid method of grading DR and DMO and is being widely used.[14]

Nonproliferative Diabetic Retinopathy or Background Diabetic Retinopathy

Nonproliferative diabetic retinopathy (NPDR) represents the early, asymptomatic stage of DR. It is characterized by increased vascular permeability, retinal ischemia, and capillary occlusion. Retinal examination shows microaneurysms, intraretinal hemorrhages, venous abnormalities such as "beading" and "looping," and intraretinal microvascular abnormalities. Other features include hard exudates due to accumulation of lipid in or under the retina and fluffy white "cotton wool spots," which are microinfarcts in the nerve fiber layer, although these are commonly a feature of preproliferative DR or DMO.[14]

Proliferative Diabetic Retinopathy

Proliferative diabetic retinopathy (PDR) is characterized by neovascularization in response to severe ischemia. New blood vessels grow into the vitreous, often at or near the optic disc or new vessels elsewhere along the vascular arcades, and are prone to bleeding. Funduscopic features include vitreous hemorrhage, vitreoretinal traction bands, retinal tears, and tractional retinal detachment. Affected individuals may experience severe vision impairment. Neovascular glaucoma (new blood vessels in the iris) is a late complication of PDR.[14]

Diabetic Macular Oedema

DMO is characterized by swelling or thickening of the macula due to subretinal and intraretinal accumulation of fluid in the macula triggered by the breakdown of the blood–retinal barrier. DMO can occur at any stage of DR and cause distortion of visual images and a decrease in visual acuity. Untreated it can lead to total loss of vision (**Fig. 1**).[14,17]

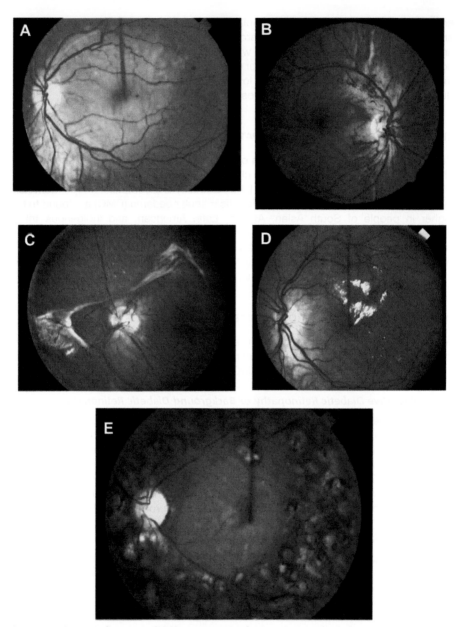

Fig. 1. Funduscopic features of different stages of DR and panretinal photocoagulation. (*A*) Nonproliferative DR (microaneurysms, dot hemorrhages. (*B*) Proliferative DR (new vessels on the disc, retinal hemorrhages). (*C*) Proliferative DR (new vessels on the disc and elsewhere, preretinal fibrosis, exudates, and retinal hemorrhages). (*D*) Diabetic maculopathy (hard exudates within the macular area, circinate hard exudates, MA, retinal hemorrhages). (*E*) Panretinal photocoagulation showing laser scars on the inferior retina and fresh laser burns on the superior retina.

RISK FACTOR CONTROL—EVIDENCE FROM CLINICAL TRIALS
Glycemic Control

The landmark DCCT (Diabetes Control and Complications Trial) and its subsequent, observational EDIC (Epidemiology of Diabetes Interventions and Complications) follow-up study in individuals with type 1 diabetes showed that intensive glycemic control reduced the development and progression of DR by 76% and 54%, respectively, over 6.5 years and diabetes-related eye surgery by 48% (95% confidence interval [CI]: 29–63, P<.001). Although, intensive glycemic control was associated with an initial worsening of DR, the beneficial "metabolic memory" effect of intensive glycemic control persisted for up to 23 years.[18]

In the seminal UKPDS study in people with type 2 diabetes, a 1% (approximately 10 mmol/mol) reduction in HbA1c equated to a 31% reduction in retinopathy. Improved glucose control showed significant ocular beneficial effects with a "legacy effect."[19] In the ACCORD eye study and its follow-up study, intensive glycemic control slowed the progression of DR compared with standard care, with a stronger treatment effect observed in individuals with mild DR. Intensive glycemic control conferred enduring protection even after ~4 years of completion of the study.[20,21]

ROLE OF GLUCOSE-LOWERING DRUGS IN DIABETIC RETINOPATHY

The newer glucose-lowering agents (sodium-glucose co-transporter-2 inhibitors and glucagon-Like peptide 1[GLP-1] receptor agonists) provide no additional benefit beyond that of improving glycemic control. In the linagliptin outcomes study (CARMELINA trial),[22] Linagliptin, a selective dipeptidyl peptidase-4 inhibitor added to usual care, significantly reduced the microvascular composite endpoint (time to retinal photocoagulation or anti-VEGF therapy for DR, vitreous hemorrhage or blindness, albuminuria progression, ESKD, greater than or equal to 50% reduction in estimated glomerular filtration rate (eGFR), and death from renal failure [hazard ratio [HR] 0.86 CI:0.78–0.95, P = .003]). Indeed, it seems that rapid improvements in glycemic control with subcutaneous semaglutide (once weekly GLP-1 receptor agonist) in the SUSTAIN 6 trial was associated with increased risk of DR and retinopathy complications.[23] Hence, it is important that physicians are alerted to the safety warning associated with the use of these drugs and monitoring for eye complications is recommended. A specific DR outcome study, the ongoing FOCUS trial, will establish the long-term effects of semaglutide on DR in subjects with type 2 diabetes.[24]

Blood Pressure Control

A systematic review by Do and colleagues reported that intensive blood pressure control is beneficial in reducing the combined outcome of DR incidence and progression (estimated risk ratio 0.78; 95% CI: 0.63–0.97), but it did not affect the 4- to 5-year progression of DR, progression to PDR or clinically significant Macular oedema (CSME), or moderate-to-severe loss of best-corrected visual acuity.[25] In the UKPDS studies, a 10 mm Hg decrement in systolic blood pressure equated to an 11% reduction in photocoagulation or vitreous hemorrhage.[19] There is some evidence that angiotensin-converting enzyme (ACE) inhibition may preferentially improve autoregulation in the retinal circulation when compared with other agents such as β-blockers.[26] A similar result was found in individuals with type 2 diabetes in the micro-HOPE study.[27] ACE inhibition may promote a hemodynamic milieu in the hypertensive, diabetic retinal circulation that serves to protect against the progression of DR.

Dyslipidemia

The FIELD study in people with type 2 diabetes showed that treatment with fenofibrate over 5 years, significantly slowed the progression of DR and reduced need for laser therapy for DMO and PDR by 31%,[28] whereas the Action to Control Cardiovascular Risk in Diabetes (ACCORD) Eye Study showed that fenofibrate and simvastatin treatment was associated with less progression of DR, although these benefits were not sustained at 4-year follow-up.[21] The mechanism of action seems to be independent of fenofibrate's lipid-lowering properties.[28]

Pregnancy

DR during pregnancy poses several challenges. Pregnant women with preexisting type 1 or type 2 diabetes (not gestational diabetes) are at a higher risk of development and progression of DR. Furthermore, the potential for DR to worsen rapidly either due to pregnancy itself, preexisting DR, or if rapid intensification of glycemic control is implemented.[29]

DIABETIC KIDNEY DISEASE

DKD suggests the presence of chronic kidney disease (CKD) due to diabetes, although the clinical spectrum can also extend to those with non-DKD or both. DKD is the global leading cause of ESKD, leading to significant morbidity and cardiovascular mortality.[30] The number of people receiving renal replacement therapy was around 2·6 million a decade ago and is likely to double by 2030.[30] However, only 10% of people with ESKD undergo hemodialysis and renal transplant therapies, whereas the remainder (~90%) succumb to cardiovascular disease or infection.[30] Large treatment gaps exist in low-income countries such as Asia and Africa where nearly 1·9 million and 432,000 people, respectively, do not receive renal replacement therapies despite needing it, which suggests the need for effective low-cost treatments and population-based prevention strategies.[31]

Pathogenesis

Metabolic and hemodynamic alterations caused by prolonged hyperglycemia, hypertension, and dyslipidemia promote inflammation, endothelial dysfunction, oxidative stress, and fibrosis.[32] Podocyte loss occurs early, followed by basement membrane thickening, mesangial expansion, reduced glomerular filtration surface density, and nodular sclerosis. Nodular glomerulosclerosis (the Kimmelstiel-Wilson lesion) of DKD is a pink hyaline material formation near the capillary loops in the glomerulus. It represents a marked increase in mesangial matrix damage as a result of nonenzymatic glycosylation of proteins. Late sequelae include arterial hyalinosis and tubulo-interstitial fibrosis.[33]

RISK FACTORS FOR DIABETIC KIDNEY DISEASE

Prolonged hyperglycemia is a strong determinant of DKD. Other associated risk factors include hypertension, smoking, obesity, physical inactivity, and dyslipidaemia.[10] Genetic susceptibility seems to be a prerequisite to the development of DKD.[34]

DIAGNOSIS

DKD is clinically defined by abnormal increase in creatinine ratio excretion with or without a reduction in glomerular filtration function (eGFR), often associated with an increase in blood pressure but without evidence of other primary causes of kidney disease.[33] The natural history of DKD includes glomerular hyperfiltration, progressive albuminuria, declining GFR, and ultimately ESKD (**Fig. 2**).

Albuminuria is diagnosed from a "spot" urine sample confirmed by 2 abnormal albuminuria creatinine ratio test results within a 3- to 6-month interval. The spectrum of albuminuria increases in severity from microalbuminuria (>2.5 mg/mmol in men; >3.5 mg/mmol in women) to macroalbuminuria (>30 mg/mmol). Microalbuminuria and macroalbuminuria are independent risk factors for cardiovascular morbidity and mortality in people with diabetes.[35] The eGFR is calculated from the abbreviated MDRD equation and is a more accurate measure of kidney function than serum creatinine. However, this may not be true in all populations. A study in India among healthy kidney donors and individuals with CKD showed that existing creatinine-based GFR estimating equations overestimate GFR by around 25%, because Indian subjects tend to have a lower protein intake and lower muscle mass.[36] Tracking an individual's creatinine level is therefore also important. The coexistence of albuminuria and CKD stages 3 to 5 is associated with a significantly increased risk of major adverse cardiovascular events independent of diabetes status.[37] Therefore, screening and monitoring with novel biomarkers such as cystatin C, which is an early predictor of DN, can also provide more accurate staging of DKD to improve health outcomes.[38]

Symptoms of DKD are usually absent until the advanced stages. Fatigue, anorexia, and swelling of the extremities are the main presenting complaints. The clinical symptoms of uremia in advanced DKD include nausea and vomiting, hiccoughs, and dysgeusia (altered taste). Signs of peripheral edema, hypertension, and concomitant presence of other microvascular complications (DR and neuropathy) can supervene.

GLYCEMIC CONTROL: EVIDENCE FROM CLINICAL TRIALS

Intensive glycemic control (HbA1c <53 mmol/mol [<7%]) offers small clinical benefits on the onset and progression of microalbuminuria but its effects on progression to

Prognosis of CKD by GFR and Albuminuria Categories KDIGO 2012				Persistent albuminuria categories Description and Range		
				A1	A2	A3
				Normal to mildly increased	Moderately Increased	Severely increased
				< 30mg/g < 3 mg/mmol	30-300 mg/g 3-30 mg/mmol	>300mg/g >30 mg/mmol
eGFR Categories ml/min/1.73m²	G1	Normal or High	≥ 90			
	G2	Mildly decreased	60-89			
Range and description	G3a	Mildly to moderately decreased	45-59			
	G3b	Moderately to severely decreased	30-44			
	G4	Severely decreased	15-29			
	G5	Kidney Failure	<15			

Green: low risk (if no other markers of kidney disease, no CKD); Yellow: moderately increased risk; Orange: high risk; Red: very high risk

Fig. 2. Prognosis of CKD by GFR and category of albuminuria. (*Adapted from* Kidney Disease: Improving Global Outcomes (KDIGO) CKD-MBD Update Work Group. KDIGO 2017 Clinical Practice Guideline Update for the Diagnosis, Evaluation, Prevention, and Treatment of Chronic Kidney Disease-Mineral and Bone Disorder (CKD-MBD) [published correction appears in Kidney Int Suppl (2011). 2017 Dec;7(3):e1]. *Kidney Int Suppl (2011).* 2017;7(1):1-59; with permission).

ESKD, death, and major cardiovascular events in people with DKD are unclear.[47] In the DCCT and EDIC studies, intensive glycemic control in people with type 1 diabetes slowed the decline in eGFR and development of albuminuria.[48] In people with type 2 diabetes, a meta-analysis by Zoungas and colleagues,[6] using patient level data from 4 large trials—UKPDS, Veteran Affairs Diabetes Trial (VADT), Action to Control Cardiovascular Risk in Diabetes (ACCORD) and Action in Diabetes and Vascular Disease: Preterax and Diamicron MR Controlled Evaluation (ADVANCE)—reported that intensive glycemic control offers a 20% risk reduction (HR 0·80, 95% CI 0·72–0·88; $P<0·0001$) for the composite of macroalbuminuria, ESKD, and death.

ROLE OF GLUCOSE-LOWERING AGENTS IN DIABETIC KIDNEY DISEASE

A dose reduction with metformin is indicated with eGFR less than 45 mL/min, and metformin should be stopped when eGFR is less than 30 mL/min.[49] People with DKD receiving dialysis are preferentially treated with insulin. However, the initial dose must be reduced by half due to reduced drug clearance. Low-dose oral sulfonylureas can be used alone or added to insulin therapy. The roles of glucose-lowering agents in DKD are summarized in **Table 1**. The specific renal outcomes of 2 SGLT-2 inhibitor studies in people with diabetes and CKD are summarized in **Table 2**.

Hypertension

Adequate blood pressure control reduces the progression of DKD. ACE inhibitors and angiotensin-receptor blockers (ARBs) reduce the incidence of moderately increased albuminuria in people with diabetes and hypertension. In addition, the use of ACE inhibitors or ARBs in people with normal blood pressure (<130/80 mm Hg) who have moderately or severely increased albuminuria stabilizes albuminuria and may reduce progression of DKD, ESKD, and death.[49] The most important trial data in people with type 1 diabetes come from the EUCLID study that randomized 530 men and women, aged 20 to 59 years, with normoalbuminuria or microalbuminuria to lisinopril.[51] Over a 2-year follow-up period, albumin excretion rate (AER) was lower by 12.7% and 49.7% in normoalbuminuric and microalbuminuric individuals, respectively (both $P = .1$). Pooled data revealed significant lowering of AER by 18.8% ($P = .03$). In people with type 2 diabetes, losartan, 50 to 100 mg, once daily was associated with a significant 28% reduction in progression to ESKD in individuals with proteinuria.[52]

Dyslipidemia

People with diabetes mellitus and CKD are at a high risk of cardiovascular events.[35] Statin therapy in DKD exerts pleiotropic effects beyond lipid lowering, including modest improvements in proteinuria, renal function, and reduced risk for major vascular events.[53]

DIABETIC NEUROPATHY

Diabetic neuropathy is a clinically diverse group of conditions that can affect both peripheral and autonomic nervous systems. Diabetic peripheral neuropathy (DPN) is the commonest form resulting in pain, reduced quality of life, gait disturbances, and depressive symptoms, in nearly 30% of affected people with type 2 diabetes.[54] Remission from pain albeit transient usually occurs when sensory deficits are complete or when metabolic control improves after a prolonged period of suboptimal metabolic control. Diabetic foot ulcers and nontraumatic lower extremity amputations that develop as a consequence of DPN have a major impact on health-related quality of life, health care utilization, and costs.[55,56] Autonomic neuropathies can cause

Table 1
Glucose-lowering agents in diabetes kidney disease

Glucose-Lowering Agent	Indications/Benefits	Clinical Trial Evidence	Dose Adjustment	Side Effects
Metformin (MF)	1. First-line agent in T2DM 2. ↑ insulin sensitivity 3. ↑ peripheral glucose uptake 4. ↓ hepatic gluconeogenesis 5. ↓ weight	1. UKPDS: intensive control with MF showed a 32% reduction in any diabetes-related endpoint, 36% for all-cause mortality in individuals with T2DM.[39] 2. MF usage in T2DM and CKD 3b is associated with lower all-cause mortality (HR 0.65; 95% CI 0.57–0.73[a]) and ESRD progression (HR 0.67; 95% CI 0.58–0.77[a]).[40]	1. Half the dose of MF if eGFR is < 45 mL/min. 2. Stop MF and do not initiate, if eGFR <30 mL/min.	Risk of lactic acidosis
Sodium glucose cotransporter 2 (SGLT-2) inhibitors	1. Useful second-line glucose-lowering agent (as add-on to MF) in T2DM and DKD. 2. ↓ renal tubular glucose reabsorption 3. ↓ weight 4. ↓ systemic blood pressure 5. ↓ intraglomerular pressure 6. ↓ albuminuria 7. ↓ reduction in GFR	1. Canagliflozin in patients with albuminuric CKD (CREDENCE study), reduced the renal composite risk of ESKD, doubling of the creatinine, or death by 34% (HR, 0.66; 95% CI, 0.53–0.81[a]); ESKD reduced by 32% (HR, 0.68; 95% CI, 0.54–0.86[a]).[41] 2. Lower risk of CV death, MI, stroke, hospitalization for heart failure.[6] 3. The EMPA-REG OUTCOME trial,[42] the CANVAS Program[43] and the DECLARE-TIMI 58 cardiovascular outcomes	Dapagliflozin, empagliflozin, and ertugliflozin should be avoided if eGFR >45 mL/min. (For each agent, use licensed dose for the specific therapeutic indication) Canagliflozin is safe at low eGFR (<45 to <30 mL/min).[41]	Risk of genitourinary infections especially candidiasis. Ketoacidosis has been reported and concomitant use of diuretics with SGLT-2 inhibitor drugs is best avoided due to the risk of dehydration.

(continued on next page)

Table 1
(continued)

Glucose-Lowering Agent	Indications/Benefits	Clinical Trial Evidence	Dose Adjustment	Side Effects
		trial[44] were RCTs in people with T2DM and CVD or CV risk factors in patients on SGLT-2 inhibitors. SGLT-2 inhibitors reduce decline in renal function with reduced progression of DKD.		
Glucagon-like peptide-1 receptor agonists (GLP-1 RAs)	1. Useful second-line glucose-lowering agent (as add-on to MF) in T2DM and DKD. 2. Stimulate glucose-dependent insulin secretion 3. ↓ weight 4. ↓systemic blood pressure 5. ↓intraglomerular pressure 6. ↓albuminuria 7. ↓reduction in GFR	1. Meta-analysis of LEADER (liraglutide), SUSTAIN-6 (semaglutide), REWIND (dulaglutide), EXSCEL (exenatide), ELIXA (lixisenatide), harmony outcomes (albiglutide), and PIONEER-6 (oral semaglutide): treatment with GLP-1 RAs reduced the composite kidney outcome (development of new-onset macroalbuminuria, decline in eGFR or increase in creatinine, ESRD, or renal death by 17% (HR0.83 [95% CI: 0.78–0.89])a [45] 2. Effects mainly driven by reduction in albuminuria.[45]	1. Avoid exenatide if eGFR <30 mL/min. 2. Liraglutide, dulaglutide, and semaglutide are not recommended with eGFR <15 mL/min. 3. Exenatide QW not recommended with eGFR <50 mL/min.[46]	Gastrointestinal side effects can occur when treatment is initiated.

Abbreviations: CVD, cardiovascular disease; HR, hazard ratio; LEADER, The Liraglutide Effect and Action in Diabetes: Evaluation of Cardiovascular Outcome Results; RCT, randomized controlled trial; REWIND, Researching Cardiovascular Events with a Weekly Incretin in Diabetes; SUSTAIN-6, ; T2DM, type 2 diabetes mellitus.

SUSTAIN-6 (Semaglutide and Cardiovascular Outcomes in Patients with Type 2 Diabetes); REWIND (Dulaglutide and cardiovascular outcomes in type 2 diabetes).

Table 2
Summary of the published sodium glucose cotransporter 2 inhibitor cardiovascular and renal outcomes trials

RCT	CREDENCE[43]	DAPA-CKD[50]
Patients Studied	DM with CKD	CKD±DM
Patients Enrolled, n (Mean Age, y)	4401 (63.0)	4304 (62)
Drug	**Canagliflozin**	**Dapagliflozin**
Dose: Daily Oral (mg)	100	10
Median Follow-up (y)	2.6	2.4
Baseline HbA1c mmol /(%)[a]	67/8.3	62/7.8
Mean DM (y)	15.8	15.0
Baseline Statin Use (%)	69	65
Baseline Prevalence of CV Disease/HF (%)	50	37.4 / 10.9
Baseline Prevalence of HF (%)	15	10.9
Outcomes[b]		
MACE Outcome (%)	−20	—
Hospitalization for HF or CV Death (%)	−31	−29
CV Death (%)	−22	—
Fatal or Nonfatal MI	Not reported	Not reported
Fatal or Nonfatal Stroke	Not reported	Not reported
All-cause Mortality (%)	0.83 (0.68–1.02)	−31
HF Hospitalization (%)	−39	—
Renal Composite End Point (%)	−30	−39
End-stage Kidney Disease (%)	−42	−36

Definition of CKD and Inclusion Criteria

CREDENCE:
1. T2 DM: ≥30 years of age; HbA1c 6.5% – 12.0%
2. eGFR: 30-89 mL/min/1.73 m^2;
3. UACR >33.9 – ≤565.6 mg/mmol
4. Stable max tolerated labelled dose of ACEi or ARB for ≥4 weeks

Exclusion criteria included: other kidney diseases, dialysis or kidney transplant; treatment with dual ACEi and ARB, direct renin inhibitor or MRA; serum K$^+$ >5.5 mmol/L; CV events within 12 weeks of screening; NYHA class IV heart failure; diabetic ketoacidosis or T1DM.

DAPA-CKD
1. T2 DM or No DM
2. ≥18 years of age
3. **eGFR ≥25 to ≤75 mL/min/1.73m^2**
4. UACR ≥ 22.6 to ≤ 565mg/mmol
5. Stable max tolerated dose of ACEi/ARB for ≥4 weeks
6.

Exclusion criteria included: T1DM, Polycystic kidney disease, lupus nephritis, ANCA-associated vasculitis, Immunosuppressive therapy ≤6 months prior to enrolment

Abbreviations: ACEi, ACE inhibitor; ANCA, antineutrophil cytoplasmic antibodies; ARB, angiotensin receptor blocker; DM, diabetes mellitus; HF, heart failure; MACE, major adverse cardiac event; NYHA, New York Heart Association; T1DM, type 1 DM; UACR, urine albumin/creatinine ratio.
[a] DM.
[b] All outcomes given as HR (95% CI).

Adapted from Das SR, Everett BM, Birtcher KK, Brown JM, Januzzi JL Jr, Kalyani RR, Kosiborod M, Magwire M, Morris PB, Neumiller JJ, Sperling LS. 2020 Expert Consensus Decision Pathway on Novel Therapies for Cardiovascular Risk Reduction in Patients With Type 2 Diabetes: A Report of the American College of Cardiology Solution Set Oversight Committee. J Am Coll Cardiol. 2020 Sep 1;76(9):1117-1145; with permission.

severe morbidity depending on the organ site of involvement and are linked to increased cardiovascular mortality.[54,56]

Pathogenesis

A unifying hypothesis for the pathogenesis of diabetic neuropathy remains elusive. It is plausible that several factors induced by the deleterious effects of hyperglycemia, nerve ischemia, segmental demyelination, and axonal degeneration of peripheral nerves acting in concert lead on to the progressive changes of DPN.[55]

RISK FACTORS FOR DIABETIC PERIPHERAL NEUROPATHY

Recognized risk factors for DPN in people with type 2 diabetes are duration of diabetes, age, glycemic control, and presence of DR.[57] Similar risk factors as well as smoking and dyslipidemia have been identified in youth with type 1 diabetes.[58]

Diagnosis

DPN or chronic distal symmetric polyneuropathy is the presence of symptoms and/or signs of peripheral nerve dysfunction in people with diabetes after the exclusion of other cause.[54] Other clinical manifestations of autonomic neuropathy include hypoglycemic unawareness, gastroparesis, constipation, diarrhea, erectile dysfunction, neurogenic bladder, and sudomotor dysfunction[54] (refer to **Table 3**).

GLYCEMIC CONTROL
Evidence from Clinical Trials

Early intensive glycemic control delays and prevents the development of clinically manifest DPN and cardiovascular autonomic neuropathy (CAN) in patients with type 1 diabetes; however, its effects in people with type 2 diabetes are modest.[60]

OTHER CONSIDERATIONS IN DIABETIC NEUROPATHY
Diabetic Foot Ulcer

Diabetic foot ulcer (DFU) is most often caused by a combined result of reduced sensation; vascular compromise; functional changes in the microcirculation; or stimulus factors such as abnormal foot anatomy, plantar callous, or ill-fitting footwear and is associated with prolonged hospitalization, significant morbidity due to increased risk of falls and loss of work productivity, and cardiovascular mortality.[54]

Risk factors for recurrence of foot include male gender, smoking, duration of diabetes previous ulceration, peripheral artery disease, and PDN.[61] The cornerstone of foot ulcer management is a multidisciplinary approach aimed at control of hyperglycemia, pressure offloading with specialized therapeutic footwear, removable devices, or total contact casts. In people with DFU and high-risk feet undergoing dialysis, Charcot foot, or prior history of amputation, the aim is not only to preserve the limb but also to reduce cardiovascular risk.[54]

PREVENTION OF MICROVASCULAR COMPLICATIONS OF DIABETES
Primary Prevention

Primary prevention of microvascular complications should address intensive management of modifiable risk factors, lifestyle modification, and system-level measures such as systematic screening, education, and awareness. A summary of screening schedules is outlined in **Table 4**. Pragmatic approaches to screening intervals are also being

Table 3
Diabetic neuropathies: classification and clinical features

Type	Symptoms	Clinical Features	Other Considerations
Generalized Neuropathies			
Hyperglycemic neuropathy	Peripheral limb tingling, numbness, pain, or hyperesthesia	As for DPN	Can occur with poor glycemic control, or rapid improvements in glycemic control
Distal symmetric sensorimotor polyneuropathy	Burning and tingling, deep aching, electric shock–like, and lancinating Exaggerated response to painful stimuli or allodynia (increased pain from an innocuous stimulus such as daytime or bedtime clothes)	Absent ankle reflexes Mild muscle weakness in both feet Loss of vibration sense, pin prick, temperature, light touch in a stocking distribution	Symptoms are typically worse at night DR or DKD may be present Treatment: antineuropathic drugs, good glycemic control
Insulin neuritis	Severe painful sensory symptoms (as descried in DPN)	Clinical signs are commonly minimal or even absent	Usually recovers in 6–12 mo
Painful neuropathy with severe weight loss	Severe painful sensory symptoms (as described in DPN)	Significant weight loss	Usually occurs in people with inadequately controlled type 1 diabetes
Focal and Multifocal Neuropathies			
Cranial neuropathies: Third, fourth, and sixth nerve palsy	Onset is abrupt. Can present with retro-orbital pain and diplopia	Third nerve palsy: ptosis, pupillary sparing	Usually recovers in 3–6 mo
Focal limb neuropathies: Carpal tunnel syndrome Ulnar neuropathy Common peroneal neuropathy	Sensorimotor symptoms, including muscle weakness depending on site of involvement	Sensorimotor signs depending on site of involvement	Decompressive surgery may be needed
Lumbosacral radiculoplexus neuropathy (previously termed diabetic amyotrophy)	Usually asymmetric; severe pain around lower back or anterior thigh Proximal weakness, weight loss	Nerve conduction shows denervation changes in affected muscle groups	Slow recovery, but muscle strength may not improve completely

(continued on next page)

Table 3
(continued)

Type	Symptoms	Clinical Features	Other Considerations
Autonomic Neuropathies			
Cardiovascular autonomic neuropathy	Postural syncope, dizziness, falls, and fatigue	Resting tachycardia is often presenting sign. Heart rate variability on lying and with deep breathing. Orthostatic hypotension	Good glycemic control; treatment of orthostatic hypotension in symptomatic individuals
Gastroparesis	Early satiety, · nausea/vomiting, bloating, · upper abdominal pain, weight loss	Delayed gastric emptying confirmed by scintigraphy, 13C breath tests, or wireless motility capsule	Treatment: dietary modifications, supplemental nutrition, antiemetic and prokinetic drugs. Surgical treatment is a last resort[59]
ED	Persistent inability to attain or maintain an erection sufficient for satisfactory sexual performance (lasting for ~6 mo) Lower urinary tract symptoms may be present	Sexual Health Inventory for Men questionnaire: used to evaluate severity of ED Assessment for hypogonadism	Treatment: replacement testosterone for hypogonadism ED treatment: psychosexual counseling, phosphodiesterase-5 inhibitors, intracorporeal or intraurethral prostaglandins, vacuum devices, penile prostheses
Sudomotor dysfunction (reduced sweating)	Dry foot with increased inflammation of the skin	Reduced normal foot odour, increased dryness, increased fissuring (especially heel areas)	Maintain hydration of dry skin (especially hyperkeratosis) with consideration of daily application of a urea-based emollient

Abbreviation: ED, erectile dysfunction.

Table 4
Screening schedule for microvascular complications in type 1 and type 2 diabetes

	Diabetic Retinopathy	Diabetic Kidney Disease	Diabetic Neuropathy
Initial screening	1. Type 1 DM: 3–5 y after diagnosis 2. Type 2 DM: at the time of diagnosis 3. Pregnant women (T1DM or T2DM) before conception and in each trimester	a. Type 1 DM: 3–5 y after diagnosis b. Type 2 DM: at the time of diagnosis	Type 1 DM: ≥5 y after diagnosis Type 2 DM: at the time of diagnosis
Screening method/examination	a. Direct or indirect ophthalmoscopy or slit-lamp examination through dilated pupils b. Retinal (fundus) photography (preferred option) c. Optical coherence tomography (OCT) scanning is a sensitive method to identify DME and can be combined with funduscopy	1. Urine albumin-creatinine ratio (ACR) 2. Estimated glomerular filtration rate (eGFR) 3. Tracking an increase in the creatinine level in individual patients	a. Pinprick sensation (small fiber) b. Vibration perception (128 Hz tuning fork); 10 g monofilament pressure sensation at the distal plantar aspect of both great toes and metatarsal joints; assessment of ankle reflex Symptom scoring systems in neuropathy Diabetic neuropathy symptom score Neuropathy impairment score Michigan neuropathy screening instrument
If microvascular complication present	1. Type 1 and type 2 diabetes: screen annually, or 2. Depending on the severity of retinopathy, monitoring intervals determined by eye specialist. 3. If there is rapid improvement in glycemic control—locally defined 4. Screen for other complications—especially DKD	ACR >3 mg/mol (urine albumin >30 mg/g creatinine) ± eGFR <60 mL/min/1.73 m² Type 1 and type 2 diabetes: screen twice a year, or depending on the severity, monitoring intervals determined by clinician Screen for other complications	a. Type 1 and type 2 diabetes: screen every year or b. Screen for other diabetes complications

(continued on next page)

Table 4
(continued)

	Diabetic Retinopathy	Diabetic Kidney Disease	Diabetic Neuropathy
If microvascular complication not present	1. Type 1 and type 2 diabetes: screen every 2 y (a new COVID-19 contingency measure for some screening services) 2. Type 2 diabetes with risk factors: annual screening only for people with long duration of diabetes ~15 y, suboptimal glycaemic control (HbA1c 64 mmol/mol (>8%), poor BP control, rapid improvement in glycaemic control 3. Screen for other complications	a. Type 1 and type 2 diabetes: screen annually b. Type 2 diabetes with risk factors: annual screening ONLY for long duration of diabetes ~15 y, suboptimal glycaemic control (HbA1c >8% or 64 mmol/mo), poor BP control, other diabetes microvascular complications c. Screen for other complications	a. Type 1 and type 2 diabetes: screen every 2 y b. Screen for other diabetes complications

Abbreviation: BP, blood pressure.

considered in many health care systems due to the COVID-19 pandemic. For example, people with stable DR can be screened at 18- to 24-month interval.[62]

Secondary Prevention

As with primary prevention, regular monitoring and aggressive management of risk factors is important to prevent and reduce the progression of dreaded complications including vision-threatening retinopathy, ESKD, painful DPN, foot ulceration, and limb (or digit) amputation.

CLINICAL CONSIDERATIONS
History Taking and Examination

A detailed history focused on duration of diabetes, smoking history, medication history (glucose-lowering agents [especially insulin], antihypertensives, lipid-lowering drugs, and aspirin), existing comorbidities, and pregnancy. Evaluation of DR should enquire about symptoms of visual impairment, floaters in the eye, presence of existing DR, assessment of visual acuity, and lens and retinal examination. Bleeding tendency due to platelet dysfunction and anemia are common in ESKD and should be monitored. An abrupt decline in eGFR or hyperkalemia should prompt exclusion of reversible conditions such as renal artery stenosis, obstructive nephropathy, and medication review for nephrotoxic drugs. Foot examination should include inspection of the skin, assessment of foot deformities, and neurologic and vascular assessment of both lower limbs. All people with diabetes, especially those with high-risk feet (eg, foot deformity), should be educated about risk factors and shown how to regularly inspect and examine their feet and refer themselves to the right health care professional according to local protocols.[63]

Recommendations for Glycemic Control

Glycemic monitoring and individualization of targets is key to the management of people with microvascular complications of diabetes. Broad principles include the following:

1. Aim for HbA1c target of less than 7% (53 mmol/mol) generally in people with microvascular complications of diabetes (note: HbA1c measurements may not be reliable in people with DKD on hemodialysis, and self-monitoring of blood glucose is also advised).[49]
2. Aim for HbA1c target of less than 6.5% (48 mmol/mol) in select empowered individuals in whom this can be achieved safely with little or no risk of hypoglycemia.
3. Aim for HbA1c target of less than 7.5% (58 mmol/mol) in older healthy adults with few coexisting comorbidities and intact cognitive and functional status.
4. Aim for HbA1c target of less than 8% (64 mmol/mol) or pursue less stringent targets in people with a history of severe hypoglycemia, long-standing diabetes, multiple coexisting comorbidities, limited life expectancy, cognitive impairment or functional dependence, or in whom stringent HbA1c targets are difficult to achieve despite optimal management.[63]

Newer glucose-lowering drugs
Although more than 50,000 subjects have been studied in various outcome trials with the use of SGLT-2 inhibitors in people with type 2 diabetes, none have specifically reported DR outcomes, and this is despite SGLT-2 inhibitors showing beneficial rates in DR progression.[23] These studies therefore draw toward the conclusion that glycemic control is of principal importance in the prevention and progression of DR. In contrast,

the body of evidence from cardiovascular outcome trials suggests that treatment with an SGLT2 inhibitor in most patients with DKD (and eGFR $\geq$ 30) results in substantial improvements in cardiorenal outcomes (refer to **Table 2**). KDIGO guidelines 2020 also recommend first-line treatment with metformin and an SGLT2 inhibitor and additional treatment as needed to achieve glycemic targets. GLP-1 agonists also demonstrate cardiorenal benefits among people with existing atherosclerotic cardiovascular disease, prevent onset of severely increased albuminuria, and preserve renal function.[49]

Recommendations for Blood Pressure Control

A blood pressure (BP) target of less than 140/90 mm Hg should be aimed for in all adults with microvascular complications of diabetes.[8] However, a tighter BP target of less than or equal to 130/80 mm Hg can be pursued in high-risk, young people with DKD with urinary albumin excretion greater than or equal to 30 mg/24 hours (urinary ACR $\geq$3). ACE inhibitors or ARBs (also, if ACE inhibitors are not tolerated) are preferred first-line agents for blood pressure control (proven benefits on reducing DKD progression).[64] Combination therapy with ACE inhibitor and ARB increases the risk of hyperkalemia and acute kidney injury and is not recommended.[65]

Management of Dyslipidemia

Weight loss with lifestyle modification and increased physical activity (if appropriate) are strongly recommended. In adults aged between 40 and 75 years, lipid lowering with a moderate-intensity statin (eg, atorvastatin, 20 mg, once daily) aiming for an LDL-cholesterol (LDL-C) target of less than 1.8 mmol/L (<70 mg/dL) or a 50% reduction from baseline (if LDL-C is between 1.8 and 3.5 mmol/L [70 and 135 mg/dL]) has beneficial effects on DR, DKD, and cardiovascular outcomes.[63] Fenofibrate may have potential benefits for people with DR and should be considered.[28]

Smoking

Smoking cessation is important to halt the progression of retinopathy. It has wider health implications and should be encouraged irrespective of the presence of diabetes or any other chronic disease.

SPECIAL SITUATIONS
Pregnancy

The ideal HbA1c target in pregnancy is 42 mmol/mol (<6%), if achieved without significant hypoglycemia.[8] Rapid, intensive glycemic control in pregnancy should be avoided. All women of child-bearing age should be counseled regarding the effects of pregnancy and ocular complications in the presence of poor glycemic control.[8] Pregnant women with preexisting diabetes should be screened for DR before conception, following the first antenatal visit and again at 28 weeks if the first assessment is normal. If any features of DR are present, additional retinal assessment should be performed at 16 to 20 weeks. Further screening in the first year of postpartum is advised.[66] Severe NPDR or PDR before pregnancy should be treated with scatter laser photocoagulation.[66] Anti-VEGF treatments for DMO during pregnancy should only be considered if the potential benefits of treatment outweigh the potential harm to the mother and/or developing fetus.[67]

TERTIARY PREVENTION

As discussed earlier, include specialist treatments as outlined in the following section.

Specialist Treatments and Other Considerations in Diabetic Retinopathy

1. Panretinal photocoagulation (PRP)

    PRP involves application of laser burns on the retinal surface, sparing the central macula. The landmark Diabetic Retinopathy Study and The Early Treatment Diabetic Retinopathy Study effectively demonstrated the benefits of scatter laser photocoagulation in patients with severe NPDR and PDR and focal laser treatment in patients with DMO.[17] PRP is indicated high-risk PDR and severe NPDR to reduce the risk of vision loss.

2. Anti-VEGF therapies

    Intravitreal anti-VEGF injection, ranibizumab, aflibercept, and bevacizumab, are evidence-based effective treatments in the management of PDR. They are effective over standard laser in patients with visual impairment due to DMO.[17] Anti-VEGF therapy may be used to inhibit neovascularization before completion of PRP or as an adjuvant to prevent the aggravation of DMO after PRP. For patients with advanced PDR, anti-VEGF therapy is recommended before vitrectomy to reduce the probability of intraoperative and postoperative hemorrhage.[17]

3. Vitrectomy: the aim of vitrectomy is to evacuate blood in the vitreous space due to vitreous hemorrhage, treat retinal detachment, and to remove the scaffolding of neovascular growth. The factors that determine the need for surgery include duration of hemorrhage, the amount of previous PRP, status of the other eye, and glycemic control.[17]

Specialist Treatments and Other Considerations in Diabetic Kidney Disease

1. Physical activity: people with DKD should incorporate moderate-intensity physical activity for at least 150 min/wk individual cardiovascular and physical tolerance.[49]

2. Diet: salt intake should be restricted to less than 2 g/d. Dietary protein intake should be approximately 0.8 g/kg body weight per day. However, people on dialysis need more dietary protein intake to prevent malnutrition.[49]

3. Blood potassium monitoring: recommended for people with DKD treated with ACE inhibitors, ARBs, or diuretics because these drugs can induce hyperkalemia or hypokalemia.[35]

4. Nephrotoxins: liberal use of nonsteroidal antiinflammatory drugs should be avoided in people with DKD.[35]

5. Hypoglycemia: people with DKD on hemodialysis are at high risk of hypoglycemia, and regular monitoring is advised. Regular inspection of feet and retinopathy screening should be undertaken.[49]

6. Metabolic abnormalities: monitoring and treatment of hypocalcemia and vitamin D deficiency with vitamin D supplements, dietary phosphate restrictions or use of phosphate binders for hyperphosphatemia, and monitoring of parathyroid hormone are important considerations in the management of people with stage 3 to 5 CKD. Chronic anemia is managed with iron replacement and erythropoietin.[32]

7. Renal replacement therapy comprises either transplantation or dialysis. A detailed discussion is out of the scope of this review. Dialysis is conventionally grouped under hemodialysis and peritoneal dialysis. Dialysis is a planned procedure and is usually started in symptomatic ESKD or in asymptomatic individuals with an eGFR of ~5 to 7 mL/min/1.73 m.[49]

Management of Neuropathic Pain in Diabetic Neuropathy

No compelling evidence exists in support of glycemic control or lifestyle management.[60] For reducing neuropathy-related pain, tricyclic antidepressants, serotonin-noradrenaline reuptake inhibitors (eg duloxetine), pregabalin, and gabapentin are strongly recommended as first-line therapies; second-line agents include lidocaine patches, capsaicin cream high-concentration patches, and tramadol; and third-line agents include strong opioids and botulinum toxin A.[54]

CRITERIA FOR SPECIALIST REFERRAL

For people with DR, specialist referral is indicated if visual acuity is less than 6/12 (20/40) or if there is symptomatic vision impairment, central macular edema (noncentral macular edema, if laser resources are available), severe nonproliferative DR, or any PD. People with diabetes and CKD should be referred to a nephrologist if eGFR is less than 30 mL/min, persistent significant albuminuria greater than or equal to $\geq$30 mg/mmol, CKD with hypertension despite use of 3 antihypertensive agents, and/or sustained decrease in eGFR of greater than or equal to 25% or ~15 mL/min in the last 12 months.[49] Referral to a neurologist for DPN should be considered for atypical or asymmetrical presentations or if motor symptoms predominate. Foot ulcers and wound care may require intervention by a podiatrist, foot surgeon, physiotherapist, and occupational therapist.[54]

DISCUSSION

Microvascular complications of diabetes both individually and collectively present a significant challenge, not only in terms of morbidity and diverse presentations but also as strong predictors of cardiovascular disease. Hence, increased awareness and education, universal access to low-cost screening, and affordable specialist treatment are important strategies in reducing the disease burden. A patient-centered approach and health care professional education strategy such as the ALPHABET strategy,[68] based on multifactorial intervention aiming for tight glycemic, blood pressure and lipid control, smoking cessation, and patient self-management education with individualized care plans, should be pursued vigorously in these high-risk individuals.[69]

In recent years, the newer glucose-lowering agents such as SGLT-2 inhibitors and GLP-1 agonists have made transformative changes in the treatment algorithm of people with type 2 diabetes at high risk of atherosclerotic disease. Early use of SGLT-2 inhibitors in DKD offers substantial renal and cardiovascular protection independent of their beneficial effects on hyperglycemia, BP, and weight loss. Other pleiotropic effects include glycosuria, natriuresis, restoring intraglomerular pressure, improvements in cardiac metabolism via shifts in fuel metabolism, and ketone oxidization as an alternative fuel to fatty acids.[70]

Although it would seem, anecdotally at least, that the evidence for the use of fenofibrate and ACE inhibitors is not widely appreciated in DR, some national guidelines do advocate the use of these agents, and in 2013, Australia became the first country in the world to approve the use of fenofibrate to reduce the progression of DR in people with type 2 diabetes.[63]

Finally, telemedicine based on digital imaging techniques, automated analyzers, and deep learning artificial systems applied to retinal image datasets in DR holds great promise for early detection and accurate treatment.

SUMMARY

The burden and costs of managing microvascular complications of diabetes are enormous to the individual and the society. Primary prevention must focus on promoting healthy eating habits, exercise and physical activity, and tobacco abstinence from an early age. Health care professionals must address risk factors specifically aiming for tight glycemic and blood pressure control with judicious use of ACE inhibitors,

ARBs, SGLT-2 inhibitors, statin, and fibrate therapies. Finally, improved technology and communication systems using innovative digitized health care systems, including diagnostic instruments and seamless data transfer, more universal screening, early aggressive risk factor management, and coordinated efforts to implement policies and programs, that promote a healthy environment, improve education, and support self-management with easy and low-cost access to specialist care are needed. The implementation of these strategies will provide greater opportunities for greater patient empowerment, reduced costs, and improved health outcomes.

CLINICAL PEARLS IN THE PREVENTION OF MICROVASCULAR COMPLICATIONS OF DIABETES

1. Multifactorial intervention including tight control of hyperglycemia, BP, dyslipidemia, and smoking cessation alongside structured patient self-management education is the cornerstone of good management to improve microvascular and cardiovascular health.
2. People with diabetes are at high risk of DR and any symptom of new visual impairment should be assessed with priority.
3. Worsening of existing DR can occur with intensive glycemic control but should not be a contraindication to achieving it. Similar effects in pregnancy and with injectable semaglutide warrants close retina monitoring.
4. SGLT2 inhibitors in people with type 2 diabetes and CKD offers substantial cardiorenal protection and must be strongly considered (with metformin) as first-line treatment.
5. Timely screening and specialist referral are important considerations in the management of people with vascular complications of diabetes.

CONFLICT OF INTEREST

W. Crasto has received lecture fees and educational grants from Sanofi-Aventis, Eli Lily, Boehringer Ingelheim, Novo Nordisk, Napp pharmaceuticals, Internis, and MSD. He has received grants in support of investigator and investigator-initiated trials from BHR pharmaceuticals. V. Patel has received lecture fees and educational grants from most large companies in diabetes care, including Sanofi-Aventis, Boehringer Ingelheim, Eli Lily, AZ, Novo Nordisk, Napp pharmaceuticals, Internis, and MSD. He has been on the Advisory Board for some of these companies. M.J. Davies has acted as consultant, advisory board member and speaker for Novo Nordisk, Sanofi-Aventis, Lilly, Merck Sharp & Dohme, Boehringer Ingelheim, Astra Zeneca and Janssen, an advisory board member for Servier and Gilead Sciences Ltd, and as a speaker for NAPP, Mitsubishi Tanabe Pharma Corporation, and Takeda Pharmaceuticals International Inc. She has received grants in support of investigator and investigator-initiated trials from Novo Nordisk, Sanofi-Aventis, Lilly, Boehringer Ingelheim, Astrazeneca, and Janssen. K. Khunti has acted as a consultant and speaker for Amgen, Astra Zeneca, Boehringer Ingelheim, Novartis, Janssen, Roche, Servier, Berlin-Chemie AG, Novo Nordisk, Sanofi-Aventis, Lilly, and Merck Sharp & Dohme. He has received grants in support of investigator and investigator-initiated trials from Novartis, Novo Nordisk, Sanofi-Aventis, Lilly, Pfizer, Janssen, Roche, Astra Zeneca Boehringer Ingelheim, and Merck Sharp & Dohme.

REFERENCES

1. International Diabetes Federation. IDF Diabetes Atlas, 9th edn Brussels, Belgium.; 2019. Available at: https://www.diabetesatlas.org. Accessed October 3, 2020.

2. Einarson TR, Acs A, Ludwig C, et al. Economic burden of cardiovascular disease in type 2 diabetes: a systematic review. Value Heal 2018. https://doi.org/10.1016/j.jval.2017.12.019.

3. Harding JL, Pavkov ME, Magliano DJ, et al. Global trends in diabetes complications: a review of current evidence. Diabetologia 2019;62(1):3–16.

4. Kosiborod M, Gomes MB, Nicolucci A, et al. Vascular complications in patients with type 2 diabetes: Prevalence and associated factors in 38 countries (the DISCOVER study program). Cardiovasc Diabetol 2018. https://doi.org/10.1186/s12933-018-0787-8.

5. Pearce I, Simó R, Lövestam-Adrian M, et al. Association between diabetic eye disease and other complications of diabetes: Implications for care. A systematic review. Diabetes Obes Metab 2019. https://doi.org/10.1111/dom.13550.

6. Zoungas S, Arima H, Gerstein HC, et al. Effects of intensive glucose control on microvascular outcomes in patients with type 2 diabetes: a meta-analysis of individual participant data from randomised controlled trials. Lancet Diabetes Endocrinol 2017. https://doi.org/10.1016/S2213-8587(17)30104-3.

7. Brownrigg JRW, Hughes CO, Burleigh D, et al. Microvascular disease and risk of cardiovascular events among individuals with type 2 diabetes: A population-level cohort study. Lancet Diabetes Endocrinol 2016. https://doi.org/10.1016/S2213-8587(16)30057-2.

8. American Diabetes Association. 2. Classification and diagnosis of diabetes: Standards of Medical Care in Diabetes-2020. Diabetes Care 2020. https://doi.org/10.2337/dc20-S002.

9. Brownlee M. The pathobiology of diabetic complications: A unifying mechanism. Diabetes 2005. https://doi.org/10.2337/diabetes.54.6.1615.

10. Fu H, Liu S, Bastacky SI, et al. Diabetic kidney diseases revisited: A new perspective for a new era. Mol Metab 2019;30:250–63.

11. Nguyen TT, Wang JJ, Wong TY. Retinal Vascular Changes in Pre-Diabetes and Prehypertension. Diabetes Care 2007;30(10). 2708 LP–2715.

12. Yau JWY, Rogers SL, Kawasaki R, et al. Global prevalence and major risk factors of diabetic retinopathy. Diabetes Care 2012. https://doi.org/10.2337/dc11-1909.

13. Liew G, Michaelides M, Bunce C. A comparison of the causes of blindness certifications in England and Wales in working age adults (16–64 years), 1999–2000 with 2009–2010. BMJ Open 2014;4(2):e004015.

14. Bhavsar AR. Diabetic retinopathy: The latest in current management. Retina 2006. https://doi.org/10.1097/01.iae.0000236466.23640.c9.

15. Zhou Y, Wang C, Shi K, et al. Relationship between dyslipidemia and diabetic retinopathy: A systematic review and meta-analysis. Medicine (Baltimore) 2018; 97(36):e12283.

16. Sailesh S. The THOR effect: thyroid hormone offsets retinopathy. J Endocrinol Thyroid Res 2018;3(1):1–9.

17. Amoaku WM, Ghanchi F, Bailey C, et al. Diabetic retinopathy and diabetic macular oedema pathways and management: UK Consensus Working Group. Eye 2020. https://doi.org/10.1038/s41433-020-0961-6.

18. Aiello LP. Diabetic retinopathy and other ocular findings in the diabetes control and complications trial/epidemiology of diabetes interventions and complications study. Diabetes Care 2014. https://doi.org/10.2337/dc13-2251.

19. Stratton IM, Cull CA, Adler AI, et al. Additive effects of glycaemia and blood pressure exposure on risk of complications in type 2 diabetes: A prospective observational study (UKPDS 75). Diabetologia 2006. https://doi.org/10.1007/s00125-006-0297-1.

20. Chew EY, Davis MD, Danis RP, et al. The effects of medical management on the progression of diabetic retinopathy in persons with type 2 diabetes: The action to control cardiovascular risk in diabetes (ACCORD) eye study. Ophthalmology 2014. https://doi.org/10.1016/j.ophtha.2014.07.019.

21. Chew EY, Lovato JF, Davis MD, et al. Persistent effects of intensive glycemic control on retinopathy in type 2 diabetes in the action to control cardiovascular risk in diabetes (ACCORD) follow-on study. Diabetes Care 2016. https://doi.org/10.2337/dc16-0024.

22. Rosenstock J, Perkovic V, Johansen OE, et al. Effect of Linagliptin vs Placebo on Major Cardiovascular Events in Adults with Type 2 Diabetes and High Cardiovascular and Renal Risk: The CARMELINA Randomized Clinical Trial. JAMA 2019. https://doi.org/10.1001/jama.2018.18269.

23. Marso SP, Bain SC, Consoli A, et al. Semaglutide and cardiovascular outcomes in patients with type 2 diabetes. N Engl J Med 2016. https://doi.org/10.1056/NEJMoa1607141.

24. EUCTR2017-003619-20-SK. A research study to look at how semaglutide compared to placebo affects diabetic eye disease in people with type 2 diabetes. 2018. Available at: http://www.who.int/trialsearch/Trial2.aspx?TrialID=EUCTR2017-003619-20-SK. Accessed October 26, 2020.

25. Do DV, Wang X, Vedula SS, et al. Blood pressure control for diabetic retinopathy. Cochrane Database Syst Rev 2015. https://doi.org/10.1002/14651858.CD006127.pub2.

26. Chaturvedi N, Sjolie AK, Stephenson JM, et al. Effect of lisinopril on progression of retinopathy in normotensive people with type 1 diabetes. The EUCLID Study Group. EURODIAB Controlled Trial of Lisinopril in Insulin-Dependent Diabetes Mellitus. Lancet 1998. https://doi.org/10.1016/s0140-6736(97)06209-0.

27. Patel V, Panja S, Venkataraman A. The HOPE Study and MICRO-HOPE Substudy. Br J Diabetes Vasc Dis 2001. https://doi.org/10.1177/14746514010010010701.

28. Effects of long-term fenofibrate therapy on cardiovascular events in 9795 people with type 2 diabetes mellitus (the FIELD study): Randomised controlled trial. Lancet 2005. https://doi.org/10.1016/S0140-6736(05)67667-2.

29. Effect of pregnancy on microvascular complications in the diabetes control and complications trial the diabetes control and complications trial research group. Diabetes Care 2000. https://doi.org/10.2337/diacare.23.8.1084.

30. Bikbov B, Purcell CA, Levey AS, et al. Global, regional, and national burden of chronic kidney disease, 1990–2017: a systematic analysis for the Global Burden of Disease Study 2017. Lancet 2020;395(10225):709–33. https://doi.org/10.1016/S0140-6736(20)30045-3.

31. Liyanage T, Ninomiya T, Jha V, et al. Worldwide access to treatment for end-stage kidney disease: A systematic review. Lancet 2015. https://doi.org/10.1016/S0140-6736(14)61601-9.

32. Lin YC, Chang YH, Yang SY, et al. Update of pathophysiology and management of diabetic kidney disease. J Formos Med Assoc 2018. https://doi.org/10.1016/j.jfma.2018.02.007.

33. Alicic RZ, Rooney MT, Tuttle KR. Diabetic kidney disease: Challenges, progress, and possibilities. Clin J Am Soc Nephrol 2017;12(12):2032–45.

34. Perkins BA, Bebu I, de Boer IH, et al. Risk Factors for Kidney Disease in Type 1 Diabetes. Diabetes Care 2019;42(5):883–90.

35. KDIGO 2017 Clinical Practice Guideline Update for the Diagnosis, Evaluation, Prevention, and Treatment of Chronic Kidney Disease–Mineral and Bone Disorder (CKD-MBD). Kidney Int Suppl 2017. https://doi.org/10.1016/j.kisu.2017.04.001.

36. Kumar V, Yadav AK, Yasuda Y, et al. Existing creatinine-based equations overestimate glomerular filtration rate in Indians. BMC Nephrol 2018. https://doi.org/10.1186/s12882-018-0813-9.
37. Currie CJ, Berni ER, Berni TR, et al. Major adverse cardiovascular events in people with chronic kidney disease in relation to disease severity and diabetes status. PLoS One 2019. https://doi.org/10.1371/journal.pone.0221044.
38. Zhou B, Zou H, Xu G. Clinical utility of serum cystatin c in predicting diabetic nephropathy among patients with diabetes mellitus: a meta-analysis. Kidney Blood Press Res 2016;41(6):919–28.
39. Turner R. Effect of intensive blood-glucose control with metformin on complications in overweight patients with type 2 diabetes (UKPDS 34). Lancet 1998. https://doi.org/10.1016/S0140-6736(98)07037-8.
40. Kwon S, Kim YC, Park JY, et al. The Long-term Effects of Metformin on Patients with Type 2 Diabetic Kidney Disease. Diabetes Care 2020. https://doi.org/10.2337/dc19-0936.
41. Perkovic V, Jardine MJ, Neal B, et al. Canagliflozin and renal outcomes in type 2 diabetes and nephropathy. N Engl J Med 2019. https://doi.org/10.1056/NEJMoa1811744.
42. Wanner C, Inzucchi SE, Lachin JM, et al. Empagliflozin and progression of kidney disease in type 2 diabetes. N Engl J Med 2016. https://doi.org/10.1056/NEJMoa1515920.
43. Neal B, Perkovic V, Mahaffey KW, et al. Canagliflozin and cardiovascular and renal events in type 2 diabetes. N Engl J Med 2017. https://doi.org/10.1056/NEJMoa1611925.
44. Mosenzon O, Wiviott SD, Cahn A, et al. Effects of dapagliflozin on development and progression of kidney disease in patients with type 2 diabetes: an analysis from the DECLARE–TIMI 58 randomised trial. Lancet Diabetes Endocrinol 2019. https://doi.org/10.1016/S2213-8587(19)30180-9.
45. Kristensen SL, Rørth R, Jhund PS, et al. Cardiovascular, mortality, and kidney outcomes with GLP-1 receptor agonists in patients with type 2 diabetes: a systematic review and meta-analysis of cardiovascular outcome trials. Lancet Diabetes Endocrinol 2019. https://doi.org/10.1016/S2213-8587(19)30249-9.
46. Yin WL, Bain SC, Min T. The effect of glucagon-like peptide-1 receptor agonists on renal outcomes in type 2 diabetes. Diabetes Ther 2020;11(4):835–44.
47. Ruospo M, Saglimbene VM, Palmer SC, et al. Glucose targets for preventing diabetic kidney disease and its progression. Cochrane Database Syst Rev 2017. https://doi.org/10.1002/14651858.CD010137.pub2.
48. De Boer IH, Sun W, Cleary PA, et al. Intensive diabetes therapy and glomerular filtration rate in type 1 diabetes. N Engl J Med 2011. https://doi.org/10.1056/NEJMoa1111732.
49. KDIGO 2020 Clinical Practice Guideline for Diabetes Management in Chronic Kidney Disease. Kidney Int 2020. https://doi.org/10.1016/j.kint.2020.06.019.
50. Heerspink HJL, Stefánsson BV, Correa-Rotter R, et al. Dapagliflozin in Patients with Chronic Kidney Disease. N Engl J Med 2020. https://doi.org/10.1056/nejmoa2024816.
51. The EUCLID Study Group. Randomised placebo-controlled trial of lisinopril in normotensive patients with insulin-dependent diabetes and normoalbuminuria or microalbuminuria. The EUCLID Study Group. Lancet 1997;349(9068):1787–92.
52. Brenner BM, Cooper ME, De Zeeuw D, et al. Effects of losartan on renal and cardiovascular outcomes in patients with type 2 diabetes and nephropathy. N Engl J Med 2001. https://doi.org/10.1056/NEJMoa011161.

53. Su X, Zhang L, Lv J, et al. Effect of statins on kidney disease outcomes: A systematic review and meta-analysis. Am J Kidney Dis 2016. https://doi.org/10.1053/j.ajkd.2016.01.016.

54. Pop-Busui R, Boulton AJM, Feldman EL, et al. Diabetic neuropathy: A position statement by the American diabetes association. Diabetes Care 2017. https://doi.org/10.2337/dc16-2042.

55. Hicks CW, Selvin E. Epidemiology of Peripheral Neuropathy and Lower Extremity Disease in Diabetes. Curr Diab Rep 2019. https://doi.org/10.1007/s11892-019-1212-8.

56. Rice JB, Desai U, Cummings AK, et al. Burden of diabetic foot ulcers for medicare and private insurers. Diabetes Care 2014;37(3):651–8. View at: Google Scholar.

57. Liu X, Xu Y, An M, et al. The risk factors for diabetic peripheral neuropathy: A meta-analysis. PLoS One 2019. https://doi.org/10.1371/journal.pone.0212574.

58. Jaiswal M, Divers J, Dabelea D, et al. Prevalence of and Risk Factors for Diabetic Peripheral Neuropathy in Youth With Type 1 and Type 2 Diabetes: SEARCH for Diabetes in Youth Study. Diabetes Care 2017;40(9):1226–32.

59. Bharucha AE, Kudva YC, Prichard DO. Diabetic Gastroparesis. Endocr Rev 2019;40(5):1318–52.

60. Callaghan BC, Little AA, Feldman EL, et al. Enhanced glucose control for preventing and treating diabetic neuropathy. Cochrane Database Syst Rev 2012. https://doi.org/10.1002/14651858.cd007543.pub2.

61. Armstrong DG, Boulton AJM, Bus SA. Diabetic foot ulcers and their recurrence. N Engl J Med 2017. https://doi.org/10.1056/NEJMra1615439.

62. Groeneveld Y, Tavenier D, Blom JW, et al. Incidence of sight-threatening diabetic retinopathy in people with Type 2 diabetes mellitus and numbers needed to screen: a systematic review. Diabet Med 2019. https://doi.org/10.1111/dme.13908.

63. 11. Microvascular complications and foot care: Standards of Medical Care in Diabete-2020. Diabetes Care 2020. https://doi.org/10.2337/dc20-S011.

64. Lewis EJ, Hunsicker LG, Bain RP, et al. The effect of angiotensin-converting-enzyme inhibition on diabetic nephropathy. N Engl J Med 1993. https://doi.org/10.1056/NEJM199311113292004.

65. Fried LF, Emanuele N, Zhang JH, et al. Combined angiotensin inhibition for the treatment of diabetic nephropathy. N Engl J Med 2013;369(20):1892–903.

66. Morrison JL, Hodgson LAB, Lim LL, et al. Diabetic retinopathy in pregnancy: a review. Clin Exp Ophthalmol 2016. https://doi.org/10.1111/ceo.12760.

67. Zhao MW, Sun YY, Xu X. The rational use of anti-vascular endothelial growth factor drugs to assist the treatment of diabetic retinopathy. Zhonghua Yan Ke Za Zhi 2019. https://doi.org/10.3760/cma.j.issn.0412-4081.2019.08.002.

68. Upreti R, Lee JD, Kotecha S, et al. Alphabet strategy for diabetes care: A checklist approach in the time of COVID-19 and beyond. World J Diabetes 2021;12(4):407–19. https://doi.org/10.4239/wjd.v12.i4.407.

69. Gæde P, Oellgaard J, Carstensen B, et al. Years of life gained by multifactorial intervention in patients with type 2 diabetes mellitus and microalbuminuria: 21 years follow-up on the Steno-2 randomised trial. Diabetologia 2016. https://doi.org/10.1007/s00125-016-4065-6.

70. Satoh H. Pleiotropic effects of SGLT2 inhibitors beyond the effect on glycemic control. Diabetol Int 2018;9(4):212–4.

Advances in Pharmacotherapeutics, Metabolic Surgery, and Technology for Diabetes

Alfredo Daniel Guerrón, MD[a], Georgia M. Davis, MD[b], Francisco J. Pasquel, MD, MPH[b],*

KEYWORDS

- Diabetes • Obesity • Diabetes technology • Metabolic surgery • GLP-1
- SGLT-2 inhibitors • CGM

KEY POINTS

- Newer drug classes with proved cardiorenal benefits are changing the paradigm of pharmacologic management of type 2 diabetes mellitus.
- Bariatric surgery options have evolved to include minimally invasive techniques with cardiometabolic benefits in type 2 diabetes mellitus.
- Continuous glucose monitoring systems with remote monitoring capabilities are improving glycemic control in patients with type 1 diabetes mellitus and type 2 diabetes mellitus.
- Automated insulin delivery systems (artificial pancreas) are consistently showing improved glycemic control in patients with type 1 diabetes mellitus.
- It is time for policy changes to help expand access to these proven therapeutic options for patients with diabetes.

INTRODUCTION

Diabetes is a highly heterogenous disease manifested by elevated glucose levels that can lead to acute (i.e. ketoacidosis) or chronic complications (microvascular and macrovascular). Strategies to improve the care of people living with diabetes have evolved significantly in the areas of pharmacotherapy, technology, and surgery. There have been significant advances in insulin formulations to simulate basal and prandial insulin action, with new glucose-responsive insulins in development.

[a] Division of Metabolic and Bariatric Surgery, Duke University, 407 Crutchfield Street, Durham, NC 27704, USA; [b] Division of Endocrinology, Emory University School of Medicine, 69 Jesse Hill Jr Drive SE, GA 30030, USA
* Corresponding author.
E-mail address: fpasque@emory.edu

Endocrinol Metab Clin N Am 50 (2021) 457–474
https://doi.org/10.1016/j.ecl.2021.05.009
endo.theclinics.com

For patients with type 2 diabetes mellitus (T2DM), there now are more than 12 classes of noninsulin agents available to help achieve glycemic control. Several of these newer classes of pharmacotherapeutic agents have effects beyond glucose reduction, including cardiorenal benefits. In addition to pharmacologic treatment advances, novel and traditional surgical techniques have shown significant benefit in obese patients with diabetes that go beyond weight reduction, including improvements in glucose metabolism and cardiovascular risk. Advances in diabetes technology also have made incredible progress, particularly in glucose monitoring and insulin delivery techniques with the integration of these technologies working toward simulating endogenous insulin secretion. This article reviews recent advances in pharmacotherapy, metabolic surgery, and technology in diabetes management, including benefits beyond improved glycemic control.

ADVANCES IN PHARMACOTHERAPY FOR DIABETES MANAGEMENT

The advancement of pharmacologic therapy for the treatment of diabetes includes development of both insulin and noninsulin agents. The rapid expansion of therapeutic options across both categories is shaping diabetes management, providing longer acting basal insulins, more rapid acting prandial insulins, and antihyperglycemic medication options with added cardiorenal benefits for the treatment of T2DM.

Advances in Insulin Therapy

Since the discovery of insulin in 1921, pharmaceutical companies have continued to develop alternative insulin formulations with the goal of minimizing postprandial glucose excursions and hypoglycemia.[1] Multiple insulin formulations are available, including human insulin (NPH and regular), rapid-acting insulin (lispro, aspart, and glulisine), ultra–rapid-acting insulin (aspart and lispro), long-acting insulins (detemir and glargine), ultra–long-acting insulins (degludec and glargine U300), inhaled insulin, and more recently weekly insulin (icodec).[1,2] The development of these different insulin formulations has afforded closer approximation of physiologic insulin secretion. One of the common fears related to insulin therapy has been for many years the incidence of overnight hypoglycemia for both patients with type 1 diabetes mellitus (T1DM) and with T2DM . Long-acting insulin formulations have shown a significant reduction in the risk of hypoglycemia along with a neutral effect on cardiovascular outcomes and cancer.[3,4] Further advances along this path include the advent of a smart insulin that is activated when glucose levels rise and deactivated when glucose levels fall. Preliminary results of these glucose-responsive insulin formulations integrated with microneedle-based transdermal insulin administration technology in animal models are very promising.[5] **Fig. 1** shows the action profiles of available insulin formulations.

Advances in Noninsulin Pharmacotherapy

For many decades, sulfonylureas and metformin have been the foundation of noninsulin therapy for the management of diabetes. The clinical development of metformin as an antidiabetic agent started in France in the late 1950s, whereas the first sulfonylurea was approved for use in Germany in the 1960s. Due to the fear of lactic acidosis observed with phenformin, however, metformin was not licensed for use in the United States until 1995.[6] In the 1970s, the United Kingdom designed the first large study looking at the effects of glycemic control beyond eliminating symptoms of hyperglycemia in patients with T2DM (UK Prospective Diabetes Study). After the results of the study, metformin emerged as the first-line medication to treat T2DM.[7] Metformin has remained a central agent in diabetes management, although the number of

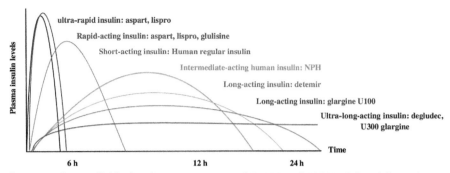

Fig. 1. Insulins available for the management of T1DM and T2DM. Colored lines show a schematic of the pharmacokinetic profiles of human insulins (NPH and regular) and insulin analogs administered subcutaneously. Additional insulin formulations include rapid-acting inhaled insulin (commercially available), weekly insulin icodec (phase 3), and smart insulins (preclinical). (*From* Cheng R, Taleb N, Stainforth-Dubois M, Rabasa-Lhoret R. The Promising Future of Insulin Therapy in Diabetes Mellitus. Am J Physiol Endocrinol Metab. 2021 Mar 15. Epub ahead of print; with permission.)

antihyperglycemic medications has grown exponentially in the last decade and discussions are reemerging about the central role of metformin in diabetes management beyond glycemic control.[8–10]

Addressing cardiovascular risk and outcomes is an important aspect of diabetes care that has resulted in several paradigm shifts in management strategies.[9,10] Thiazolidinediones had a short period of success in the diabetes treatment arena until a meta-analysis showed a potential increase in the risk of cardiovascular outcomes.[11] Even though the risk of atherosclerotic cardiovascular disease (ASCVD) events may be lowered with pioglitazone, the class lost significant attention with the confirmation of increased heart failure and fracture risk.[12] As a result, the Food and Drug Administration (FDA) added regulations in 2007 to ensure the cardiovascular safety of new antihyperglycemic agents in people with diabetes. New trials would be powered to demonstrate noninferiority in major adverse cardiovascular events (MACEs), such as nonfatal myocardial infarction, nonfatal stroke, and cardiovascular death. Several large cardiovascular outcomes trials (CVOTs) were conducted demonstrating noninferiority in cardiovascular endpoints for dipeptidyl peptidase-4 (DPP-4) inhibitors, glucagon-like peptide-1 (GLP-1) receptor analogs, and sodium glucose cotransporter type 2 (SGLT-2) inhibitors.[9] Reproducible findings from these CVOTs have shown not only a reduction in MACEs with GLP-1 receptor analogs[13–18] and SGLT-2 inhibitors[19,20] but also incredible benefits of SGLT-2 inhibitors in reducing heart failure admissions in patients with heart failure with reduced ejection fraction (HFrEF)[21–23] and slowing the progression of kidney disease in those with proteinuria.[24,25] **Table 1** shows results of landmark clinical trials evaluating cardiorenal benefits of SGLT-2 inhibitors beyond MACEs.[22–25] GLP-1 receptor analogs now are the preferred agents for patients with high ASCVD risk or established ASCVD, whereas SGLT-2 inhibitors are preferred in those with HFrEF or diabetic kidney disease. Ongoing trials with dapagliflozin (DELIVER [Dapagliflozin Evaluation to Improve the LIVEs of Patients With PReserved Ejection Fraction Heart Failure] [NCT03619213]) and empagliflozin (EMPEROR-Preserved [NCT03057951]) are evaluating the role of these SGLT-2 inhibitors in patients with HFpEF. In addition, the use of SGLT-2 inhibitors has expanded to nondiabetic patients with heart failure or significant proteinuria with reproducible favorable cardiovascular outcomes in these populations (**Table 2**. Although the use

Table 1
Cardiovascular and renal outcomes (beyond major adverse cardiovascular events) in trials studying sodium glucose cotransporter 2 inhibitors in patients with and without diabetes

	Trials Focused on Renal Outcomes (Patients with Proteinuria)		Trials Focused on Heart Failure Outcomes (Patients with Low Ejection Fraction)	
	CREDENCE[25]	DAPA-CKD[24]	DAPA-HF[22]	EMPEROR HF[23]
Proportion without diabetes	0%	32%	58%	50%
Median follow-up	2.6 y	2.4 y	1.5 y	1.3 y
Primary outcome components	HD, GFR<15, Cr × 2, renal or CV death	50% GFR reduction, ESKD, renal or CV death	CV death, urgent visit or hospitalization for HF	CV death or hospitalization for HF
Primary outcome (HR [95% CI])	**0.80 (0.67–0.95)**	**0.61 (0.51–0.72)**	**0.74 (0.65–0.85)**	**0.75 (0.65–0.86)**
Renal composite outcome (worsening GFR, ESKD, renal death)	**0.66 (0.53–0.81)**	**0.56 (0.45–0.68)**	0.71 (0.44–1.16)	**0.50 (0.32–0.77)[a]**
ESKD (HD or GFR <15)	**0.68 (0.54–0.86)**	**0.64 (0.50–0.82)**		
CV death or hospitalizations for HF	**0.69 (0.57–0.83)**	**0.71 (0.55–0.92)**	**0.75 (0.65–0.85)**	**0.75 (0.65–0.86)**
CV death	0.78 (0.61–1.00)	0.81 (0.58–1.12)	**0.82 (0.69–0.98)**	0.92 (0.75–1.12)
Hospitalizations for HF	**0.61 (0.47–0.80)**	Not reported	**0.70 (0.59–0.83)**	**0.69 (0.59–0.81)**
All-cause mortality	0.83 (0.68–1.02)	**0.69 (0.53–0.88)**	**0.83 (0.71–0.97)**	0.92 (0.77–1.10)
Fatal or nonfatal stroke	Not an endpoint	Not an endpoint	Not an endpoint	Not an endpoint
Fatal or nonfatal MI	Not an endpoint	Not an endpoint	Not an endpoint	Not an endpoint

Abbreviations: CREDENCE, Canagliflozin and Renal Events in Diabetes with Established Nephropathy Clinical Evaluation; DAPA-CKD, Dapagliflozin and Prevention of Adverse Outcomes in Chronic Kidney Disease; DAPA-HF, Dapagliflozin and Prevention of Adverse Outcomes in Heart Failure; EMPEROR-Reduced, Empagliflozin Outcome Trial in Patients with Chronic Heart Failure and a Reduced Ejection Fraction.
Cr, creatinine; CV, cardiovascular; ESKD, end-stage kidney disease; GFR, glomerular filtration rate; HD hemodialysis; HF, heart failure; HR, hazard ratio; MI, myocardial infarction.
Bold numbers represent statistically significant effect estimate.
[a] Composite renal outcome (chronic dialysis or renal transplantation or a profound, sustained reduction in the estimated GFR).

Table 2
Pros and cons of commonly used antidiabetic agents after metformin for patient with type 2 diabetes mellitus

	Sulfonylureas	Thiazolidinediones (Pioglitazone)	Dipeptidyl Peptidase 4 Inhibitors	Sodium Glucose Cotransporter Type 2 Inhibitors	Glucagon-like Peptide-1 Receptor Analogs	Insulin
Efficacy	++	++	+	++	+++	+++
Weight	↑↑	↑↑	—	↓	↓↓↓	↑↑
Hypoglycemia	↑↑	—	—	—	—	↑↑
Heart failure	?	↑	*	↓↓↓	—	?
ASCVD	?↓	↓	—	↓	↓↓↓	—
Kidney Disease	→	→	→	↓↓↓	↓	→
Cost	$	$	$$$	$$$$	$$$$	$$$
Additional considerations	CV risk with older SU, avoid in elderly	Bone loss, macular edema (pioglitazone)	Pancreatitis, heart failure potential with some agents (*saxagliptin/alogliptin)	Mycotic infections, euglycemic DKA, AKI, amputations?	Gastrointestinal adverse effects, retinopathy (semaglutide)?	Hypokalemia

Abbreviations: $, low; $$$, moderate; $$$$, high; +, low; ++, moderate; +++, high; AKI, acute kidney injury; CV, cardiovascular; DKA, diabetic ketoacidosis; SU, sulfonylureas.

of thiazolidinediones largely was abandoned due to heart failure risk, interest in using pioglitazone to improve liver biochemical and histologic parameters in patients with nonalcoholic steatohepatitis (NASH) has emerged.[26,27] One of the most promising drug class is a novel dual glucose-dependent insulinotropic polypeptide and GLP-1 receptor agonist, which appears to have superior efficacy (up to 9 of 10 patients reaching hemoglobin [Hb]A$_{1C}$ <7%) compared with one of the most potent GLP-1 receptor agonists.[28,29] These newer agents (incretin-based agents), associated with significant weight loss, are also are gaining significant attention for the management of obesity and NASH.

The potential for additional benefits beyond glycemic control of available and upcoming agents reminds us that the diverse pathophysiologic derangements present in T2DM raise opportunities for individualized pharmacotherapy in patients with other cardiometabolic comorbidities (NASH, ASCVD, and heart failure). Further developments in precision medicine may allow further individualization of drug therapy.[30]

ADVANCES IN METABOLIC SURGERY

More than 50 operations have been tried for the surgical management of obesity in the past 6 decades, evolving from open techniques to minimally invasive surgery with the innovation of laparoscopy, robotics, and most recently endoluminal therapies.[31] Similarly, the specialty has evolved from bariatric surgery, denoting mere manipulation of the gastrointestinal tract to induce weight loss to metabolically active surgery mediating improvements in glycemia, cardiometabolic benefits, chronic illness improvement, and becoming a bridge to organ transplantation.[32–35] Despite the increasing numbers of obesity and the existence of a safe and efficient solution, only 0.01% of the world's population underwent bariatric surgery in 2013[36] and fewer than 1% of the 24 million US adults eligible for bariatric surgery actually received it every year.[37] Several surgical options are now available for the treatment of obesity. In the United States, the most performed bariatric procedure is the sleeve gastrectomy (SG), which represented 61.4% of the bariatric procedures in 2018.[38]

It is important to emphasize that the current practice of metabolic surgery is exceedingly safe compared with previous experience. Early postoperative death occurs in 1 in 1000 patients and risk of all complications has reached an all-time low of 2% to 5%.

Types of Bariatric/Metabolic Surgical Procedures

From an anatomic point of view regarding the mechanism by which weight loss is achieved, surgical procedures may be classified as restrictive or hypoabsorptive. Restrictive procedures are those in which the size of the stomach is reduced, thus creating an early feeling of satiety, whereas hypoabsorptive procedures are those in which a portion of the small intestine is bypassed, decreasing the quantity of nutrients absorbed. Some techniques combine both mechanisms to accomplish greater weight loss, however, the addition of resections and intestinal anastomoses to the surgical procedure increases its complexity and, therefore, its risk of complications, such as leaks and internal hernias.[39–41] Different bariatric surgeries are displayed in **Fig. 2**. Minimally invasive techniques now are the standard of care for bariatric patients. Leaving aside endoscopic sleeve gastroplasty, which is performed via upper endoscopy, laparoscopic and robotic approaches have shown excellent results and are noninferior to one another.

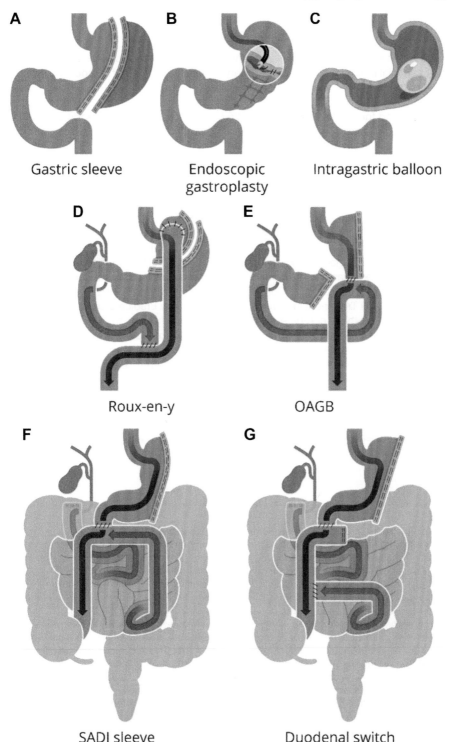

Fig. 2. Metabolic surgery techniques. (*A*) SG: a purely restrictive procedure that has gained popularity due to its technical simplicity and low incidence of complications.[86] (*B*)

Impact of Bariatric/Metabolic Surgery on Diabetes

The term, *metabolic surgery*, was implemented after numerous studies demonstrated the beneficial outcomes of bariatric surgery in obese patients with associated comorbidities. In 1991, a National Institutes of Health (NIH) consensus statement recommended consideration of bariatric surgery for patients with a body mass index (BMI) above 40 kg/m^2 and for patients with a BMI of 35.0 kg/m^2 to 39.9 kg/m^2 in addition to high-risk comorbid conditions, such as severe T2DM, life-threatening cardiopulmonary problems, or physical problems that interfere with daily life.[42] The second Diabetes Surgery Summit, endorsed by almost 50 international scientific societies, refined these recommendations to include consideration of metabolic and bariatric surgery in subjects with BMI of 30.0 kg/m^2 to 34.9 kg/m^2 with persisting hyperglycemia despite optimal lifestyle and medication regimens, regardless of additional comorbidities. These BMI thresholds should be reduced by 2.5 kg/m^2 for Asian patients.[32,43]

Remission of T2DM after metabolic surgery has been addressed by relevant randomized controlled trials, which revealed higher remission rates after surgery than those seen with intensive medical therapy alone. The exact mechanism by which bariatric/metabolic surgery leads to the remission of diabetes and additional cardiometabolic benefits is not fully elucidated.[44] Some of the most relevant randomized controlled trials were the Surgical Treatment and Medications Potentially Eradicate Diabetes Efficiently (STAMPEDE),[45] which compared intensive medical therapy to Roux-en-Y gastric bypass (RYGB) or SG. Within a 5-year follow-up, 29% of the patients who underwent RYGB and 23% who underwent SG achieved HbA$_{1C}$ level less than 6%, whereas only 5% who underwent medication therapy alone were able to achieve this goal. Calorie Reduction or Surgery: Seeking to Reduce Obesity and Diabetes Study (CROSSROADS)[46] was a similar RCT comparing medical therapy to RYGB, which showed remission rates of 6% and 60% respectively, although it had a shorter follow-up of 1 year. The most recent RCT with the largest follow-up of 10 years is the study by Mingrone and colleagues,[47] which compared medical management to RYGB or biliopancreatic diversion (BPD) with duodenal switch (DS) at a single center. In this study,

←————————————————————————————

Endoscopic sleeve gastroplasty: intraluminal suturing device to reduce gastric capacity. (*C*) Intragastric balloon device: balloon in the gastric lumen reduces stomach capacity and stimulates mechanoreceptors ultimately leading to satiety[87]; its major pitfall is weight regain after removal. (*D*) RYGB: combined restrictive and malabsorptive technique. The procedure implies the division of the stomach, creating a small gastric pouch and a large gastric remnant. A gastrojejunal anastomosis then is performed, allowing for the future alimentary content to transit from the gastric pouch into the small intestine.[88] (*E*) Minigastric bypass (one anastomosis gastric bypass [OAGB]): this is a single anastomotic bypass in which a longer gastric pouch with a vertical, antecolic, omega-loop gastrojejunostomy is performed, proposed as a simpler (noninferior) alternative to RYGB. This technique has raised apprehension regarding the potential risk of biliary reflux, although this has not been described in the current data. Prospective trials with long-term follow-up are awaited to better clarify this.[89,90] (*F*) Single-anastomosis duodeno-ileal bypass (SADI sleeve), similar to BPD but with a 1-loop Billroth II–like reconstruction. (*G*) BPD/DS: this technique combines SG with the section and closure of a duodenal stump and gastroileal and ileoileal anastomosis. The suggested length of the common channel is 200 cm to 250 cm to prevent serious malabsorptive complications[91] It historically has been regarded as the best procedure for patients with BMI greater than 50 kg/m^2 (superobese). (*Illustrated by* Megan Llewellyn, MSMI, CMI; copyright Duke University; with permission under a CC BY-ND 4.0 license).

5.5% of the patients in the medical treatment arm achieved sustained remission after 10-year, compared with 25% in the RYGB group and 50% in BPD/DS group.

After these outstanding results, efforts were directed to elaborate a predictor of diabetes remission according to the characteristics of the patients, the severity of diabetes, and the type of surgery. DiaRem is a scoring tool to predict the probability of remission of diabetes after RYGB, based on 4 independent risk factors: age, insulin use, HbA$_{1C}$, and type of antidiabetic medication.[48] A later version, DiaRem2,[48,49] incorporated the duration of diabetes to the score. Similarly, the ABCD score followed 4 risk factors (age, BMI, C-peptide level, and duration of diabetes).[50] Aminian and colleagues[51] designed the individualized metabolic surgery (IMS) score from a large cohort of patients with long-term follow-up (approximately 7 years) to determine the procedure associated with the highest remission of diabetes (available at https://riskcalc.org/Metabolic_Surgery_Score/. The investigators reported 3 severity categories of T2DM for evidence-based procedure selection. For mild diabetes (IMS score <25) both RYGB and SG can achieve high remission rates and for moderate scores (IMS score 25–95) remission is significantly higher after RYGB (60%) versus only 25% after SG. For those with severe diabetes, remission is less likely (approximately 12%) and a lower risk procedure (SG) was suggested. Given that the described models generally were limited to few surgical options, the DiaRem score was expanded to include a wider variety of patient characteristics, such as race and ethnicity, as well as BPD/DS.[52] In this cohort (N = 602 with >1 year follow -up), BPD/DS displayed the higher odds of diabetes remission.

To summarize, these scores show that disease severity indicators (ie, regimen complexity [insulin use] and duration of diabetes) are the strongest predictors of diabetes remission in patients undergoing metabolic surgery.

ADVANCES IN DIABETES TECHNOLOGY

Significant progress in the field of diabetes technology has dramatically shaped diabetes management strategies for those with both T1DM and T2DM, particularly over the past decade. The current focus of these interventions surrounds glycemic control in existing diabetes, although certain technologies may be applicable to diabetes diagnostics and prevention.

Advances in Glucose Monitoring

Glucose monitoring modalities have seen significant transformations over the past two decades. Capillary fingerstick glucose monitoring has been the mainstay of diabetes management for much of this time, with a more recent uptake in the use of continuous glucose monitoring (CGM) technology. The use of CGM has expanded rapidly over the past 3 years to 5 years, and more recently in the setting of the COVID-19 pandemic. Contrasting the well-known method of fingerstick glucose monitoring, CGM employs a small subcutaneous sensor that provides estimated glucose values every few minutes. This technology affords patients closer monitoring of glucose values, often combined with predictive alerts for impending hypoglycemic and hyperglycemic events.

Over the past 10 years, CGM technology transformed to become more affordable and user-friendly. Early CGM systems often required frequent calibrations using fingerstick glucose values to maintain accuracy, with advancements in this area significantly reducing or eliminating the number of required calibrations.[53–55] CGM systems currently available for personal use include both real-time (RT) CGM and flash glucose monitoring. RT-CGM provides users with continuous glucose values and trends via transmission to a device reader or smartphone combined with alerts set to monitor for hypoglycemia, hyperglycemia, and rates of change in glucose trends. Flash glucose monitoring provides the same glucose and trend data but requires moving a device (reader or smartphone) over the sensor (scanning) before values can be visualized. Newer versions of flash CGM recently have incorporated alert capabilities even in the absence of scanning. Although clinical trials investigating the use of CGM in previous years had been mostly in those with T1DM, it has been shown to improve glycemic control in both T1DM and T2DM. Maiorino and colleagues[56] conducted a recent meta-analysis of trials with RT-CGM and flash glucose monitoring in those with T1DM and T2DM to evaluate changes in glycemic control with CGM use. Even though the results showed only a modest overall reduction HbA_{1C} with the use of CGM, this improvement in glycemic control was accompanied by other favorable changes in glycemic control metrics, including (1) increased time in target glucose range [time-in-range (TIR)], (2) less time in hypoglycemic and hyperglycemic ranges, and (3) decreased glycemic variability.[56] Improvements in overall glycemic control evidenced by HbA_{1C} and TIR without a compensatory increase in hypoglycemia and glycemic variability with the use of CGM represent a significant clinical achievement in diabetes management for those requiring insulin therapy.

Furthermore, improvements in accuracy, usability, and affordability of CGM continue to advance the field of glucose monitoring. The development of accurate and reliable glucose sensing technologies has built the foundation for the evolution of other advanced diabetes technologies and remote glucose monitoring capabilities.

From Insulin Pumps to the Artificial Pancreas

Insulin delivery devices have seen a similar transformation, with the advent of insulin pen injectors to the first insulin pump in 1963. Although the first commercially available insulin pump came to market in the 1970s, more widespread commercial use did not occur until the 1990s, with the emergence of smart pumps.[57] As both glucose monitoring and insulin delivery devices continued to advance, so did their integrated use. The concurrent use of CGM with either multiple daily insulin injections or insulin pump therapy, also referred to as sensor-augmented pump (SAP) therapy, was the first step in device integration. The next level of integration involved direct communication between the CGM sensor and the insulin delivery device, allowing for the automatic modification of insulin delivery based on CGM glucose values without requiring user intervention. The first development in this area of CGM pump cross-talk was the ability of the insulin pump to suspend infusion once the CGM threshold for low glucose was met.[58] As communication between CGM and pump technology continued to progress, insulin delivery was able to be suspended prior to hitting threshold hyperglycemia with the use of CGM glucose trend data.[59,60]

The evolution and integration of these devices has been on an incredible trajectory over the past decade. The overarching goal of recreating physiologic insulin secretion with the use of these devices is often referred to as artificial pancreas technology, also called closed-loop or automated insulin delivery (AID). In this level of integration, algorithm-based communications between insulin pump and CGM automatically modulate insulin delivery to maximize time in target glucose range. The first hybrid closed-loop system, the Medtronic (Medtronic, Inc, Minneapolis, MN) 670G, received FDA approval in 2017.[61] Subsequent approval of the Tandem (San Diego, CA) t:slim X2 pump with the Control-IQ algorithm occurred in 2019,[61] with other systems currently in development. Significant improvement in glycemic control metrics without an increase in hypoglycemia risk has been established with the use of closed-loop or AID in those with T1DM. A meta-analysis by Pease and colleagues[62] showed consistent improvement in TIR with closed-loop insulin delivery compared with other methods of glucose monitoring and insulin delivery, including SAP therapy.[60] Limited data exist on the use of this technology for the treatment of T2DM, but studies are ongoing (NCT04617795).

As algorithms within these AID systems continue to advance, so does the probability of achieving desired glycemic control with fewer untoward glycemic excursions. Access to this technology capable of providing such glycemic control can have a profound impact on quality of life, a priority metric that always must be considered as diabetes management strategies move forward. Existing limitations surrounding formal approval of AID systems have inspired movements within the diabetes community to create open-source do-it-yourself closed-loop systems operating outside of FDA regulations.[63] The #WeAreNotWaiting movement developed out of a common goal to improve access to glycemic control data and diabetes management technologies that could translate to better clinical outcomes and quality of life.[63]

Advances in Remote Diabetes Care

During the coronavirus disease 2019 (COVID-19) pandemic, a rapid acceleration in the use of multiple technologies occurred to address limitations in personal protective equipment and to reduce the exposure risk to severe acute respiratory syndrome coronavirus 2 (SARS-CoV-2).[64–69] In health systems with electronic health records (EHRs) with remote access, rapid electronic consults were implemented with some centers improvising population health management approaches to care for large populations of patients with diabetes remotely.[70] In addition, the FDA did not object to the use of CGM to monitor glucose levels remotely in patients with COVID-19.[71,72] Given the lack of experience or accuracy inpatient data, a hybrid approach (CGM with periodic confirmatory point-of-care testing) has been recommended to ensure reliable glucose values.[69,73] A schematic on the emergent implementation strategies is shown in **Fig. 3**. The technology allows remote monitoring. Continuous data can be obtained if a receiver or smartphone is within 20 ft for G6 sensors (Dexcom, San Diego, CA) or via intermittent flashing with the FreeStyle Libre (Abbott, Chicago, IL).[74] Limited information is available on the use of AID with remote monitoring during COVID-19[75] and more information is needed to understand efficacy, safety, barriers to implementation, and costs, before recommending this technology in the hospital.[74]

Evolution of Glycemic Control Metrics

HbA_{1C} has been a longstanding metric for evaluation of glycemic control with associated glycemic control targets associated with the prevention of microvascular complications.[76,77] Despite its widespread use, HbA_{1C} does not provide a comprehensive assessment of glycemic control patterns important in diabetes management. The wealth of glucose data generated by CGM use created a need for standardized CGM-specific glycemic control metrics.[78] In 2017, an expert consensus was convened to define core CGM glycemic control metrics in order to provide guidance on effective use and interpretation of CGM data for clinical management.[79] Consensus recommendations included percent time in target glucose ranges, adjusted for special populations (ie, pregnancy and high hypoglycemia risk), and the standardization of core CGM data presentation and visualization using the Ambulatory Glucose Profile for interpretation.[79] Already, data supporting the use of TIR as a valid outcome measure in relation to the development of microvascular complications have been

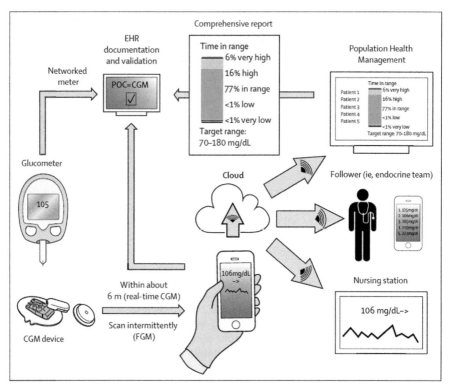

Fig. 3. Remote glucose monitoring during COVID-19. RT-CGM or flash glucose monitoring data are transmitted via Bluetooth from the sensor to a receiver or smartphone. From a smartphone, sensor glucose data can be transferred to the cloud (via cellular signal or WiFi) and from there to RT followers (caregivers and telemetry) as well as to dashboard software (eg, LibreView or Dexcom CLARITY) for comprehensive assessment of multiple patients. Comprehensive glucose reports can be scanned and uploaded to the chart. Additional implementation information, scientific literature, and links are available at covidindiabetes.org. FGM, flash glucose monitoring; POC, point-of-care. (*From* Pasquel FJ, Lansang MC, Dhatariya K, et al. Management of diabetes and hyperglycaemia in the hospital. Lancet Diabetes Endocrinol 2021;9(3):174–88; with permission of Elsevier, Inc.)

reported.[80] As glycemic control data continue to expand, new glycemic control metrics associated with meaningful changes in clinical outcomes are likely to emerge.

OPPORTUNITIES FOR CHANGE

After decades of development of newer medications, surgical procedures, and technologies, it has become clear that such interventions can meaningfully improve the care of patients living with diabetes beyond glucose control. Unfortunately, dramatic inequalities in glycemic control and access to health care and these advancing therapies exist across racial, ethnic, and socioeconomic backgrounds, where often more affluent people are able to buy better health care services and secure better health outcomes.[81] Many of those who may not have had a voice have joined the conversation through social media platforms. Social movements, such as #insulin4all,[82] #WeAreNotWaiting,[83] #OpenAPS,[84] and #BeyondA1c,[85] are raising awareness in the diabetes community to accelerate policy changes. The authors hope such policies allow for medical, surgical, and technological advances to reach the larger community to optimize glycemic control, clinical outcomes, and quality of life.

CLINICS CARE POINTS

- It is important to assess baseline cardiovascular and renal disease and risk factors when choosing antihyperglycemic agents for the treatment of type 2 diabetes, as newer agents may modify this risk.
- Metabolic surgical techniques assist not only with weight loss, but also in improving glycemic control and may also provide cardiometabolic benefit.
- The use of continuous glucose monitoring is rapidly expanding and becoming more reliable and accessible for the treatment of both type 1 and type 2 diabetes.
- The integration of insulin pump therapy with continuous glucose monitoring, also called automated insulin delivery, is becoming more accessible and has been shown to improve outcomes in new glycemic control metrics (ie, time-in-range), specifically in those with type 1 diabetes.

DISCLOSURE

ADG has received personal fees from Gore, Medtronic, Phenomix, Levita, and Biom'up. GMD is supported partially by the NIH under award number 1K23DK122199 to 01A1 and has received research support from Insulet. FJP has received research support from Dexcom, Merck, and Insulet, and consulting fees from Boehringer Ingelheim, AstraZeneca, Eli Lilly and Co, and Merck outside the submitted work. FJP is supported partially by the NIH under award numbers 1K23GM128221-01A3 and P30DK111024-05S1.

REFERENCES

1. Cheng R, Taleb N, Stainforth-Dubois M, et al. The promising future of insulin therapy in diabetes mellitus. Am J Physiol Endocrinol Metab 2021;320(5):E886–90.
2. Rosenstock J, Bajaj HS, Janež A, et al. Once-weekly insulin for type 2 diabetes without previous insulin treatment. N Engl J Med 2020;383(22):2107–16.
3. Investigators OT, Gerstein HC, Bosch J, et al. Basal insulin and cardiovascular and other outcomes in dysglycemia. N Engl J Med 2012;367(4):319–28.
4. Marso SP, McGuire DK, Zinman B, et al. Efficacy and safety of degludec versus glargine in type 2 diabetes. N Engl J Med 2017;377(8):723–32.
5. Yu J, Wang J, Zhang Y, et al. Glucose-responsive insulin patch for the regulation of blood glucose in mice and minipigs. Nat Biomed Eng 2020;4(5):499–506.
6. Pasquel FJ, Hinedi Z, Umpierrez GE, et al. Metformin-associated lactic acidosis. Am J Med Sci 2015;349(3):263–7.
7. Effect of intensive blood-glucose control with metformin on complications in overweight patients with type 2 diabetes (UKPDS 34). Lancet 1998;352(9131):854–65.
8. Nathan DM. Some answers, more controversy, from UKPDS. United Kingdom prospective diabetes study. Lancet 1998;352(9131):832–3.

9. Marx N, Davies MJ, Grant PJ, et al. Guideline recommendations and the positioning of newer drugs in type 2 diabetes care. Lancet Diabetes Endocrinol 2021;9(1):46–52.

10. Cosentino F, Grant PJ, Aboyans V, et al. 2019 ESC guidelines on diabetes, prediabetes, and cardiovascular diseases developed in collaboration with the EASD. Eur Heart J 2020;41(2):255–323.

11. Nissen SE, Wolski K. Effect of rosiglitazone on the risk of myocardial infarction and death from cardiovascular causes. N Engl J Med 2007;356(24):2457–71.

12. Kernan WN, Viscoli CM, Furie KL, et al. Pioglitazone after ischemic stroke or transient ischemic attack. N Engl J Med 2016;374(14):1321–31.

13. Marso SP, Bain SC, Consoli A, et al. Semaglutide and cardiovascular outcomes in patients with type 2 diabetes. N Engl J Med 2016;375(19):1834–44.

14. Husain M, Birkenfeld AL, Donsmark M, et al. Oral semaglutide and cardiovascular outcomes in patients with type 2 diabetes. N Engl J Med 2019;381(9):841–51.

15. Gerstein HC, Colhoun HM, Dagenais GR, et al. Dulaglutide and cardiovascular outcomes in type 2 diabetes (REWIND): a double-blind, randomised placebo-controlled trial. Lancet 2019;394(10193):121–30.

16. Holman RR, Bethel MA, Mentz RJ, et al. Effects of once-weekly exenatide on cardiovascular outcomes in type 2 diabetes. N Engl J Med 2017;377(13):1228–39.

17. Hernandez AF, Green JB, Janmohamed S, et al. Albiglutide and cardiovascular outcomes in patients with type 2 diabetes and cardiovascular disease (Harmony Outcomes): a double-blind, randomised placebo-controlled trial. Lancet 2018; 392(10157):1519–29.

18. Marso SP, Daniels GH, Brown-Frandsen K, et al. Liraglutide and cardiovascular outcomes in type 2 diabetes. N Engl J Med 2016;375(4):311–22.

19. Zinman B, Wanner C, Lachin JM, et al. Empagliflozin, cardiovascular outcomes, and mortality in type 2 diabetes. N Engl J Med 2015;373(22):2117–28.

20. Neal B, Perkovic V, Mahaffey KW, et al. Canagliflozin and cardiovascular and renal events in type 2 diabetes. N Engl J Med 2017;377(7):644–57.

21. Kosiborod M, Cavender MA, Fu AZ, et al. Lower risk of heart failure and death in patients initiated on sodium-glucose cotransporter-2 inhibitors versus other glucose-lowering drugs: the CVD-REAL study (comparative effectiveness of cardiovascular outcomes in new users of sodium-glucose cotransporter-2 inhibitors). Circulation 2017;136(3):249–59.

22. McMurray JJV, Solomon SD, Inzucchi SE, et al. Dapagliflozin in patients with heart failure and reduced ejection fraction. N Engl J Med 2019;381(21):1995–2008.

23. Packer M, Anker SD, Butler J, et al. Cardiovascular and renal outcomes with empagliflozin in heart failure. N Engl J Med 2020;383(15):1413–24.

24. Heerspink HJL, Stefansson BV, Correa-Rotter R, et al. Dapagliflozin in patients with chronic kidney disease. N Engl J Med 2020;383(15):1436–46.

25. Perkovic V, Jardine MJ, Neal B, et al. Canagliflozin and renal outcomes in type 2 diabetes and nephropathy. N Engl J Med 2019;380(24):2295–306.

26. Belfort R, Harrison SA, Brown K, et al. A placebo-controlled trial of pioglitazone in subjects with nonalcoholic steatohepatitis. N Engl J Med 2006;355(22):2297–307.

27. Cusi K, Orsak B, Bril F, et al. Long-term pioglitazone treatment for patients with nonalcoholic steatohepatitis and prediabetes or type 2 diabetes mellitus: a randomized trial. Ann Intern Med 2016;165(5):305–15.

28. Lilly News release. Tirzepatide achieved superior A1C and body weight reductions across all three doses compared to injectable semaglutide in adults with type 2 diabetes. Available at: https://investor.lilly.com/news-releases/news-

release-details/tirzepatide-achieved-superior-a1c-and-body-weight-reductions. Accessed March 23, 2021.

29. Frias JP, Nauck MA, Van J, et al. Efficacy and safety of LY3298176, a novel dual GIP and GLP-1 receptor agonist, in patients with type 2 diabetes: a randomised, placebo-controlled and active comparator-controlled phase 2 trial. Lancet 2018; 392(10160):2180–93.

30. Zeng Z, Huang S-Y, Sun T. Pharmacogenomic studies of current antidiabetic agents and potential new drug targets for precision medicine of diabetes. Diabetes Ther 2020;11(11):2521–38.

31. Buchwald H, Buchwald JN. Metabolic (bariatric and nonbariatric) surgery for type 2 diabetes: a personal perspective review. Diabetes Care 2019;42(2): 331–40.

32. Vidal J, Corcelles R, Jimenez A, et al. Metabolic and bariatric surgery for obesity. Gastroenterology 2017;152(7):1780–90.

33. Aminian A, Nissen SE. Success (but unfinished) story of metabolic surgery. Diabetes Care 2020;43(6):1175–7.

34. Daniel Guerron A, Portenier DD. Patient selection and surgical management of high-risk patients with morbid obesity. Surg Clin North Am 2016;96(4):743–62.

35. Guerron AD, Ortega CB, Lee HJ, et al. Asthma medication usage is significantly reduced following bariatric surgery. Surg Endosc 2019;33(6):1967–75.

36. Angrisani L, Santonicola A, Iovino P, et al. Bariatric surgery worldwide 2013. Obes Surg 2015;25(10):1822–32.

37. ASMBS. Obesity in America. 2018. Available at: https://asmbs.org/resources/obesity-in-america. Accessed March 23, 2021.

38. ASMBS. Estimate of bariatric surgery numbers, 2011-2019 2021. Available at: https://asmbs.org/resources/obesity-in-america. Accessed March 23, 2021.

39. Zhao H, Jiao L. Comparative analysis for the effect of Roux-en-Y gastric bypass vs sleeve gastrectomy in patients with morbid obesity: evidence from 11 randomized clinical trials (meta-analysis). Int J Surg 2019;72:216–23.

40. Zhang Y, Wang J, Sun X, et al. Laparoscopic sleeve gastrectomy versus laparoscopic Roux-en-Y gastric bypass for morbid obesity and related comorbidities: a meta-analysis of 21 studies. Obes Surg 2015;25(1):19–26.

41. Svane MS, Madsbad S. Bariatric surgery - effects on obesity and related co-morbidities. Curr Diabetes Rev 2014;10(3):208–14.

42. Gastrointestinal surgery for severe obesity. Proceedings of a National Institutes of Health Consensus Development Conference. March 25-27, 1991, Bethesda, MD. Am J Clin Nutr 1992;55(2 Suppl):487S–619S.

43. Rubino F, Nathan DM, Eckel RH, et al. Metabolic surgery in the treatment algorithm for type 2 diabetes: a joint statement by international diabetes organizations. Diabetes Care 2016;39(6):861–77.

44. Iqbal Z, Adam S, Ho JH, et al. Metabolic and cardiovascular outcomes of bariatric surgery. Curr Opin Lipidol 2020;31(4):246–56.

45. Schauer PR, Bhatt DL, Kirwan JP, et al. Bariatric surgery versus intensive medical therapy for diabetes - 5-year outcomes. N Engl J Med 2017;376(7):641–51.

46. Cummings DE, Arterburn DE, Westbrook EO, et al. Gastric bypass surgery vs intensive lifestyle and medical intervention for type 2 diabetes: the CROSS-ROADS randomised controlled trial. Diabetologia 2016;59(5):945–53.

47. Mingrone G, Panunzi S, De Gaetano A, et al. Metabolic surgery versus conventional medical therapy in patients with type 2 diabetes: 10-year follow-up of an open-label, single-centre, randomised controlled trial. Lancet 2021;397(10271): 293–304.

48. Still CD, Wood GC, Benotti P, et al. Preoperative prediction of type 2 diabetes remission after Roux-en-Y gastric bypass surgery: a retrospective cohort study. Lancet Diabetes Endocrinol 2014;2(1):38–45.

49. Still CD, Benotti P, Mirshahi T, et al. DiaRem2: incorporating duration of diabetes to improve prediction of diabetes remission after metabolic surgery. Surg Obes Relat Dis 2019;15(5):717–24.

50. Lee WJ, Hur KY, Lakadawala M, et al. Predicting success of metabolic surgery: age, body mass index, C-peptide, and duration score. Surg Obes Relat Dis 2013;9(3):379–84.

51. Aminian A, Brethauer SA, Andalib A, et al. Individualized metabolic surgery score: procedure selection based on diabetes severity. Ann Surg 2017;266(4): 650–7.

52. Guerron AD, Perez JE, Risoli T Jr, et al. Performance and improvement of the DiaRem score in diabetes remission prediction: a study with diverse procedure types. Surg Obes Relat Dis 2020;16(10):1531–42.

53. Bailey T, Bode BW, Christiansen MP, et al. The performance and usability of a factory-calibrated flash glucose monitoring system. Diabetes Technol Ther 2015; 17(11):787–94.

54. Shah VN, Laffel LM, Wadwa RP, et al. Performance of a factory-calibrated real-time continuous glucose monitoring system utilizing an automated sensor applicator. Diabetes Technol Ther 2018;20(6):428–33.

55. Wadwa RP, Laffel LM, Shah VN, et al. Accuracy of a factory-calibrated, real-time continuous glucose monitoring system during 10 days of use in youth and adults with diabetes. Diabetes Technol Ther 2018;20(6):395–402.

56. Maiorino MI, Signoriello S, Maio A, et al. Effects of continuous glucose monitoring on metrics of glycemic control in diabetes: a systematic review with meta-analysis of randomized controlled trials. Diabetes Care 2020;43(5):1146–56.

57. Kesavadev J, Saboo B, Krishna MB, et al. Evolution of insulin delivery devices: from syringes, pens, and pumps to DIY artificial pancreas. Diabetes Ther 2020; 11(6):1251–69.

58. Bergenstal RM, Welsh JB, Shin JJ. Threshold insulin-pump interruption to reduce hypoglycemia. N Engl J Med 2013;369(15):1474.

59. Beato-Vibora PI, Quiros-Lopez C, Lazaro-Martin L, et al. Impact of sensor-augmented pump therapy with predictive low-glucose suspend function on glycemic control and patient satisfaction in adults and children with type 1 diabetes. Diabetes Technol Ther 2018;20(11):738–43.

60. Forlenza GP, Li Z, Buckingham BA, et al. Predictive low-glucose suspend reduces hypoglycemia in adults, adolescents, and children with type 1 diabetes in an at-home randomized crossover study: results of the PROLOG trial. Diabetes Care 2018;41(10):2155–61.

61. Medtronic press release. Medtronic Initiates U.S. Launch of World's First Hybrid Closed Loop System for Type 1 Diabetes. Available at: https://newsroom. medtronic.com/node/13701/pdf. Accessed March 24, 2021.

62. Pease A, Lo C, Earnest A, et al. Time in range for multiple technologies in type 1 diabetes: a systematic review and network meta-analysis. Diabetes Care 2020; 43(8):1967–75.

63. Kesavadev J, Srinivasan S, Saboo B, et al. The do-it-yourself artificial pancreas: a comprehensive review. Diabetes Ther 2020;11(6):1217–35.

64. Pasquel FJ, Umpierrez GE. Individualizing inpatient diabetes management during the coronavirus disease 2019 pandemic. J Diabetes Sci Technol 2020. 1932296820923045.

65. Reutrakul S, Genco M, Salinas H, et al. Feasibility of inpatient continuous glucose monitoring during the COVID-19 pandemic: early experience. Diabetes Care 2020;43(10):e137–8.

66. Shehav-Zaltzman G, Segal G, Konvalina N, et al. Remote glucose monitoring of hospitalized, quarantined patients with diabetes and COVID-19. Diabetes Care 2020;43(7):e75–6.

67. Ushigome E, Yamazaki M, Hamaguchi M, et al. Usefulness and safety of remote continuous glucose monitoring for a severe COVID-19 patient with diabetes. Diabetes Technol Ther 2021;23(1):78–80.

68. Agarwal S, Mathew J, Davis GM, et al. Continuous glucose monitoring in the intensive care unit during the COVID-19 pandemic. Diabetes Care 2021;44(3): 847–9.

69. Davis GM, Faulds E, Walker T, et al. Remote continuous glucose monitoring with a computerized insulin infusion protocol for critically ill patients in a COVID-19 medical ICU: proof of concept. Diabetes Care 2021;44(4):1055–8.

70. Jones MS, Goley AL, Alexander BE, et al. Inpatient transition to virtual care during COVID-19 pandemic. Diabetes Technol Ther 2020;22(6):444–8.

71. Dexcom press release. Fact sheet for healthcare providers: use of Dexcom continuous glucose monitoring systems during the COVID-19 pandemic. Available at: https://www.dexcom.com/hospitalfacts. Accessed March 23, 2020.

72. Abbott press release. Available at: https://abbott.mediaroom.com/2020-04-08-Abbotts-FreeStyle-R-Libre-14-Day-System-Now-Available-in-U-S-for-Hospitalized-Patients-with-Diabetes-During-COVID-19-Pandemic.   Accessed March 23, 2021.

73. Galindo RJ, Aleppo G, Klonoff DC, et al. Implementation of continuous glucose monitoring in the hospital: emergent considerations for remote glucose monitoring during the COVID-19 pandemic. J Diabetes Sci Technol 2020. 1932296820932903.

74. Pasquel FJ, Lansang MC, Dhatariya K, et al. Management of diabetes and hyperglycaemia in the hospital. Lancet Diabetes Endocrinol 2021;9(3):174–88.

75. Hamdy O, Gabbay RA. Early observation and mitigation of challenges in diabetes management of COVID-19 patients in critical care units. Diabetes Care 2020;43(8):e81–2.

76. Stratton IM, Adler AI, Neil HA, et al. Association of glycaemia with macrovascular and microvascular complications of type 2 diabetes (UKPDS 35): prospective observational study. BMJ 2000;321(7258):405–12.

77. The effect of intensive treatment of diabetes on the development and progression of long-term complications in insulin-dependent diabetes mellitus. N Engl J Med 1993;329(14):977–86.

78. Danne T, Nimri R, Battelino T, et al. International consensus on use of continuous glucose monitoring. Diabetes Care 2017;40(12):1631–40.

79. Battelino T, Danne T, Bergenstal RM, et al. Clinical targets for continuous glucose monitoring data interpretation: recommendations from the international consensus on time in range. Diabetes Care 2019;42(8):1593–603.

80. Beck RW, Bergenstal RM, Riddlesworth TD, et al. Validation of time in range as an outcome measure for diabetes clinical trials. Diabetes Care 2019;42(3):400–5.

81. Emanuel EJ, Gudbranson E, Van Parys J, et al. Comparing health outcomes of privileged US citizens with those of average residents of other developed countries. JAMA Intern Med 2021;181(3):339.

82. Conner F, Pfiester E, Elliott J, et al. Unaffordable insulin: patients pay the price. Lancet Diabetes Endocrinol 2019;7(10):748.

83. Omer T. Empowered citizen 'health hackers' who are not waiting. BMC Med 2016;14(1).
84. Litchman ML, Lewis D, Kelly LA, et al. Twitter analysis of #OpenAPS DIY artificial pancreas technology use suggests improved A1C and quality of life. J Diabetes Sci Technol 2019;13(2):164–70.
85. Need for regulatory change to incorporate beyond A1C glycemic metrics. Diabetes Care 2018;41(6):e92–4.
86. Yang P, Chen B, Xiang S, et al. Long-term outcomes of laparoscopic sleeve gastrectomy versus Roux-en-Y gastric bypass for morbid obesity: results from a meta-analysis of randomized controlled trials. Surg Obes Relat Dis 2019;15(4):546–55.
87. Tate CM, Geliebter A. Intragastric balloon treatment for obesity: review of recent studies. Adv Ther 2017;34(8):1859–75.
88. Landin M, Sudan R. This is how we do it: laparoscopic Roux-en-Y gastric bypass. J Laparoendosc Adv Surg Tech A 2020;30(6):619–22.
89. Mahawar KK, Kumar P, Carr WR, et al. Current status of mini-gastric bypass. J Minim Access Surg 2016;12(4):305–10.
90. De Luca M, Tie T, Ooi G, et al. Mini gastric bypass-one anastomosis gastric bypass (MGB-OAGB)-IFSO position statement. Obes Surg 2018;28(5):1188–206.
91. Conner J, Nottingham JM. Biliopancreatic diversion with duodenal switch. StatPearls; 2020.

Ethnic Disparities in Diabetes

Nasser Mikhail, MD[a], Soma Wali, MD[b], Arleen F. Brown, MD, PhD[b,*]

KEYWORDS

- Ethnicity • Disparities • Diabetes • Obesity • Prevention • Treatment
- Lifestyle changes

KEY POINTS

- Racial/ethnic disparities in diabetes persist and are driven by individual, health system, and social factors.
- Obesity is a key driver of excess type 2 diabetes among minorities, but racial/ethnic minority patients may have higher burden of diabetes and prediabetes at lower body mass index (BMI) than Whites; one contributor may be higher rates of visceral adiposity at a given BMI, particularly for Asian subgroups.
- Behavioral, social, health system, and neighborhood factors contribute to disparities in diabetes and obesity.
- Multilevel (patient, provider, health system, and/or community) interventions that promote weight loss and lifestyle change have been shown to prevent or reduce obesity and may prove to be crucial to control the diabetes epidemic among minorities.
- Metformin and sodium-glucose cotransporter 2 inhibitors are drugs of choice for initial medical management of diabetes among minorities with type 2 diabetes mellitus.

INTRODUCTION

The World Health Organization defines equity as the absence of avoidable, unfair, or remediable differences among groups of people, whether those groups are defined socially, economically, demographically, or by other means of stratification.[1] Health equity implies a fair opportunity to attain one's full health. Unfortunately, marked racial/ethnic disparities in the United States exist for almost all aspects of diabetes and its care. Minority groups experience higher diabetes incidence and prevalence, worse metabolic control, and more complications. The causes of these disparities are complex; however, individual, health care system, social, and community-level

Funded by: NCATS UL1TR001881; NHLBI 1U01HL142109; NHLBI 1UG3 HL154302.
[a] Endocrinology Division, Department of Medicine, Olive View-UCLA Medical Center, David-Geffen-UCLA School of Medicine, Sylmar, CA 91342, USA; [b] Department of Medicine, Olive View-UCLA Medical Center, David-Geffen-UCLA School of Medicine, Sylmar, CA 91342, USA
* Corresponding author. UCLA GIM and HSR, 1100 Glendon Avenue, Suite 850, Los Angeles, CA 90024.
E-mail address: abrown@mednet.ucla.edu

Endocrinol Metab Clin N Am 50 (2021) 475–490
https://doi.org/10.1016/j.ecl.2021.05.006
0889-8529/21/© 2021 Elsevier Inc. All rights reserved.

endo.theclinics.com

factors all contribute to both heightened risk of diabetes and poorer outcomes. The disproportionately high rates of infection and mortality associated with COVID-19 among Latinos, African Americans, Native Americans, and racial/ethnic minority groups, particularly those with diabetes, obesity, and other chronic conditions, underscore the pervasive and destructive consequences of these inequities.[2–4] This article provides an update on racial/ethnic disparities in diabetes in the United States and describes evidence-based strategies for diabetes prevention and treatment among minority adults. We use the same terminology for each racial/ethnic group (eg, African American vs Black; Hispanic vs Latino) as in the corresponding reference.

DISPARITIES IN DIABETES PREVALENCE

Evidence from the National Health and Nutrition Examination Surveys (NHANES) between 2011 and 2016 indicate that the age- and sex-adjusted prevalence of total diabetes (diagnosed and undiagnosed) was 12.1% for non-Hispanic White, 20.4% for non-Hispanic Black, 22.1% for Hispanic, and 19.1% for non-Hispanic Asian adults (overall P<.001).[5] The prevalence of undiagnosed diabetes generally followed similar pattern: 3.9% for non-Hispanic White, 5.2% for non-Hispanic Black, 7.5% for Hispanic, and 7.5% for non-Hispanic Asian adults (overall P<.001).[5] Marked heterogeneity in diabetes prevalence is observed within the same ethnic group (**Table 1**). Among

Table 1
Estimated prevalence of diabetes, diagnosed and undiagnosed, in the United States among persons aged 20 y or older among different ethnic groups

Ethnic Group	[a]Prevalence of Diabetes (95% Confidence Interval)
A. Non-Hispanic Whites	12.1% (11.0–13.4)
B. Non-Hispanic Blacks	20.4% (18.8–22.1)
C. Hispanics	22.1% (19.6–24.7)
Hispanic subgroups	
1. Mexican	24.6% (21.6–27.6)
2. Puerto-Rican	21.7% (14.6–28.8)
3. Cuban/Dominican	20.5% (13.7–27.3)
4. [b]Central American	19.3% (12.4–26.1)
5. [c]South American	12.3% (8.5–16.2)
D. Non-Hispanic Asians	19.1% (16.0–21.1)
Non-Hispanic Asian subgroup	
1. [d]East Asian	14.0% (9.5–18.4)
2. [e]South Asian	23.3% (15.6–30.9)
3. [f]Southeast Asian	22.4% (15.9–28.9)

[a] Weighted age- and sex-adjusted (95% confidence interval).
[b] Central America: Costa Rica, Guatemala, Honduras, Nicaragua, Panama, Salvador.
[c] South America: Argentina, Chile, Columbia, Ecuador, Paraguay, Peru, Uruguay, Venezuela.
[d] East Asia: China, Japan, Korea.
[e] South Asian: India, Pakistan, Sri Lanka, Bangladesh, Nepal, Bhutan.
[f] Southeast Asia: Philippines, Vietnam, Cambodia, Thailand, Indonesia, Malaysia, Singapore.
Adapted from Cheng YJ, Kanaya AM, Araneta MRG, et al. Prevalence of Diabetes by Race and Ethnicity in the United States, 2011-2016. JAMA. 2019;322(24):2389-2398; with permission.

Hispanic subgroups, prevalence ranged from 12.3% for South Americans to 24.6% for Mexican Americans. There are limited population-based data on Native Hawaiian and Other Pacific Islander (NHOPI) communities; however, estimates suggest a 19% prevalence of diabetes.[6]

DISPARITIES AND TRENDS IN DIABETES INCIDENCE

After a steady increase in diabetes incidence in adults from 1990 to 2007, data from National Health Interview Survey (NHIS) demonstrated a decline in incident diabetes between 2008 and 2017.[7] However, this decrease in incidence was driven primarily by non-Hispanic Whites (annual percentage change was -5.1%, $P = .002$) followed by Asians (annual percentage change -3.4%, $P = .06$), whereas incidence rates among Hispanics and non-Hispanic Blacks did not decrease.[7] In fact, the latest age-adjusted data for 2017 to 2018 indicated that incidence of diagnosed diabetes in adults was highest in Hispanics (9.7 per 1000 persons), followed by non-Hispanic Blacks (8.2 per 1000 persons), and Asians (7.4 per 1000 persons), whereas non-Hispanic Whites had the lowest incidence (5.0 per 1000 persons).[8]

PREVALENCE OF PREDIABETES

The most recent National Diabetes Statistics Report showed that 34.5% of all US adults had prediabetes (defined as hemoglobin A1c [HbA1c] 5.7% to <6.5%, or fasting plasma glucose 100 to <126 mg/dL, or 2-hour postprandial plasma glucose 140 to <200 mg/dL).[8] The prevalence of prediabetes was stable from 2005 to 2008 and 2013 to 2016 and did not differ substantially by race/ethnicity or education: 31.0% among Whites, 36.8% among non-Hispanic Blacks, 36.1% among Hispanics, and 33.0% among Asians.[8] Screening for prediabetes in asymptomatic adults is recommended for adults of any age who are overweight or obese (body mass index [BMI] $\geq$25 kg/m^2 or $\geq$23 kg/m^2 in Asian Americans) and have one or more additional risk for diabetes. The BMI cutoff point of 23 kg/m2 for Asian American subgroups due to increased risk at lower BMI.[9]

Disparities in Diabetes in Youth

According to SEARCH for Diabetes in Youth, a population-based registry study, incidence of both type 1 and type 2 diabetes is increasing in persons younger than 20 years.[10] From 2002 to 2015, the annual relative percent increase was 1.9% and 4.8% in type 1 and type 2 diabetes, respectively.[10] As in the adult population, there were clear racial/ethnic differences in the rate of increase of diabetes among youth.[10] In type 1 diabetes, the steepest increase in incidence was among Asians/Pacific Islanders (4.4% per year), followed by Hispanics (4.0% per year), then Blacks (2.7%/ year), and finally Whites 0.7% per year.[10] In type 2 diabetes, similar order was observed. Thus, the fastest increase was among Asians/Pacific Islanders (7.7% per year), followed by Hispanics (6.5% per year), Blacks (6.0%/year), American Indians (3.7% per year), and finally Whites (0.7% per year). Reasons for the increase in type 1 diabetes are unclear; however, the increased incidence in type 2 diabetes is likely due to the increase in obesity in US youths, particularly among minority youth.[11]

DISPARITIES IN PREVALENCE OF GESTATIONAL DIABETES

In 2016, the unadjusted national prevalence of gestational diabetes was 6%.[12] The lowest prevalence was observed among non-Hispanic Blacks (4.8%), followed by non-Hispanic Whites (5.3%), then Hispanics (6.6%), then American Indians/Native

Alaskans, and highest in Asians (11.1%).[12] Although the prevalence of gestational diabetes is lowest among Black women, their risk of subsequent type 2 diabetes was higher than that of all other racial/ethnic groups,[13] and the adjusted hazard ratio of developing diabetes after gestational diabetes was 7.6 for Black women and 4.4 for White women (P = .028).[13]

DISPARITIES IN GLYCEMIC CONTROL

Studies have consistently shown that diabetes control, as reflected by HbA1c concentrations, is worse in Black and Hispanic patients compared with Whites. In a national cohort of persons older than 65 years enrolled in Medicare Advantage Health plans in 2011, Ayanian and colleagues examined the proportions of patients with HbA1c levels $\leq$9.0%.[14] They found this goal was achieved by 84.0%, 80.6%, and 74.6% among White, Hispanic, and Black enrollees, respectively (P<.001 for the difference between any 2 groups).[14] The racial/ethnic gap in HbA1c continues to widen. Analysis of NHANES conducted between 2003 and 2014 showed worsening of glycemic control among African American and Mexican American patients with type 2 diabetes, whereas corresponding values tended to improve among White patients.[15] It should be emphasized, however, that the difference in HbA1c levels between Black and White persons may be attributed in part to racial/ethnic differences in glycation of hemoglobin.[16] Thus, on average, HbA1c levels are 0.4% points (95% confidence interval [CI], 0.2%–0.6% percentage points) higher among Blacks than those among White individuals for a given mean blood glucose concentrations.[16]

TRENDS AND DISPARITIES IN DIABETES CARE IN THE UNITED STATES

Serial analysis of the NHANES data between 2005 and 2016 suggests that diabetes care has not significantly improved during that period.[17] Only 23% to 25% of patients met the composite goal of targets for HbA1c (<7–8.5%, depending on age and complications), blood pressure (<140/90 mm Hg), low-density lipoprotein cholesterol (<100 mg/dL), and no smoking.[17] These proportions did not change between 2005 and 2016, and racial/ethnic disparities persist.[17] For example, from 2013 to 2016, 25% of non-Hispanic White patients attained the diabetes care composite goal, compared with only 14% of non-Hispanic Blacks and 18% of Hispanic patients.[17]

DISPARITIES IN DIABETES-RELATED COMPLICATIONS

In general, racial/ethnic minorities have more frequent macrovascular and microvascular diabetes complications than Whites.[18,19] In 2010, incidence (cases per 10,000) of end-stage renal disease (ESRD) was more than double in Blacks (36.6) compared with Whites (16.0).[18] Corresponding rates for lower extremity amputation were 40.0 versus 20.4, for stroke 63.1 versus 39.0, and for hyperglycemic death 2.2 versus 1.4. A notable exception was the incidence of acute myocardial infarction, which was lower in Blacks than in Whites, 32.5 versus 37.5, respectively.[18] No corresponding data regarding Hispanic patients were reported.[18] However, findings from settings in which patients receive uniform medical coverage suggest that incidence rates for many of these complications among Black, Asian, and Latino patients are comparable to or lower than those for Whites.[20] The notable exception was ESRD, with adjusted hazard ratios relative to Whites (95% CI) of 2.03 (1.62–2.54; P<.001) for Black patients; 1.85 (1.40–2.43; P<.001) for Asian patients; and 1.46 (1.10–1.93; P = .004) for Latino patients.[21] Hospitalizations due to diabetic ketoacidosis (DKA) increased by 38% overall between 2005 to 2006 and 2013 to 2014 but vary substantially by race and ethnicity. The highest increase in hospitalizations for DKA was among Hispanics (+58.1%), followed by Blacks (+26.9%), and Whites (+18.5%).[9,21] There are also disparities in rates of hypoglycemia: Hypoglycemia requiring health care services is more common in Blacks (4.7%) and Hispanics (3.6%) than in Whites (2.9%).[22]

Both race/ethnicity and the presence of a diabetes diagnosis are important risk factors for hospitalization and death from the 2019 novel coronavirus disease 2019 (COVID-19).[23] Having type 2 diabetes is an important risk factor for hospitalization and severe outcomes regardless of race/ethnicity, and there is emerging evidence of disparities in diabetes complications.[24] In a recent study of 180 patients with type 1 diabetes and laboratory-confirmed COVID-19 from 52 clinical sites across the United States, Black patients had higher odds of presenting with DKA than Whites (odds ratio [OR] = 3.7 [95% CI 1.4, 10.6]).[25]

DISPARITIES IN DIABETES-RELATED MORTALITY

Mansour and colleagues reported significant ethnic disparities in mortality in patients with diabetes who participated in NHANES surveys during 1999 to 2010.[26] Follow-up of this cohort revealed that all-cause and cardiovascular (CV) mortality decreased in all ethnic groups with diabetes. However, the magnitude of reduction in CV mortality significantly differed between various ethnic groups.[26] Thus, Whites experienced the largest reduction in CV mortality from 20.4% down to 14.5%, followed by non-Hispanic Blacks from 20.6% to 16.3%, whereas Hispanics had only a marginal reduction from 18.4% to 17.5%.[26] Similarly, a recent analysis of NHIS conducted from 1997 to 2017 showed a significant decline in CV complications among White patients only, but no change among Black or Hispanic patients.[27] Taken together, while mortality rates decreased in patients with diabetes overall, the least mortality reduction was observed among Hispanics and non-Hispanic Blacks. This finding is in accordance with NHANES data mentioned previously showing that diabetes care during 2005 to 2016 was worst among minorities.[17]

CAUSES OF RACIAL/ETHNIC DIABETES DISPARITIES
Obesity and Visceral Adiposity

Causes of high prevalence of diabetes in minorities are multifactorial (**Box 1**).[28] The obesity epidemic is a main driver of diabetes, particularly among racial/ethnic

---

Box 1
Causes of racial/ethnic diabetes disparities

1. Obesity and visceral adiposity

2. Unhealthy diet

3. Food insecurity

4. Sedentary lifestyle

5. Acculturation (in some immigrant groups)

6. Low socioeconomic and educational levels

7. Low health literacy

8. Limited English language proficiency

9. Neighborhood factors: poor-quality housing, lack of safe areas for exercise, grocery stores selling high-caloric food and beverages.

minorities. Non-Hispanic Black adults have the highest prevalence of obesity, and Mexican Americans have the highest annual increase in obesity and in waist circumference.[11] Similarly, there has been a steady increase in obesity in US youths (2–19 years) among non-Hispanic Blacks and Mexican Americans, but a recent decline was observed among non-Hispanic Whites.[11] By 2030, it is predicted that severe obesity defined as BMI $\geq$35 kg/m^2 will be highest among non-Hispanic Blacks 31.7% (95% CI, 29.9–33.4), followed by Hispanics 24.5% (95% CI, 22.8–26.2), and non-Hispanic Whites 23.4% (95% CI 22.1–24.8).[29] Although less population-based data are available, evidence suggests that NHOPI obesity rates approach 50%, and rates of diabetes far exceed those in US population overall.[6,30]

The association between obesity and diabetes varies for different racial/ethnic groups. The Patient Outcomes Research To Advance Health Literacy (PORTAL) multisite study examined the association between diabetes and BMI in adults in three integrated health systems.[31] They found higher burden of diabetes and prediabetes at lower BMIs for African American, Hispanic, Asian, and Hawaiian/Pacific Islander patients when compared with Whites. Many Asian American groups, including South Asians and Filipinos, have higher rates of visceral adiposity at a given BMI, which appears to be associated with higher risk of diabetes at younger ages and lower BMI than other groups.[32–35]

Health behaviors

Dietary factors and physical inactivity are risk factors both for developing type 2 diabetes and for inadequate control among those with diabetes.[36–38] High-sugar and high-fat diets are associated with poorer outcomes, and although some traditional diets may be protective,[39] cultural factors, language barriers, and literacy levels can contribute to difficulty adhering to dietary recommendations. Several racial/ethnic groups have lower rates of physical activity, including non-Hispanic Blacks, Native Americans, and Alaska Natives. Ethnic differences in medication adherence have also been identified as a contributor to suboptimal glycemic control among African Americans and Latinos.[40]

Acculturation and immigration

Acculturation, the adoption of attitudes, customs, and values of the prevailing culture of a new society,[41] has been associated with lifestyle changes that may contribute to obesity and type 2 diabetes in some immigrant populations and may be protective for others. For example, among Japanese American men who were more adherent to a Japanese lifestyle in the Honolulu Heart Program, rates of diabetes were lower.[39] In the Multi-Ethnic Study of Atherosclerosis (MESA), acculturation, measured by factors such as place of birth, language, diet, and exercise patterns, was not associated with diabetes prevalence for Chinese Americans or Mexican-origin Hispanics; however, among non–Mexican-origin Hispanics, higher diabetes prevalence was observed in those with the highest levels of acculturation, prevalence ratio (PR) 2.49 (95% CI, 1.14–5.44).[42] This relationship was partially mediated by BMI and diet. Recent evidence on African immigrants, who represent one of the fastest growing immigrant groups in the United States,[43] suggests complex associations between immigration and acculturation. Using data from the NHIS, Turkson-Ocran reported that age-standardized diabetes prevalence was significantly lower in African immigrants than in US-born African Americans, 7% and 10%, respectively (P<.01).[43] Moreover, compared with US-born African Americans, African immigrants who had lived in the United States for 10 or more years were significantly less likely to have diabetes, with a PR of 0.61 (95% CI, 0.43–0.79), hypertension (PR, 0.69%; 95% CI, 0.61–0.78), overweight/obesity (PR, 0.87; 95% CI, 0.77–0.96), or physical inactivity (PR, 0.21%; 95% CI, 0.15–0.28).[43] Hence, African immigrants seem to have a healthier metabolic profile than African Americans.

Social disparities

There is a complex interplay between type 2 diabetes disparities and several social factors, including low individual socioeconomic status (eg, education and income),[8] food insecurity,[44,45] low health literacy and numeracy,[46] communication and language barriers,[47] and neighborhood socioeconomic status. We highlight selected social disparities and their interplay in the following sections.

Limited English proficiency and language concordance. Among patients in the Kaiser Permanente Northern California Diabetes Registry, nonadherence to newly prescribed medications was higher among both Limited English Proficient (LEP) Latino patients and English-speaking Latinos relative to Whites. Among LEP Latinos, the relative risk was 1.36 for oral medications (95% CI, 1.31–1.41) and 1.49 for insulin (95% CI, 1.32–1.69; P<.05). Among English-speaking Latinos, the relative risk was 1.23 for oral medications (95% CI, 1.19–1.27) and 1.28 for insulin (95% CI, 1.23–1.39; P<.05).[47] It is important to note that patients included in these analyses were all insured in the same system of care. Furthermore, among the LEP patients, these associations were independent of provider language concordance.

Food insecurity. Food insecurity, defined as limited food access due to cost, is more common among minority patients and has been associated with poorer glycemic control. In longitudinal analyses of patients in a primary care network in Massachusetts, food insecurity was associated with higher HbA1c (increase of 0.6%; 95% CI, 0.4%–0.8%; P<.0001) over an average 3-year follow-up.[48]

Neighborhood factors. Several studies have suggested that neighborhood environments are associated with diabetes prevalence, incidence, and outcomes.[49] Minority communities, particularly Black neighborhoods, were more likely to be characterized by food deserts, poor-quality housing, and fewer resources for physical activity and exercise.[50] Analysis of US Counties using data from 2013 indicates that counties with higher unemployment, higher poverty, and longer commutes had higher incidence rates than counties with lower levels. By contrast, counties with more exercise opportunities, access to healthy food, and primary care physicians had fewer diabetes cases. In analyses that used data from MESA, communities with better neighborhood resources, for example, grocery stores, parks, and recreational facilities that support physical activity and healthy diets, had a 38% lower incidence of type 2 diabetes.[51] Although the physical environment has long been associated with diabetes, obesity, and physical activity, there is little empirical evidence on whether policy interventions to modify the built environment can improve outcomes from diabetes and its complications.[48,52]

Genetic factors

Genetic factors for diabetes susceptibility contribute similarly to diabetes risk across race/ethnicities.[28] Few studies, however, have had adequate diversity and sample size to quantify the contributions of genetic factors to racial/ethnic differences in diabetes prevalence. In addition, many of these genetic associations may be confounded by environmental exposures that contribute to disease susceptibility. To date, there is little evidence that genetic differences play a major role in racial/ethnic diabetes disparities.[53]

PREVENTION OF DIABETES AMONG MINORITY GROUPS
Lifestyle Changes

Weight loss strategies, including diet and exercise, are essential to prevent or delay onset of diabetes. In the Diabetes Prevention Program (DPP) trial, which included 3234 multiethnic individuals at high risk for diabetes, participants were randomized to a lifestyle-modification program, metformin, or placebo.[36] After an average follow-up of 2.8 years, incidence of diabetes was reduced by 58% and 31% by lifestyle changes and metformin, respectively, compared with placebo.[36] Subgroup analyses of the DPP showed that lifestyle intervention tended to be more effective among minority groups with 61% to 71% reduction in incidence of diabetes compared with 51% reduction among White subjects.[54] The success of the DPP led to culturally tailored adaptations for Hispanics,[54,55] American Indians/Alaska Natives,[56] and African Americans,[57] including faith-based lifestyle interventions in African American churches.[58] These adaptations generally achieved limited or partial success because of short duration of follow-up, high attrition rates, and female preponderance.[54–58]

Metformin

Although metformin was inferior to lifestyle changes in prevention of diabetes in the DPP,[36] its use in this setting may be considered when lifestyle changes are not feasible or successful. In the DPP, metformin appears more effective in reduction of new-onset diabetes among minorities than among Whites.[36] African Americans had a 44% reduction in new-onset diabetes, followed by Hispanics with a 31% reduction, and Whites 24% reduction.[36] In addition, the American Diabetes Association recommends consideration of metformin for patients with prediabetes, especially those with BMI $\geq$35 kg/m^2, those younger than 60 years, or women with a history of gestational diabetes.[59] It is unclear whether these BMI criteria apply.

Neighborhood and Diabetes Incidence

Experimental evidence from the Moving to Opportunity and Tranquility housing mobility study examined the impact of moving to a lower poverty community for residents of public housing projects. After an average of 10 to 15 years of follow-up among 4498 families (approximately 85% African American or Latina women with children), among those who received housing vouchers to reside in a low-poverty area compared with those who did not receive a voucher, incidence of diabetes was 22% lower (95% CI, 31.1%-35.5%), and incidence of obesity was 13% lower (95% CI, 14.4%- 17.7%).[50]

MANAGEMENT OF DIABETES AMONG RACIAL/ETHNIC MINORITIES
Lifestyle Intervention

In the "The Action for Health in Diabetes (Look Ahead)" trial, 5145 (36% minorities, 40% men) overweight or obese participants with type 2 diabetes were randomized to intensive lifestyle intervention and a control group of diabetes support and education.[60] The objective of the lifestyle intervention was loss of 10% of body weight with decreased caloric and fat intake and increased physical activity.[60] After a mean follow-up of 8 years, female patients from all ethnic groups had similar weight loss.[60] Among men, there was a trend toward less weight loss among African American and Hispanic men compared with Whites.[60] A more recent randomized trial conducted in Illinois evaluated culturally tailored diet changes and increase in physical activity in low-income African American patients with type 2 diabetes.[61] Compared with standard care group, HbA1c levels were significantly lower at 6 months, but the difference was no longer significant at 12 and 18 months.[61]

The ADA recommends diabetes self-management education (DSME) in all patients with diabetes. The goal of DSME is to increase the patient's self-efficacy to manage diet, physical activity, glucose monitoring, and stress management.[62] In one meta-analysis of 20 randomized trials of African Americans and Hispanics, DSME programs resulted in modest but significant HbA1c reduction of 0.31% (95% CI, −0.48% to −0.14%) compared with standard care.[63] However, another meta-analysis of eight African American studies did not find any significant impact of DSME in improving HbA1c values.[64] Overall, data suggest that long-term lifestyle intervention adopted in the Look Ahead trial is generally effective in all ethnic groups.[60]

Drug Therapy for Treatment of Diabetes Among Minorities

Metformin

In analyses of electronic health record data, metformin was associated with better HbA1c control for African Americans (n = 7429) than for Whites (n = 8783) (0.9% and 0.4%, respectively, $P<.001$ for the interaction between metformin exposure and race).[65] These results are generally in agreement with those of the DPP showing superior efficacy of metformin in prevention of diabetes among African Americans (44% reduction of new-onset diabetes vs placebo).[36] In addition, a subgroup analysis from the DPP showed that African American subjects with prediabetes treated with metformin have significantly greater decrease in fasting plasma glucose concentrations than Whites up to 2 years after intervention.[66]

Sodium-glucose cotransporter type 2 inhibitors

Sodium-glucose cotransporter 2 (SGLT2) inhibitors are effective, safe, and easy to administer (once a day orally). They have the added benefits of reducing systolic blood pressure and body weight. SGLT2 inhibitors significantly decrease CV and renal events in patients with type 2 diabetes and high CV risk.[67,68] Although these agents are well suited for treatment of type 2 diabetes in racial/ethnic minorities, these groups remain underrepresented in the major trials of SGLT2 inhibitors.[69] However, evidence indicates that the SGLT2 inhibitors empagliflozin and dapagliflozin decrease incidence of CV events in all ethnic groups, including Black patients that constituted approximately 5% of the study populations.[67,68] In a recent randomized trial formed exclusively of African Americans with type 2 diabetes and hypertension, empagliflozin reduced HbA1c levels by 0.78%, mean ambulatory systolic blood pressure by 8.4 mm Hg, and body weight by 1.2 kg compared with placebo after 6 months.[70]

Glucagon-like peptide-1 receptor agonists

Similar to SGLT2 inhibitors, glucagon-like peptide-1 receptor (GLP-1) agonists decreased weight, systolic blood pressure, and CV events in patients with type 2 diabetes and established CV disease.[71] Secondary analysis of phase III trials showed that glycemic efficacy, weight reduction, and safety of the GLP-1 agonist liraglutide are generally similar between African American, Latino/Hispanic, and White patients.[72,73] In the LEADER trial in which Blacks constituted 8.3% of the study population, CV benefits of liraglutide were similar for all racial groups.[71] As with insulin for type 2 diabetes, cost and the requirement for subcutaneous administration may be barriers to use by low-income or minority adults.[74,75]

Addressing Social Determinants of Health

There are limited data on the impact of intervening on the social factors on diabetes outcomes. Patient-provider communication is a critical element in health care provision. Interventions to improve diabetes management among LEP patients have demonstrated improvements in glycemic control.[76] In one study, Latino patients who switched from language-discordant to language-concordant primary care physician had significant improvement in their glycemic control.[77] Enhancing the use of interpreters and efforts aiming at standardization of Medical Spanish in Medical Schools may enhance communication and trust between physicians and LEP Latino patients.[78] Another promising area of investigation is the impact of social needs screening (eg, for food insecurity, housing, transportation) and referral on disparities in diabetes outcomes. The importance of social factors for patients with diabetes and their contribution to health inequities are well documented,[79,80] but there are limited data on whether screening and referral for food or housing insecurity, transportation needs, safety, or other social risk factors is associated with improvement in glycemic control or other components of diabetes care. However, several systematic reviews demonstrate that interventions with community health workers (CHWs)—a lay health worker who is a trusted member, and/or has a close understanding, of the community served.[81] CHWs can take on many different roles, including coordination with the health care system, visit accompaniment, home visits, social support, patient education, social needs screening and linkage to services, and advocacy. In these varied roles, CHWs have been shown to improve clinical and social outcomes among underserved Black, Latino, and Asian adults with diabetes. Diabetes outcomes associated with CHW involvement in care include improved diabetes knowledge and self-care behaviors and modest improvement in glycemic control.[81–90]

SUMMARY AND CURRENT NEEDS

Racial/ethnic disparities in diabetes incidence, prevalence, metabolic control, complications, and mortality are profound and persistent. The gap in incidence of type 2 diabetes between Whites and many minority groups has widened.[5,7,8,10] Obesity has been a main driver of the increase in diabetes incidence, particularly among racial/ethnic minority populations[11]; it is also important to recognize the role of metabolic disease in nonobese individuals. Evidence from randomized controlled trials demonstrates that weight loss, increased physical activity, and medications are effective in preventing and managing diabetes among all racial groups.[36] There is also recognition that strategies to target the obesity and diabetes epidemics must also incorporate social, health system, and community factors that influence these conditions. Rigorous multilevel research can help to address the many gaps in our understanding of diabetes disparities. We need to expand the diversity of behavioral, pharmaceutical, and other clinical trials. High-quality data are needed to better understand patterns of diabetes in the heterogeneous subgroups that make up Latino, Asian, NHOPI, and immigrant populations. More data are also needed on the equity impact of polices at the local, state, and federal levels, for example, to limit the impact of sugar-sweetened beverages, refined carbohydrates, and processed meats. Applying an equity framework in the design, implementation, and analysis of clinical, social, and policy interventions is of critical importance to understanding variation in the effectiveness of these strategies.

CLINICS CARE POINTS

- Screen for prediabetes and diabetes in minority groups if body mass index (BMI) is ≥ 25 kg/m^2 (or ≥ 23 kg/m^2 in Asian Americans). Tailored screening at even lower BMIs may be indicated for some racial/ethnic groups.
- Lifestyle changes are effective in patients with diabetes and in adults with prediabetes to prevent or delay onset of diabetes for individuals of all ethnicities.

- Effective diabetes prevention and treatment should incorporate strategies to address social determinants of health, such as language discordance, low health literacy, food insecurity, and community-level barriers to healthy lifestyle and evidence-based clinical care.
- Metformin is the initial drug of choice for diabetes. It may have superior efficacy among African Americans.
- In addition to their antidiabetic effects, sodium-glucose cotransporter 2 inhibitors and glucagon-like peptide-1 receptor agonists are useful for treatment of diabetes among African Americans and Hispanics as they reduce systolic blood pressure, body weight, and cardiovascular events.

ACKNOWLEDGMENTS

The authors are grateful to Mr Armen Carapetian and Mr Rishabh Shah for their professional assistance with literature.

DISCLOSURE

The authors have no disclosures.

REFERENCES

1. World Health Organization. Health equity 2020. Available at: http://wwwwho.int./topics/health_equity/en/. Accessed June 1, 2020.
2. Yancy CW. COVID-19 and African Americans. JAMA 2020;323(19):1891–2.
3. Gu T, Mack JA, Salvatore M, et al. Characteristics associated with racial/ethnic disparities in COVID-19 outcomes in an academic health care system. JAMA Netw Open 2020;3(10):e2025197.
4. Ko JY, Danielson ML, Town M, et al. Risk Factors for COVID-19-associated hospitalization: COVID-19-Associated Hospitalization Surveillance Network and Behavioral Risk Factor Surveillance System. Clin Infect Dis 2021;72(11):e695–703. https://doi.org/10.1093/cid/ciaa1419.
5. Cheng YJ, Kanaya AM, Araneta MRG, et al. Prevalence of diabetes by race and ethnicity in the United States, 2011-2016. JAMA 2019;322(24):2389–98.
6. Grandinetti A, Kaholokula JK, Theriault AG, et al. Prevalence of diabetes and glucose intolerance in an ethnically diverse rural community of Hawaii. Ethn Dis 2007;17(2):250–5.
7. Benoit SR, Hora I, Albright AL, et al. New directions in incidence and prevalence of diagnosed diabetes in the USA. BMJ Open Diabetes Res Care 2019;7(1):e000657.
8. Centers for Disease Control and Prevention. National diabetes Statistics Report, 2020. Atlanta (GA): Centers for Disease Control and Prevention, U.S. Depart of Health and Human Services; 2020.
9. Hsu WC, Araneta MR, Kanaya AM, et al. BMI cut points to identify at-risk Asian Americans for type 2 diabetes screening. Diabetes Care 2015;38(1):150–8.
10. Mayer-Davis EJ, Dabelea D, Lawrence JM. Incidence Trends of Type 1 and Type 2 Diabetes among Youths, 2002-2012. N Engl J Med 2017;377(3):301.
11. Wang Y, Beydoun MA, Min J, et al. Has the prevalence of overweight, obesity and central obesity levelled off in the United States? Trends, patterns, disparities, and future projections for the obesity epidemic. Int J Epidemiol 2020;49(3):810–23.

12. Deputy NP, Kim SY, Conrey EJ, et al. Prevalence and Changes in Preexisting Diabetes and Gestational Diabetes Among Women Who Had a Live Birth - United States, 2012-2016. MMWR Morb Mortal Wkly Rep 2018;67(43):1201–7.
13. Xiang AH, Li BH, Black MH, et al. Racial and ethnic disparities in diabetes risk after gestational diabetes mellitus. Diabetologia 2011;54(12):3016–21.
14. Ayanian JZ, Landon BE, Newhouse JP, et al. Racial and ethnic disparities among enrollees in Medicare Advantage plans. N Engl J Med 2014;371(24):2288–97.
15. Smalls BL, Ritchwood TD, Bishu KG, et al. Racial/Ethnic Differences in Glycemic Control in Older Adults with Type 2 Diabetes: United States 2003-2014. Int J Environ Res Public Health 2020;17(3):950.
16. Bergenstal RM, Gal RL, Connor CG, et al. Racial differences in the relationship of glucose concentrations and hemoglobin A1c Levels. Ann Intern Med 2017; 167(2):95–102.
17. Kazemian P, Shebl FM, McCann N, et al. Evaluation of the Cascade of Diabetes Care in the United States, 2005-2016. JAMA Intern Med 2019;179(10):1376–85.
18. Gregg EW, Li Y, Wang J, et al. Changes in diabetes-related complications in the United States, 1990-2010. N Engl J Med 2014;370(16):1514–23.
19. Luo H, Bell RA, Garg S, et al. Trends and racial/ethnic disparities in diabetic retinopathy among adults with diagnosed diabetes in North Carolina, 2000-2015. N C Med J 2019;80(2):76–82.
20. Karter AJ, Ferrara A, Liu JY, et al. Ethnic disparities in diabetic complications in an insured population. JAMA 2002;287(19):2519–27.
21. Kalla Vyas A, Oud L. Temporal patterns of hospitalizations for diabetic ketoacidosis in children and adolescents. PLoS One 2021;16(1):e0245012.
22. Lopez JM, Bailey RA, Rupnow MF. Demographic disparities among medicare beneficiaries with type 2 diabetes mellitus in 2011: diabetes prevalence, comorbidities, and hypoglycemia events. Popul Health Manag 2015;18(4):283–9.
23. Guo W, Li M, Dong Y, et al. Diabetes is a risk factor for the progression and prognosis of COVID-19. Diabetes Metab Res Rev 2020;e3319. https://doi.org/10. 1002/dmrr.3319.
24. Manohar J, Abedian S, Martini R, et al. Social and Clinical Determinants of COVID-19 Outcomes: Modeling Real-World Data from a Pandemic Epicenter. medRxiv 2021. https://doi.org/10.1101/2021.04.06.21254728.
25. Ebekozien O, Agarwal S, Noor N, et al. Inequities in Diabetic Ketoacidosis Among Patients With Type 1 Diabetes and COVID-19: Data From 52 US Clinical Centers. J Clin Endocrinol Metab 2021;106(4):e1755–62.
26. Mansour O, Golden SH, Yeh HC. Disparities in mortality among adults with and without diabetes by sex and race. J Diabetes Complications 2020;34(3):107496.
27. Chiou T, Tsugawa Y, Goldman D, et al. Trends in Racial and Ethnic Disparities in Diabetes-Related Complications, 1997-2017. J Gen Intern Med 2020;35(3): 950–1.
28. Golden SH, Brown A, Cauley JA, et al. Health disparities in endocrine disorders: biological, clinical, and nonclinical factors–an Endocrine Society scientific statement. J Clin Endocrinol Metab 2012;97(9):E1579–639.
29. Ward ZJ, Bleich SN, Cradock AL, et al. Projected U.S. State-Level Prevalence of Adult Obesity and Severe Obesity. N Engl J Med 2019;381(25):2440–50.
30. Mau MK, Sinclair K, Saito EP, et al. Cardiometabolic health disparities in native Hawaiians and other Pacific Islanders. Epidemiol Rev 2009;31:113–29.
31. Zhu Y, Sidell MA, Arterburn D, et al. Racial/Ethnic Disparities in the Prevalence of Diabetes and Prediabetes by BMI: Patient Outcomes Research To Advance

Learning (PORTAL) Multisite Cohort of Adults in the U.S. Diabetes Care 2019; 42(12):2211–9.

32. Bakker LE, Sleddering MA, Schoones JW, et al. Pathogenesis of type 2 diabetes in South Asians. Eur J Endocrinol 2013;169(5):R99–114.

33. Narayan KM, Aviles-Santa L, Oza-Frank R, et al. Report of a National Heart, Lung, And Blood Institute Workshop: heterogeneity in cardiometabolic risk in Asian Americans In the U.S. Opportunities for research. J Am Coll Cardiol 2010; 55(10):966–73.

34. Sohal T, Sohal P, King-Shier KM, et al. Barriers and Facilitators for Type-2 Diabetes Management in South Asians: A Systematic Review. PLoS One 2015; 10(9):e0136202.

35. Spanakis EK, Golden SH. Race/ethnic difference in diabetes and diabetic complications. Curr Diab Rep 2013;13(6):814–23.

36. Knowler WC, Barrett-Connor E, Fowler SE, et al. Reduction in the incidence of type 2 diabetes with lifestyle intervention or metformin. N Engl J Med 2002; 346(6):393–403.

37. Neuenschwander M, Ballon A, Weber KS, et al. Role of diet in type 2 diabetes incidence: umbrella review of meta-analyses of prospective observational studies. BMJ 2019;366:l2368.

38. Yeh HC, Duncan BB, Schmidt MI, et al. Smoking, smoking cessation, and risk for type 2 diabetes mellitus: a cohort study. Ann Intern Med 2010;152(1):10–7.

39. Huang B, Rodriguez BL, Burchfiel CM, et al. Acculturation and prevalence of diabetes among Japanese-American men in Hawaii. Am J Epidemiol 1996;144(7): 674–81.

40. Heisler M, Faul JD, Hayward RA, et al. Mechanisms for racial and ethnic disparities in glycemic control in middle-aged and older Americans in the health and retirement study. Arch Intern Med 2007;167(17):1853–60.

41. Perez-Escamilla R. Acculturation, nutrition, and health disparities in Latinos. Am J Clin Nutr 2011;93(5):1163S–7S.

42. Kandula NR, Diez-Roux AV, Chan C, et al. Association of acculturation levels and prevalence of diabetes in the multi-ethnic study of atherosclerosis (MESA). Diabetes Care 2008;31(8):1621–8.

43. Turkson-Ocran RN, Nmezi NA, Botchway MO, et al. Comparison of Cardiovascular Disease Risk Factors Among African Immigrants and African Americans: An Analysis of the 2010 to 2016 National Health Interview Surveys. J Am Heart Assoc 2020;9(5):e013220.

44. Walker RJ, Campbell JA, Egede LE. Differential impact of food insecurity, distress, and stress on self-care behaviors and glycemic control using path analysis. J Gen Intern Med 2019;34(12):2779–85.

45. Walker RJ, Grusnick J, Garacci E, et al. Trends in Food Insecurity in the USA for individuals with prediabetes, undiagnosed diabetes, and diagnosed diabetes. J Gen Intern Med 2019;34(1):33–5.

46. Cavanaugh KL. Health literacy in diabetes care: explanation, evidence and equipment. Diabetes Manag (Lond) 2011;1(2):191–9.

47. Fernandez A, Schillinger D, Warton EM, et al. Language barriers, physician-patient language concordance, and glycemic control among insured Latinos with diabetes: the Diabetes Study of Northern California (DISTANCE). J Gen Intern Med 2011;26(2):170–6.

48. Berkowitz SA, Karter AJ, Corbie-Smith G, et al. Food Insecurity, Food "Deserts," and Glycemic Control in Patients With Diabetes: A Longitudinal Analysis. Diabetes Care 2018;41(6):1188–95.

49. Cunningham SA, Patel SA, Beckles GL, et al. County-level contextual factors associated with diabetes incidence in the United States. Ann Epidemiol 2018; 28(1):20–25 e22.

50. Schootman M, Andresen EM, Wolinsky FD, et al. The effect of adverse housing and neighborhood conditions on the development of diabetes mellitus among middle-aged African Americans. Am J Epidemiol 2007;166(4):379–87.

51. Auchincloss AH, Mujahid MS, Shen M, et al. Neighborhood health-promoting resources and obesity risk (the multi-ethnic study of atherosclerosis). Obesity (Silver Spring) 2013;21(3):621–8.

52. Amuda AT, Berkowitz SA. Diabetes and the Built Environment: Evidence and Policies. Curr Diab Rep 2019;19(7):35.

53. Golden SH, Yajnik C, Phatak S, et al. Racial/ethnic differences in the burden of type 2 diabetes over the life course: a focus on the USA and India. Diabetologia 2019;62(10):1751–60.

54. Van Name MA, Camp AW, Magenheimer EA, et al. Effective translation of an intensive lifestyle intervention for hispanic women with prediabetes in a community health center setting. Diabetes Care 2016;39(4):525–31.

55. McCurley JL, Gutierrez AP, Gallo LC. Diabetes Prevention in U.S. Hispanic Adults: A Systematic Review of Culturally Tailored Interventions. Am J Prev Med 2017;52(4):519–29.

56. Jiang L, Johnson A, Pratte K, et al. Long-term Outcomes of Lifestyle Intervention to Prevent Diabetes in American Indian and Alaska Native Communities: The Special Diabetes Program for Indians Diabetes Prevention Program. Diabetes Care 2018;41(7):1462–70.

57. Sattin RW, Williams LB, Dias J, et al. Community Trial of a Faith-Based Lifestyle Intervention to Prevent Diabetes Among African-Americans. J Community Health 2016;41(1):87–96.

58. Berkley-Patton J, Bowe Thompson C, Bauer AG, et al. A Multilevel Diabetes and CVD Risk Reduction Intervention in African American Churches: Project Faith Influencing Transformation (FIT) Feasibility and Outcomes. J Racial Ethn Health Disparities 2020;7(6):1160–71.

59. American Diabetes A. 3. Prevention or Delay of Type 2 Diabetes: Standards of Medical Care in Diabetes-2020. Diabetes Care 2020;43(Suppl 1):S32–6.

60. West DS, Dutton G, Delahanty LM, et al. Weight loss experiences of african american, hispanic, and non-hispanic white men and women with type 2 diabetes: the look AHEAD Trial. Obesity (Silver Spring) 2019;27(8):1275–84.

61. Lynch EB, Mack L, Avery E, et al. Randomized Trial of a Lifestyle Intervention for Urban Low-Income African Americans with Type 2 Diabetes. J Gen Intern Med 2019;34(7):1174–83.

62. Powers MA, Bardsley J, Cypress M, et al. Diabetes self-management education and support in type 2 diabetes. Diabetes Educ 2017;43(1):40–53.

63. Ricci-Cabello I, Ruiz-Perez I, Rojas-Garcia A, et al. Characteristics and effectiveness of diabetes self-management educational programs targeted to racial/ethnic minority groups: a systematic review, meta-analysis and meta-regression. BMC Endocr Disord 2014;14:60.

64. Cunningham AT, Crittendon DR, White N, et al. The effect of diabetes self-management education on HbA1c and quality of life in African-Americans: a systematic review and meta-analysis. BMC Health Serv Res 2018;18(1):367.

65. Williams LK, Padhukasahasram B, Ahmedani BK, et al. Differing effects of metformin on glycemic control by race-ethnicity. J Clin Endocrinol Metab 2014;99(9): 3160–8.

66. Zhang C, Zhang R. More effective glycaemic control by metformin in African Americans than in Whites in the prediabetic population. Diabetes Metab 2015; 41(2):173–5.
67. McMurray JJV, Solomon SD, Inzucchi SE, et al. Dapagliflozin in patients with heart failure and reduced ejection fraction. N Engl J Med 2019;381(21):1995–2008.
68. Zinman B, Wanner C, Lachin JM, et al. Empagliflozin, cardiovascular outcomes, and mortality in type 2 diabetes. N Engl J Med 2015;373(22):2117–28.
69. Hoppe C, Kerr D. Minority underrepresentation in cardiovascular outcome trials for type 2 diabetes. Lancet Diabetes Endocrinol 2017;5(1):13.
70. Ferdinand KC, Izzo JL, Lee J, et al. Antihyperglycemic and Blood Pressure Effects of Empagliflozin in Black Patients With Type 2 Diabetes Mellitus and Hypertension. Circulation 2019;139(18):2098–109.
71. Marso SP, Daniels GH, Brown-Frandsen K, et al. Liraglutide and Cardiovascular Outcomes in Type 2 Diabetes. N Engl J Med 2016;375(4):311–22.
72. Davidson JA, Orsted DD, Campos C. Efficacy and safety of liraglutide, a once-daily human glucagon-like peptide-1 analogue, in Latino/Hispanic patients with type 2 diabetes: post hoc analysis of data from four phase III trials. Diabetes Obes Metab 2016;18(7):725–8.
73. Shomali ME, Orsted DD, Cannon AJ. Efficacy and safety of liraglutide, a once-daily human glucagon-like peptide-1 receptor agonist, in African-American people with Type 2 diabetes: a meta-analysis of sub-population data from seven phase III trials. Diabet Med 2017;34(2):197–203.
74. Lipska KJ, Ross JS, Van Houten HK, et al. Use and out-of-pocket costs of insulin for type 2 diabetes mellitus from 2000 through 2010. JAMA 2014;311(22):2331–3.
75. Herkert D, Vijayakumar P, Luo J, et al. Cost-Related Insulin Underuse Among Patients With Diabetes. JAMA Intern Med 2019;179(1):112–4.
76. Njeru JW, Wieland ML, Kwete G, et al. Diabetes Mellitus Management Among Patients with Limited English Proficiency: A Systematic Review and Meta-Analysis. J Gen Intern Med 2018;33(4):524–32.
77. Parker MM, Fernandez A, Moffet HH, et al. Association of Patient-Physician Language Concordance and Glycemic Control for Limited-English Proficiency Latinos With Type 2 Diabetes. JAMA Intern Med 2017;177(3):380–7.
78. Ortega P, Diamond L, Aleman MA, et al. Medical Spanish Standardization in U.S. Medical Schools: Consensus Statement From a Multidisciplinary Expert Panel. Acad Med 2020;95(1):22–31.
79. de Wit M, Trief PM, Huber JW, et al. State of the art: understanding and integration of the social context in diabetes care. Diabet Med 2020;37(3):473–82.
80. Frier A, Devine S, Barnett F, et al. Utilising clinical settings to identify and respond to the social determinants of health of individuals with type 2 diabetes-A review of the literature. Health Soc Care Community 2020;28(4):1119–33.
81. Norris SL, Chowdhury FM, Van Le K, et al. Effectiveness of community health workers in the care of persons with diabetes. Diabet Med 2006;23(5):544–56.
82. Hunt CW, Grant JS, Appel SJ. An integrative review of community health advisors in type 2 diabetes. J Community Health 2011;36(5):883–93.
83. Little TV, Wang ML, Castro EM, et al. Community health worker interventions for Latinos with type 2 diabetes: a systematic review of randomized controlled trials. Curr Diab Rep 2014;14(12):558.
84. Shah M, Kaselitz E, Heisler M. The role of community health workers in diabetes: update on current literature. Curr Diab Rep 2013;13(2):163–71.

85. Islam N, Nadkarni SK, Zahn D, et al. Integrating community health workers within Patient Protection and Affordable Care Act implementation. J Public Health Manag Pract 2015;21(1):42–50.

86. Centers for Disease Control and Prevention. Addressing Chronic Disease Through Community Health Workers: A Policy and Systems-Level Approach. Atlanta, GA: 2015. Available at: https://www.cdc.gov/dhdsp/docs/chw_brief.pdf. Accessed June 16, 2021.

87. National Association of Chronic Disease Directors. Community programs linked to clinical services – community health workers: reimbursement/advocacy. 2020. Available at: https://www.cdc.gov/dhdsp/pubs/docs/chw_evidence_assessment_report.pdf.

88. Egbujie BA, Delobelle PA, Levitt N, et al. Role of community health workers in type 2 diabetes mellitus self-management: A scoping review. PLoS One 2018;13(6): e0198424.

89. Palmas W, March D, Darakjy S, et al. Community Health Worker Interventions to Improve Glycemic Control in People with Diabetes: A Systematic Review and Meta-Analysis. J Gen Intern Med 2015;30(7):1004–12.

90. Gary TL, Batts-Turner M, Yeh HC, et al. The effects of a nurse case manager and a community health worker team on diabetic control, emergency department visits, and hospitalizations among urban African Americans with type 2 diabetes mellitus: a randomized controlled trial. Arch Intern Med 2009;169(19):1788–94.

Diabetes in Youth
A Global Perspective

Anna R. Kahkoska, MD, PhD[a],*, Dana Dabelea, MD, PhD[b]

KEYWORDS

- Diabetes • Obesity • Epidemiology • Management • Complications
- Youth and young adults

KEY POINTS

- Although diabetes in youth was previously thought to be primarily type 1 diabetes, the incidence of type 2 diabetes in increasing among youth and has become a major form of pediatric diabetes.
- The incidence of both type 1 and type 2 diabetes is increasing, with disproportional increases among non-White youth in the United States. Incidence estimates from low- and middle-income countries are based on limited data, but suggest increasing incidence worldwide.
- Management of diabetes in youth is centered around maintaining glycemic control to prevent acute and chronic complications. New technology and pharmacologic treatment modalities are rapidly emerging.
- Diabetes in youth is a serious disease, and tight glycemic control is difficult to attain over childhood and into young adulthood.

INTRODUCTION

Diabetes in children and adolescents is now acknowledged to be a complex disorder with heterogeneity in its etiology, pathogenesis, clinical presentation, and outcomes. The majority of pediatric diabetes is classified into 1 of 2 broad categories according to physiologic framework established by the American Diabetes Association in 1997[1]: type 1 diabetes (T1D), an absolute deficiency of insulin usually owing to autoimmune destruction of the β-cells, and type 2 diabetes (T2D), a combination of insulin resistance and relative insulin deficiency.[2,3] Until recently, diabetes diagnosed in children and adolescents was almost entirely considered to be T1D, but T2D has recently

[a] Department of Nutrition, University of North Carolina at Chapel Hill, McGavran-Greenberg Hall 2205A, Chapel Hill, NC 27599, USA; [b] Lifecourse Epidemiology of Adiposity and Diabetes (LEAD) Center, Colorado School of Public Health, University of Colorado School of Medicine, Anschutz Medical Campus, 13001 East 17th Avenue, Box B119, Room W3110, Aurora, CO 80045, USA
* Corresponding author.
E-mail address: anna_kahkoska@med.unc.edu

Endocrinol Metab Clin N Am 50 (2021) 491–512
https://doi.org/10.1016/j.ecl.2021.05.007
0889-8529/21/© 2021 Elsevier Inc. All rights reserved.

endo.theclinics.com

emerged among youth with obesity and in high-risk ethnic populations.[4,5] Although there are other forms of diabetes that affect youth, including genetic defects of β-cell function, genetic defects of insulin action, and a variety of secondary forms of diabetes,[3,6] this article focuses on the most common forms of pediatric diabetes: T1D and T2D in youth.

PRESENTATION AND CLASSIFICATIONS OF DIABETES IN YOUTH

Categories of diabetes in youth are distinguished by characteristic clinical presentations and are summarized in **Table 1**.

Type 1 Diabetes

T1D is caused by immune-mediated β-cell destruction leading to insulin deficiency. Symptoms appear when approximately 90% of pancreatic β-cells are destroyed,[7] are usually rapid in onset, and include polyuria, polydipsia, weight loss, abdominal symptoms, headaches, and ketoacidosis. Insulin is necessary for survival.[8] The autoimmune destruction of the β-cells is mediated by T cells and accompanied by the formation of autoantibodies such as those against the 65KD isoform of glutamic acid decarboxylase, those against the zinc transporter 8, insulinoma–associated-2 antibodies, insulin autoantibodies, and islet cell autoantibodies. These antibodies are present before the appearance of clinical disease and predict disease development.[9–11] The presence of each antibody at diagnosis varies with age of onset, race/ethnicity, and sex,[12–14] but 1 or more autoantibodies are typically present at diagnosis with T1D in 80% to 90% of affected children.[8]

Type 2 Diabetes

The current view is that T2D in youth is primarily characterized by insulin resistance detected at the level of skeletal muscle, liver, and adipose tissues with a failure of β-cell compensation and a relative insulin deficiency.[8] However, the exact sequence of metabolic changes leading to dysglycemia and ultimately youth-onset T2D remains unknown. For example, increasing evidence supports the possibility, at least in subsets of individuals at risk of T2D, that hyper-responsiveness of the islet β-cell to a hostile environment drives hyperinsulinemia; this may be the upstream culprit of excessive weight gain, insulin resistance, subsequent β-cell failure, and the development of T2D.[15,16] Although the extent to which children progress through stages of obesity, insulin resistance, and glucose intolerance to T2D is not fully understood, it seems that the pathway to disease and the clinical evolution of the disease, once diagnosed, are much shorter and less predictable in children than in adults, comprising a different and more aggressive pathophysiologic process.[17] For example, the TODAY trial found that youth with T2D showed a more rapid decrease in insulin sensitivity and β-cell function compared with adults, with decreased response to metformin and rosiglitazone treatment.[18]

Pediatric patients with T2D are overweight or obese (body mass index ≥85th percentile for age and sex), and comorbidities such as hypertension and dyslipidemia can be present at diagnosis. Often there is a strong family history in first- and second-degree family members. Weight loss at diagnosis is less common than in T1D, and acanthosis nigricans is frequently identified on physical examination. Patients usually present with evidence of residual β-cell function, although no standardized cutoffs exist for insulin or C-peptide levels. These patients typically lack evidence of autoimmunity. Ketosis is less common than in T1D because individuals with T2D usually produce enough insulin to

Table 1
Classical presentation of diabetes in youth

	T1D	T2D	Monogenic Diabetes
Age at onset or presentation	Bimodal; Age 4–6 y, Age 10–14 y	Post-pubertal	Before age 25 y
Autoantibodies	Present	Absent	Absent
Weight status	Usually normal weight; increasing prevalence of overweight or obesity	Overweight or obesity common (>90%)	Usually normal weight; increasing prevalence of overweight or obesity
Insulin resistance	Less common	Present	Absent
Risk of diabetic ketoacidosis	High	Low	Low
Endogenous insulin production (C-peptide level)	Low	Detectable	Detectable
Family history of diabetes	Infrequent (10%–15%)	Frequent (90%)	Frequent, usually multiple generations

Autoantibodies include for GADA, IA-2A, ZnT8-A
Monogenic diabetes includes neonatal diabetes and mitochondrial diabetes arising from single-gene mutations in HNF1-alpha, HNF4-alpha or glucokinase.

Abbreviation: GADA, glutamic acid decarboxylase; IA-2, insulinoma–associated-2 antibodies.
Adapted from Shah AS, Nadeau KJ. The changing face of paediatric diabetes. Diabetologia. 2020 Apr;63(4):683-691; with permission.

prevent lipolysis. Insulin may or may not be required at diagnosis or for long-term treatment of hyperglycemia, but insulin is typically not required for survival.[8]

EPIDEMIOLOGY
Type 1 Diabetes

Approximately 98,200 children under the age of 15 years and 128,900 youth under the age of 20 years are estimated to develop T1D annually worldwide.[19] The incidence and prevalence of T1D varies greatly between different countries, and within countries, between different ethnic populations (**Fig. 1**).[3,20] An increase in the incidence of T1D has been observed globally in recent decades, with a disproportionately greater increase in those under the age of 5 years[21,22] and in developing countries or those undergoing recent economic transition.[21,23] There is also variation in temporal trends in global incidence of T1D in youth, with evidence for a plateau in incidence in some countries in recent years, as well as cyclical trends.[3] The most recent data on incidence per 100,000 population per year showed that Finland (62.3), Sweden (43.2), and Kuwait (41.7) have the highest incidence rates of T1D among youth 0 to 14 years.[24] In Asia, the incidence of T1D is very low; for example, approximately 2 per 100,000 person-years in Japan,[25] 3.1 per 100,000 in China,[26] and approximately 5 per 100,000 in Taiwan.[27] In the United States, nationally representative data from the SEARCH for Diabetes in Youth study showed that the incidence of T1D is increasing,[5] with the highest rates of increase among Hispanic White youth compared with non-Hispanic White youth (4.2% vs 1.2%).[5]

Data on the incidence of T1D in low- and middle-income countries (LMIC) are limited. Available estimates are highly variable across the globe but suggest a

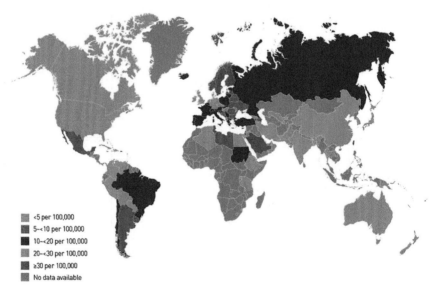

Fig. 1. Age-sex standardized incidence rates (per 100,000 population per annum) of T1D in children and adolescents aged 0 to 14 years. Estimates are directly standardized where possible, with countries shaded according to their rate. (*From* Patterson CC, Karuranga S, Salpea P, et al. Worldwide estimates of incidence, prevalence and mortality of type 1 diabetes in children and adolescents: Results from the International Diabetes Federation Diabetes Atlas. *Diabetes research and clinical practice.* 2019;157:107842; with permission.)

temporal increase since 1990, particularly among younger age ranges (ie, 0–4 years).[28] In particular, data are sparse from African and South East Asian countries; the need for enhanced epidemiologic surveys and research in these and other LMIC has been emphasized.[19,28]

By way of prevalence, there are an estimated 600,900 children under 15 years and 1,110,1000 youth under 20 years living with T1D worldwide.[19] More than one-quarter of the prevalent cases occur in Europe, followed by 20% on the North American continent.[19] In most Western countries, T1D accounts for more than 90% of childhood and adolescent diabetes, whereas across the lifespan, T1D accounts for 5% to 10% of individuals with diabetes.[3] The International Diabetes Federation offers an interactive resource that displays T1D estimates in children and adolescents and offers data for download, including incidence and prevalence estimates from countries worldwide.[24,29] Within the United States, the prevalence of T1D was shown to be highest among White youth and lowest in American Indian youth, with prevalence rates of 2.55 per 1000 (95% confidence interval, 2.48–2.62) versus 0.35 per 1000 (95% confidence interval, 0.26–0.47), respectively.[30]

Looking ahead, the EURODIAB study projected that between 2005 and 2020, the number of new cases with T1D in European children aged less than 5 years will double, and the prevalence in those aged 14 years old or less will increase by 70%.[21] In the United States alone, projections based on SEARCH data suggest that number of youth with T1D age younger than 20 years may increase by 23% by 2050, even if the incidence of T1D remains stable, with even greater increases is incidence continues to increase.[31] As noted elsewhere in this article, one challenge to estimating global incidence and prevalence rates is that nationwide, population-based prospective registries are typically only conducted in well-resourced countries, limiting representation from lower resources settings.[19]

Type 2 Diabetes

Compared with childhood T1D, population-based epidemiologic data are more limited[3]; therefore, the burden of T2D in youth is more difficult to estimate. Estimations are further challenged by the relative rarity and the limited standard clinical and epidemiologic definitions.[20] Despite this circumstance, evidence from the past 20 years strongly suggests that T2D is becoming more common,[32] particularly in high-risk indigenous populations.[33,34]

Epidemiologic estimates of the incidence of T2D in children and adolescents have ranged from 1 to 51 in 1000.[4] Increasing incidence rates for T2D in pediatric patients have been reported in the United States, Canada, Japan, Austria, the UK, and Germany.[35–37] In the United States, the SEARCH study, one of the few population-based studies of childhood T2D that exist, estimated that the annual number of newly diagnosed youth with T2D is approximately 3700.[38] Other studies estimate that T2D may now account for 20% to 50% of new-onset diabetes cases in specific pediatric populations within the United States.[39,40]

Although the worldwide incidence of T2D in children and adolescents vary substantially among countries, age categories, and ethnic groups,[41] the incidence seems to be consistently highest among youth of non-White origin and other indigenous populations.[5,42] Within the United States, the SEARCH study has provided comprehensive estimates of incidence of pediatric T2D in all major racial ethnic groups, showing that in 2002 to 2005, the rates of T2D (per 100,000 per year) were the highest among American Indian youth (20.5 and 35.3 for ages 10–14 and 15–19 years, respectively), followed by African American (20.8 and 17.0 respectively), Asian and Pacific Islanders (11.6 and 12.6), and Hispanic youth (11.2 and 12.0), and were low (3.3 and 4.1) among non-Hispanic Whites.[38] Of note, the highest incidence rates of (screen-detected) T2D in youth were reported by the Pima Indian study: 330 per 100,000 per year.[43] Data from LMIC are extremely limited, particularly with regard to African, South American, and Asian countries.[41]

Fig. 2 summarizes global prevalence estimates of T2D in youth. Overall, the prevalence patterns mirror the incidence patterns, where T2D seems to affect disproportionately minority racial/ethnic groups, especially African Americans, South and East Asians, Pacific Island Natives, and American Indians/First Nation peoples.[44–49] In the United States, SEARCH estimated that 19,147 children/youth had T2D in 2009, with the highest prevalence among American Indian and African American youth.[50] Gaps in prevalence data to represent LMIC mirror those for the incidence data, where estimates from these countries remain limited to date.[41]

SEARCH data projects that by 2050, even at current incidence rates, the number of youth with T2D may increase by almost 50%, whereas if the incidence of T2D increases, there may be more than a 4-fold increase in the number of youth with T2D.[31] Worldwide, with increasing levels of obesity and physical inactivity among children and adolescents in many countries, T2D in childhood and adolescence has the potential to become a global public health issue.[24]

ETIOLOGY AND RISK FACTORS
Type 1 Diabetes

It is accepted that the etiology of T1D is multifactorial; however, the specific roles for the immune system, genetic susceptibility, and environmental factors in the pathogenic processes underlying T1D remain unclear. Diabetes-associated autoantibodies, which are serologic markers of β-cell autoimmunity, include GAD, IA2, insulin autoantibodies, and ZnT8.[51] Genetic susceptibility plays a large role in T1D with the HLA genotypes (DR and DQ genes) explaining approximately 40% to 50% of T1D risk.[52] The remaining genetic risk for T1D can be attributed to the other non-HLA genes or loci that are involved in, or contribute to, immune regulation in the pancreatic β-cells.[53,54] However, studies exploring potential temporal changes in the frequency and/or

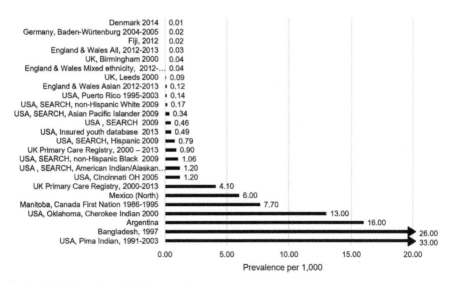

Fig. 2. Global burden of T2D in youth.

distribution of HLA genotypes associated with T1D susceptibility found a decreasing frequency of high-risk HLA genotypes over time in individuals diagnosed with T1D,[55–58] which may suggest an increasing role for environmental factors in the etiology.[7]

Several environmental factors have been implicated in the disease etiology and are thought to operate through a variety of mechanisms, including triggering an autoimmune response, overloading the β-cells and promoting apoptosis, or, as proposed more recently, through alterations in the intestinal microbiome (**Table 2**). Although the exact environmental triggers (infective, nutritional, and/or chemical) that initiate pancreatic β-cell destruction remain largely unknown, the process usually begins months to years before the manifestation of clinical symptoms.[59–61] Notably, the hygiene hypothesis proposes that the decreasing early life exposure to infectious agents in Westernized societies has led to an impairment in the maturation of the immune system, thus permitting an increased occurrence of immune-mediated disorders, including T1D.[62] The accelerator[63] and the overload hypotheses[64] both propose that environmental risk factors prevalent in contemporary societies may accelerate the onset of T1D to affect younger children by increasing the demand for insulin production and thus overloading the β-cells. Novel insights may soon be available from longitudinal, collaborative efforts such as The Environmental Determinants of Diabetes in the Young (TEDDY) study, that follow children at risk for T1D from birth onwards.[65]

Type 2 Diabetes

The etiology of T2D includes contribution by genetic and physiologic components, lifestyle factors such as excess energy intake, insufficient physical activity, and increased sedentary behavior[4]; the resulting pathogenesis of T2D is variable between individuals.[66] The current view is that peripheral insulin resistance is a key feature that occurs early in the disease course, and initially is compensated by increased insulin secretion reflected in hyperinsulinemia.[66] Sustained hyperglycemia over time results in β-cell exhaustion and declining insulin secretion and glucose toxicity. However, T2D is a heterogeneous disease, as recently reported by studies of adult-onset diabetes from Scandinavia, where distinct pathophysiologic subgroups were identified by cluster analysis,[67] including one characterized by obesity, severe hyperinsulinemia, and insulin resistance and another by severe insulin deficiency. Similar research in youth-onset T2D is, at best, limited, but urgently needed, to build foundational knowledge regarding the sequence of metabolic abnormalities leading to obesity, dysglycemia and T2D, which is the necessary first step for the development of efficient, targeted and precise prevention and treatment approaches.

Although many studies show a strong family history among affected youth, with 45% to 80% having at least 1 parent with diabetes and 74% to 100% having a first- or second-degree relative with T2D,[33] there are very limited data on genes associated with early-onset T2D.[68] However, family history does not always imply a genetic cause, because factors such as similar environmental influences within families and the effects of the intrauterine environment on the offspring also demand consideration, as described in **Table 2**.

MANAGEMENT OF DIABETES IN YOUTH

There are comprehensive pediatric- and adolescent-specific guidelines for care.[17] As in adults, the management of both T1D and T2D is centered around keeping blood glucose levels in near-normal ranges to delay or prevent the development of cardiovascular disease risk factors and diabetes-related complications.[17] Medical standards

Table 2
Risk factors and key evidence for the development of T1D and T2D in youth; information

Diabetes Type	Risk Factor	Summary of Evidence
T1D	Genetics	Genetic susceptibility is determined by multiple genes. HLA genotype confers approximately 30%–50% of risk. The remaining genetic risk for T1D can be attributed to the other non-HLA genes or loci identified that contribute model to small effects on disease risk.
	Viral infections, childhood immunizations, ad early life immune exposure to infectious agents	Viral infections may trigger autoimmunity and accelerate the autoimmune destruction of β-cells in genetically susceptible individuals, including enterovirus infection during pregnancy, infancy, childhood, and adulthood, although prospective data remains mixed. Data for other viruses are limited. Large population-based studies have found no associations between childhood immunizations and the development of T1D.
	Early life diet	Breastfeeding and early exposure to cows' milk have been extensively studied, suggesting both a protective effect of breastfeeding, as well as little or no association. Positive associations between early exposure to solid foods, such as cereals or gluten-containing foods, and risk of T1D have been reported. Overfeeding early in life might lead to accelerated weight gain, resulting in β-cell overload and failure.
	Early life growth	US and European cohort studies have shown that children who later developed T1D have faster growth trajectories or weight gain in the first years of life. Some studies have demonstrated an inverse association between age at T1D diagnosis and childhood body mass index.

T2D		
	Genetics	There is often strong family history among affected youth, specific genetic factors have yet to be deterministically identified.
	Obesity, diet, and physical activity	As in adults,[120-124] the recent increase in T2D in youth is believed to have paralleled the increasing prevalence of overweight worldwide. Obesity is linked to increased fast food or consumption of high sugar/high-fat diets, with concurrent decrease in physical activity levels.
	Socioeconomic status	As in adults, youth with T2D are more likely to be from lower socioeconomic backgrounds, which may reflect higher prevalence of obesity.
	Early life factors	There is a U- or J-shaped relationship between birth weight and adult obesity and metabolic disease, demonstrating that both a nutritionally limited or excessive in utero environment can lead to postnatal obesity and T2D later in life. Exposure to maternal diabetes in utero is a significant risk factor for obesity, impaired glucose tolerance and T2D in youth. However, breastfeeding seems to be protective against later development obesity and T2D.
	Endocrine disrupting chemicals	There is moderate evidence for a relationship between exposure to dichlorodiphenyldichloroethylene (p,p′-DDE) and diabetes development.[125] Data from humans on other EDCs, such as bisphenol A, phthalates and perfluorinated chemicals, are limited, as are studies among youth specifically.

Adapted from Dabelea D, Hamman RF, Knowler WC. Chapter 15: Diabetes in Youth. In: Cowie CC, Casagrande SS, Menke A et al., eds. Diabetes in America. 3rd ed. Bethesda (MD): National Institute of Diabetes and Digestive and Kidney Diseases (US); 2018; with permission.

of care also emphasize individualized care considering patient factors and preferences in the selection of clinical goals and approaches, with special attention to integrating culturally sensitive and developmentally appropriate self-management education and tools.[17] It is recommended that a new diagnosis of diabetes in youth prompt screening for comorbidities, including celiac disease and thyroid disease among youth with T1D and cardiovascular disease risk factors or components of metabolic syndrome among youth with T2D.[17] Youth should also undergo screening for subclinical or early complications of diabetes,[17,69] with prompt intervention upon positive findings,[70] including psychosocial well-being.[17,71]

In this age range, diabetes care providers must work closely with youth and their families to foster supportive home and school[72] environments for self-management.[17] Additionally, toward the end of adolescence, pediatric care providers should work with adult care providers to facilitate the transition from pediatric to adult care, which typically occurs in early adulthood and represents a critical period for other major life transitions and shifting responsibilities of diabetes care.[17]

Type 1 Diabetes

The T1D self-management regime includes monitoring blood glucose, dosing insulin, measuring and regulating carbohydrates, and responding to episodes of hypoglycemia with appropriate intake of rapid-acting carbohydrate.[73] Blood glucose monitoring can be accomplished with frequent blood glucose checks or the use of newly developed continuous glucose monitoring (CGM) systems,[74] which have shown considerable uptake in recent years, particularly in pediatric populations.[75] In a departure from previous years, the updated 2021 American Diabetes Association Standards of Care now recommend that CGM systems be considered for all children and adolescents with T1D given the evidence for an association between CGM system use, adherence, and clinical outcomes.[76]

For insulin replacement, care guidelines recommend intensive insulin therapy that consists of multiple-dose insulin injections (3–4 injections/d of basal and prandial insulin) or insulin pump therapy.[17,77] In recent years, a number of novel diabetes devices and technologies have emerged,[78] including sensor-augmented pump therapy ranging from low-glucose suspend, to predictive low-glucose suspend, to hybrid closed loop systems.[79] These technologies have shown benefit in pediatric and adolescent populations with regard to improved glycemic control with decreased hypogycemia.[80–84] It is likely that these technological advances in the diabetes treatment landscape, and particularly the fully automated insulin delivery systems, will transform day-to-day diabetes management in the coming years by decreasing the burden of glucose monitoring and insulin dosing.

Optimal nutrition and monitoring of carbohydrate intake is an important component of the recommended treatment plan for youth with diabetes,[17,74] although the literature on specific diets for T1D, including low and very low carbohydrate diets, is mixed and lacking in rigorous, randomized studies. It is also recommended that youth and adolescents with T1D engage in regular physical activity after receiving appropriate education on blood glucose management strategies to avoid exercise-related glucose disturbances.[17,85] Finally, noninsulin adjuvants have recently been evaluated in combination with insulin to improve glycemic control in the setting of T1D, including amylin analogues, metformin, sodium glucose cotransporter-2 inhibitors, and glucagon-like peptide-1 receptor agonists.[86]

Specific to the management of pediatric T1D versus the majority of adult cases is the careful individualization of hemoglobin A1c (HbA1c) targets to avoid hypoglycemia, which may be more common in this age range owing to erratic patterns in exercise and food intake. In general, an HbA1c goal of less than 7% is appropriate for many children, but less stringent targets (ie, HbA1c of <7.5%) are appropriate for those with frequent hypoglycemia, hypoglycemia unawareness, or the inability to access or use blood glucose monitoring technology regularly. In general, lower targets may be appropriate for youth if they do not lead to more frequent hypoglycemia or during the honeymoon period shortly after diagnosis.[17]

Given the increasing burden of childhood diabetes in LMIC, recent clinical practice guidelines have provided additional references for diabetes care in low-resource settings. There are unique challenges to diabetes management in these settings, including high out-of-pocket expenses, which may be cost prohibitive, a limited availability of insulin and other diabetes supplies, suboptimal home management equipment, food scarcity, social deprivation, and discrimination or stigma.[87] International programs such as Life for a Child, Changing Diabetes in Children, and Insulin for Life have focused on providing critical resources for diabetes management to youth with T1D in LMIC. Other efforts have developed a framework for T1D management, including insulin therapy, blood glucose monitoring, HbA1c testing, screening for complications, diabetes education, and multidisciplinary team care according to the tiers of resources that are available.[88]

Type 2 Diabetes

As with T1D, comprehensive diabetes self-management education and support are central to providing clinical care among new-onset T2D in childhood, as well as in longstanding disease.[17] Long-term weight management is also central to the management of pediatric T2D, which can be achieved through healthy diet and regular physical activity, which comprise first-line approaches in this pouation.[17,89] As in youth without diabetes, best practices for weight management emphasize the selection of weight-oriented strategies that are tailored to the individual child and family, including dietary goals, physical activity, the home environment, and other self-management behaviors.[90] Compared with T1D, where all youth must initiate insulin replacement therapy as soon as possible after diagnosis, pharmacologic management of T2D varies according to clinical features and includes metformin, liraglutide, and insulin treatment.[17,89,91] Care providers should refer to the algorithm depicted in the most recent American Diabetes Association consensus guidelines for an approach to new-onset diabetes in youth with overweight and obesity.[17] Evidence for best pharmacologic practices remains limited and has focused on metformin. Metabolic surgery is indicated for the treatment of T2D in adolescents with a body mass index of greater than 35 kg/m^2, uncontrolled glycemia, and/or significant comorbidities after treatment with other lifestyle and pharmacologic interventions.[17] Limited evidence suggests benefits associated with bariatric surgery,[92] but more randomized control trials are needed, particularly among adolescents and young adults with T2D.[17] In addition, there may be a role for technological advances such as CGM systems, insulin pumps, and automated insulin delivery systems, particularly among advanced T2D requiring aggressive glycemic control; the need for these treatment modalities will likely vary case by case.

OUTCOMES AND COMPLICATIONS OF DIABETES
Glycemic Control

Youth with diabetes show variable degrees of suboptimal glycemic control as measured by HbA1c, which can vary considerably after onset of disease through puberty and into early adulthood. In the US-based SEARCH study, 17% of youth with T1D had an

HbA1c of 9.5% or greater, as did 27% of youth with T2D.[93] Poor glycemic control was associated with increasing age, as well as a longer duration of for both diabetes types.[93] Over the course of development, data from youth with T1D demonstrate elevated HbA1c levels that peak to greater than 9.0% in 17-year-olds and remain elevated at greater than 8.0% until a mean age of 30 years.[94] Poorer glycemic control during early adulthood or from childhood to young adulthood has been attributed to a lack of continuity in diabetes-related clinical care as well as changes in self-care as children and adolescents with T1D grow into adulthood. Longitudinal data from pediatric T2D are limited.[95–97] Unfortunately, there is a substantial body of evidence of health inequity that affects glycemic control outcomes, including significant race-based disparities.[93,98] A number of sociodemographic risk factors, including lower socioeconomic status, lower parental educational attainment, less parental involvement in diabetes management, and impaired family dynamics, have also been identified.

Although some evidence suggests that glycemic control may be improving over the past 1 to 3 decades in the United States, Europe, and Australia,[99–101] other studies have shown no change across 19 countries[102] and even increases in mean HbA1c in the most recent US-based clinical T1D Exchange Registry.[103] Altogether, these data suggest that HbA1c remains unacceptably high among youth, which increases the risk for complications as they age into adulthood, as discussed elsewhere in this article.

In general, clinical outcomes are known to be consistently worse in LMIC, particularly where essential resources and diabetes supplies may be limited.[88,104,105] These differences are most starkly represented by higher mortality rates compared with well-resourced countries,[106] but data also suggest poorer glycemic control and more frequent complications.[19,88,107]

Complications

Sustained hyperglycemia in diabetes is linked to the development of chronic complications of the disease, which represent the major source of morbidity and mortality. The benefits of intensive insulin therapy for the prevention of long-term microvascular and microvascular complications of T1D were demonstrated by the Diabetes Control and Complications Trial (DCCT),[108,109] with persistent benefit more than 30 years later.[110,111] In youth and adolescents, multiple studies have corroborated that the risk for these outcomes is associated with glycemic control.[20]

Data on both acute and chronic complications among youth with T1D and have been reviewed comprehensively and discussed extensively elsewhere,[20] including microvascular complications (ie, diabetic retinopathy, nephropathy, peripheral neuropathy, and cardiac autonomic neuropathy) and cardiovascular disease risk factors or markers of subclinical cardiovascular disease (ie, hypertension, dyslipidemia, obesity and insulin resistance, arterial stiffness, carotid intima medial thickness, and coronary artery calcification). In short, diabetes diagnosed in childhood and adolescence remains a leading cause of nephropathy, retinopathy, neuropathy, and coronary and peripheral vascular disease later in life; it is now recognized that these complications emerge early in disease duration[111] and often co-occur.[112,113] **Fig. 3** shows a subset of major diabetes complications in US youth and adolescents by diabetes type.

In children and adolescents with T1D, acute complications such as diabetic ketoacidosis and hypoglycemia are more common than chronic complications and carry a greater risk of morbidity and mortality, particularly severe hypoglycemia.[114] More recently, early and subclinical cardiovascular disease has emerged as a major clinical concern as the prevalence of overweight and obesity grows within this patient population.[115] Although less common than in T1D, youth with T2D can also present in diabetic ketoacidosis, with reported frequencies from 8% to 29%.[20] Youth with T2D

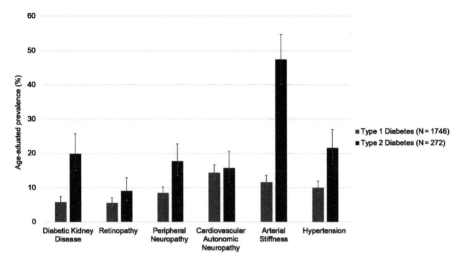

Fig. 3. Age-adjusted prevalence of complications in youth-onset diabetes by type. (*Data from* Dabelea D, Stafford JM, Mayer-Davis EJ, et al. Association of type 1 diabetes vs type 2 diabetes diagnosed during childhood and adolescence with complications during teenage years and young adulthood. *Jama.* 2017;317(8):825-835.)

seem to have a consistently and significantly greater prevalence of comorbidities than their peers with T1D (see **Fig. 3**).[111] As noted elsewhere in this article, the prevalence of complications seems to be higher among youth in LMIC owing to suboptimal glycemic control resulting from inadequate or unstable resources for diabetes management.[88] Finally, emerging data from the coronavirus disease 2019 pandemic suggest that infection with severe acute respiratory syndrome coronavirus 2 may be associated with an increase in diabetic ketoacidosis in both adult and pediatric populations,[116–118] although more studies are needed to untangle to mechanistic framework for this association.

Mortality

Mortality rates are approximately 2 to 5 times higher for youth with T1D compared with the general population, secondary to acute complications[114]; these data have been reviewed and discussed elsewher.[20] Mortality rates seem to be higher for females than males and for non-White versus White youth, although the overall rates may be improving over time.[20] An analysis by World Bank income groups from the IDF Diabetes Atlas showed that although the majority of T1D cases occur in the high-income and upper-middle-income countries, the majority of deaths are in the low-income and lower-middle-income countries.[19] Data on mortality among youth with T2D are comparatively quite limited but seem to be similarly inflated 2 to 3 times higher than the general population and related to the duration of disease.[20]

CHALLENGES AND OPPORTUNITIES

There exist opportunities to better characterize diabetes in youth and transform knowledge to evidence-based interventions to prevent and diagnose the disease earlier or improve management and outcomes to prevent complications. First, more robust data are needed on the epidemiology of T1D and T2D in youth across the globe, particularly in lower resource settings. The initiation of sustainable surveillance systems for pediatric diabetes will be maximally informative if they are designed as population-based rather than clinic-based efforts and incorporate tools to differentiate childhood T1D from T2D. By way of etiology and risk factors, data from novel, large-scale prospective efforts such as the TEDDY Study are expected to yield insights into whether or how recent changes in exposures to such risk factors may be responsible for the steady increase in T1D worldwide.[65] Longitudinal prebirth cohort studies may yield insights into T2D in particular.[20] Finally, an increasing amount of genetic data may also help to elucidate high-risk markers to identity at-risk youth for both types of diabetes screening. As the field continues to inform on the role of environmental exposures, their biologic signatures and pathways, the causal associations or mechanisms that are identified may represent robust targets for novel interventions to prevent or delay the onset of childhood diabetes.

In the meantime, new treatment options, including diabetes devices for T1D and noninsulin pharmacologic options for T2D, are currently under study among youth and adolescents and offer the potential to decrease the incidence and prevalence of complications. It is critical that changes to treatment based on these new data are made accessible and equitable to youth around the world, including those in low-resource or underserved locations.

Changes in epidemiology underscore that, as there are more youth are diagnosed with T1D or T2D, particularly early in life, these populations will have a longer duration of exposure to an altered metabolic milieu, increasing the risk of acute complications, chronic microvascular and macrovascular complications, and other comorbidities. In particular, the development of higher levels of cardiovascular risk factors and preclinical cardiovascular disease among youth with diabetes and the potential future impact on morbidity and mortality pose special challenges.

Contemporary large-scale translational and epidemiologic studies in youth with diabetes to understand these outcomes are lacking, primarily owing to the lack of common standardized protocols and validated surrogate end points that can be compared across studies. Future studies are needed urgently, in addition to the development and validation of the effects of prevention programs on the development and burden of complications and mortality.

There exist significant health disparities in pediatric diabetes, made apparent from global mortality differences in lower-middle-income countries versus upper-middle-income countries, as well as racial/ethnic differences within the specific countries. Interventions to address disparities will be central to improving outcomes among children and adolescents with diabetes within specific geographic populations and across the globe, requiring collaboration from multiple clinical and community stakeholders to be effective.

Finally, from a global health care system perspective, the increasing prevalence of diabetes in youth, coupled with the need for high-quality disease management may place a large demand on health care costs.[8,119] Although increasing understanding of the multifactorial etiology of childhood diabetes and its complications will hopefully translate into improved strategies for care or prevention of these disease, the future impact of childhood diabetes should not be underestimated; for this reason, the conduction and translation of high-quality research in this field should be prioritized to meet and address the clinical and public health challenges related to the growing population of youth with diabetes.

SUMMARY

- The incidence and prevalence of T1D and T2D are increasing worldwide, along with a significant burden of complications, which seem to emerge earlier than previously believed. More population-based, prospective cohorts are needed to accurately characterize incidence, prevalence and trends in pediatric diabetes burden, short- and long-term morbidity and mortality across the world.

- New data may yield insights into etiologic risk factors for both T1D and T2D; both diseases are multifactorial with contribution from genetics as well as environmental or lifestyle factors.
- New treatment modalities are emerging, particularly for T1D, which may aid in glycemic management and decrease risk for acute and chronic complications of diabetes.

CLINICS CARE POINTS

- Diabetes in youth necessitates early and aggressive intervention to prevent morbidity and mortality associated with both acute and chronic complications. Research is underway to identify and offer approaches to intervene on risk factors for the disease and complications.

- The clinical care of diabetes must be tailored to an individual child or adolescent, including goals and modalities of treatment, such that it is sustainable, developmentally appropriate, and culturally sensitive. Ensuring that individuals have access to vital diabetes supplies is essentially, particularly in low resource settings common in LMIC.

- Care must also be considered in the context of where the child spends time (ie, home, school), integrate other individuals who will share diabetes responsibility or have influence on key behavioral aspects of management, and anticipate the transition from pediatric to adult care providers in early adulthood.

DISCLOSURE

A.R. Kahkoska is supported by the National Institute of Diabetes and Digestive and Kidney Diseases of the National Institutes of Health under Award Number F30DK113728. The content is solely the responsibility of the authors and does not necessarily represent the official views of the National Institutes of Health. A.R. Kahkoska has received financial support from Novo Nordisk for travel to present data in 2019.

REFERENCES

1. Association AD. Report of the expert committee on the diagnosis and classification of diabetes mellitus. Diabetes Care 1997;20(7):1183–97.
2. Association AD. 2. Classification and diagnosis of diabetes: standards of medical care in diabetes-2020. Diabetes Care 2020;43(Suppl 1):S14.
3. Mayer-Davis EJ, Kahkoska AR, Jefferies C, et al. ISPAD Clinical Practice Consensus Guidelines 2018: definition, epidemiology, and classification of diabetes in children and adolescents. Pediatr Diabetes 2018;19:7–19.
4. Pulgaron ER, Delamater AM. Obesity and type 2 diabetes in children: epidemiology and treatment. Curr Diabetes Rep 2014;14(8):508.
5. Mayer-Davis EJ, Lawrence JM, Dabelea D, et al. Incidence trends of type 1 and type 2 diabetes among youths, 2002–2012. N Engl J Med 2017;376(15):1419–29.
6. Hattersley AT, Greeley SA, Polak M, et al. ISPAD Clinical Practice Consensus Guidelines 2018: the diagnosis and management of monogenic diabetes in children and adolescents. Pediatr Diabetes 2018;19(Suppl 27):47–63.

7. Insel RA, Dunne JL, Atkinson MA, et al. Staging presymptomatic type 1 diabetes: a scientific statement of JDRF, the Endocrine Society, and the American Diabetes Association. Diabetes care 2015;38(10):1964–74.

8. Association AD. Diagnosis and Classification of Diabetes Mellitus. Diabetes Care 2013;36(Supplement 1):S67–74.

9. Barker JM, Barriga KJ, Yu L, et al. Prediction of autoantibody positivity and progression to type 1 diabetes: Diabetes Autoimmunity Study in the Young (DAISY). J Clin Endocrinol Metab 2004;89(8):3896–902.

10. Wasserfall CH, Atkinson MA. Autoantibody markers for the diagnosis and prediction of type 1 diabetes. Autoimmun Rev 2006;5(6):424–8.

11. Yu L, Boulware DC, Beam CA, et al. Zinc transporter-8 autoantibodies improve prediction of type 1 diabetes in relatives positive for the standard biochemical autoantibodies. Diabetes Care 2012;35(6):1213–8.

12. Pihoker C, Gilliam LK, Hampe CS, et al. Autoantibodies in Diabetes. Diabetes 2005;54(suppl_2):S52–61.

13. Graham J, Hagopian WA, Kockum I, et al. Genetic effects on age-dependent onset and islet cell autoantibody markers in type 1 diabetes. Diabetes 2002;51(5):1346–55.

14. Vermeulen I, Weets I, Asanghanwa M, et al. Contribution of antibodies against IA-2 and zinc transporter 8 to classification of diabetes diagnosed under 40 years of age. Diabetes Care 2011;34(8):1760–5.

15. Nolan CJ, Prentki M. Insulin resistance and insulin hypersecretion in the metabolic syndrome and type 2 diabetes: time for a conceptual framework shift. Diabetes and Vascular Disease Research 2019;16(2):118–27.

16. Malone JI, Hansen BC. Does obesity cause type 2 diabetes mellitus (T2DM)? Or is it the opposite? Pediatric diabetes 2019;20(1):5–9.

17. Association AD. 13. Children and adolescents: standards of medical care in diabetes– 2020. Diabetes Care 2020;43(Supplement 1):S163–82.

18. Narasimhan S, Weinstock RS. Youth-onset type 2 diabetes mellitus: lessons learned from the TODAY study. Mayo Clin Proc 2014;89(6):806-16.

19. Patterson CC, Karuranga S, Salpea P, et al. Worldwide estimates of incidence, prevalence and mortality of type 1 diabetes in children and adolescents: results from the International Diabetes Federation Diabetes Atlas. Diabetes Res Clin Pract 2019;157:107842.

20. Dabelea D, Hamman RF, Knowler WC. Diabetes in Youth. In: Cowie CC, Casagrande SS, Menke A, et al, editors. Diabetes in America. 3rd edition. Bethesda (MD): National Institute of Diabetes and Digestive and Kidney Diseases (US); 2018.

21. Patterson CC, Dahlquist GG, Gyurus E, et al. Incidence trends for childhood type 1 diabetes in Europe during 1989-2003 and predicted new cases 2005-20: a multicentre prospective registration study. Lancet 2009;373(9680):2027–33.

22. Gyurus EK, Patterson C, Soltesz G. Twenty-one years of prospective incidence of childhood type 1 diabetes in Hungary–the rising trend continues (or peaks and highlands?). Pediatr Diabetes 2012;13(1):21–5.

23. Sipetic S, Maksimovic J, Vlajinac H, et al. Rising incidence of type 1 diabetes in Belgrade children aged 0-14 years in the period from 1982 to 2005. J Endocrinol Invest 2013;36(5):307–12.

24. Federation. ID, IDF Diabetes Atlas teB. Available at: https://www.diabetesatlas.org.BAa. Accessed March 18, 2021.

25. Tajima N, Morimoto A. Epidemiology of childhood diabetes mellitus in Japan. Pediatr Endocrinol Rev 2012;10(Suppl 1):44–50.
26. Zhao Z, Sun C, Wang C, et al. Rapidly rising incidence of childhood type 1 diabetes in Chinese population: epidemiology in Shanghai during 1997-2011. Acta Diabetol 2014;51(6):947–53.
27. Lin WH, Wang MC, Wang WM, et al. Incidence of and mortality from Type I diabetes in Taiwan from 1999 through 2010: a nationwide cohort study. PLoS One 2014;9(1):e86172.
28. Adeloye D, Chan KY, Thorley N, et al. Global and regional estimates of the morbidity due to type I diabetes among children aged 0-4 years: a systematic review and analysis. J Glob Health 2018;8(2):021101.
29. Federation ID. Diabetes Data Portal IDF Diabetes Atlas 9th Edition 2019.
30. Dabelea D, Mayer-Davis EJ, Saydah S, et al. Prevalence of type 1 and type 2 diabetes among children and adolescents from 2001 to 2009. JAMA 2014; 311(17):1778–86.
31. Imperatore G, Boyle JP, Thompson TJ, et al. Projections of type 1 and type 2 diabetes burden in the U.S. population aged <20 years through 2050: dynamic modeling of incidence, mortality, and population growth. Diabetes Care 2012; 35(12):2515–20.
32. Zeitler P, Fu J, Tandon N, et al. ISPAD Clinical Practice Consensus Guidelines 2014. Type 2 diabetes in the child and adolescent. Pediatr Diabetes 2014; 15(Suppl 20):26–46.
33. Dabelea D, Pettitt DJ, Jones KL, et al. Type 2 diabetes mellitus in minority children and adolescents. An emerging problem. Endocrinol Metab Clin North Am 1999;28(4):709–29.
34. Kitagawa T, Mano T, Fujita H. The epidemiology of childhood diabetes mellitus in Tokyo metropolitan area. Tohoku J Exp Med 1983;141(Suppl):171–9.
35. Reinehr T. Type 2 diabetes mellitus in children and adolescents. World J Diabetes 2013;4(6):270.
36. Chen L, Magliano DJ, Zimmet PZ. The worldwide epidemiology of type 2 diabetes mellitus—present and future perspectives. Nat Rev Endocrinol 2012; 8(4):228.
37. Cizza G, Brown R, Rothe K. Rising incidence and challenges of childhood diabetes. A mini review. J Endocrinol Invest 2012;35(5):541.
38. Group TWGftSfDiYS. Incidence of Diabetes in Youth in the United States. JAMA 2007;297(24):2716–24.
39. Hannon TS, Rao G, Arslanian SA. Childhood obesity and type 2 diabetes mellitus. Pediatrics 2005;116(2):473–80.
40. Program DiCAWGotNDE. An update on type 2 diabetes in youth from the National Diabetes Education Program. Pediatrics 2004;114(1):259–63.
41. Farsani SF, Van Der Aa M, Van Der Vorst M, et al. Global trends in the incidence and prevalence of type 2 diabetes in children and adolescents: a systematic review and evaluation of methodological approaches. Diabetologia 2013;56(7): 1471–88.
42. Fagot-Campagna A, Pettitt D, Engelgau M, et al. Williamson DF, Narayan KM: type 2 diabetes among North American children and adolescents: an epidemiologic review and a public health perspective. J Pediatr 2000;136:664–72.
43. Pavkov ME, Hanson RL, Knowler WC, et al. Changing patterns of type 2 diabetes incidence among Pima Indians. Diabetes Care 2007;30(7):1758–63.

44. Savage PJ, Bennett PH, Senter RG, et al. High prevalence of diabetes in young Pima Indians: evidence of phenotypic variation in a genetically isolated population. Diabetes 1979;28(10):937–42.

45. Dabelea D, Hanson RL, Bennett PH, et al. Increasing prevalence of Type II diabetes in American Indian children. Diabetologia 1998;41(8):904–10.

46. Dean H. NIDDM-Y in First Nation children in Canada. Clin Pediatr (Phila) 1998; 37(2):89–96.

47. Scott CR, Smith JM, Cradock MM, et al. Characteristics of youth-onset noninsulin-dependent diabetes mellitus and insulin-dependent diabetes mellitus at diagnosis. Pediatrics 1997;100(1):84–91.

48. Neufeld ND, Raffel LJ, Landon C, et al. Early presentation of type 2 diabetes in Mexican-American youth. Diabetes Care 1998;21(1):80–6.

49. Macaluso CJ, Bauer UE, Deeb LC, et al. Type 2 diabetes mellitus among Florida children and adolescents, 1994 through 1998. Public Health Rep 2002;117(4): 373–9.

50. Hamman RF, Pettitt D, Dabelea D, et al. Estimates of the Burden of Diabetes in United States Youth in 2009. Diabetes 2012;61(Suppl 1):A355.

51. Watkins RA, Evans-Molina C, Blum JS, et al. Established and emerging biomarkers for the prediction of type 1 diabetes: a systematic review. Transl Res 2014;164(2):110–21.

52. Pociot F, McDermott MF. Genetics of type 1 diabetes mellitus. Genes Immun 2002;3(5):235–49.

53. Sepe V, Loviselli A, Bottazzo GF. Genetics of type 1A diabetes. N Engl J Med 2009;361(2):211.

54. Barrett JC, Clayton DG, Concannon P, et al. Genome-wide association study and meta-analysis find that over 40 loci affect risk of type 1 diabetes. Nat Genet 2009;41(6):703–7.

55. Gillespie KM, Bain SC, Barnett AH, et al. The rising incidence of childhood type 1 diabetes and reduced contribution of high-risk HLA haplotypes. Lancet 2004; 364(9446):1699–700.

56. Vehik K, Hamman RF, Lezotte D, et al. Trends in high-risk HLA susceptibility genes among Colorado youth with type 1 diabetes. Diabetes Care 2008; 31(7):1392–6.

57. Fourlanos S, Varney MD, Tait BD, et al. The rising incidence of type 1 diabetes is accounted for by cases with lower-risk human leukocyte antigen genotypes. Diabetes Care 2008;31(8):1546–9.

58. Hermann R, Knip M, Veijola R, et al. Temporal changes in the frequencies of HLA genotypes in patients with Type 1 diabetes–indication of an increased environmental pressure? Diabetologia 2003;46(3):420–5.

59. Verge CF, Gianani R, Kawasaki E, et al. Prediction of type I diabetes in first-degree relatives using a combination of insulin, GAD, and ICA512bdc/IA-2 autoantibodies. Diabetes 1996;45(7):926–33.

60. Skyler JS, Krischer JP, Wolfsdorf J, et al. Effects of oral insulin in relatives of patients with type 1 diabetes: The Diabetes Prevention Trial–Type 1. Diabetes Care 2005;28(5):1068–76.

61. Ziegler AG, Rewers M, Simell O, et al. Seroconversion to multiple islet autoantibodies and risk of progression to diabetes in children. JAMA 2013;309(23): 2473–9.

62. Gale EA. A missing link in the hygiene hypothesis? Diabetologia 2002;45(4): 588–94.

63. Wilkin TJ. The accelerator hypothesis: weight gain as the missing link between type I and type II diabetes. Diabetologia 2001;44(7):914–22.
64. Dahlquist G. Can we slow the rising incidence of childhood-onset autoimmune diabetes? The overload hypothesis. Diabetologia 2006;49(1):20–4.
65. Group TS. The Environmental Determinants of Diabetes in the Young (TEDDY) study: study design. Pediatr Diabetes 2007;8(5):286–98.
66. Kahn SE, Cooper ME, Del Prato S. Pathophysiology and treatment of type 2 diabetes: perspectives on the past, present, and future. Lancet 2014;383(9922): 1068–83.
67. Ahlqvist E, Storm P, Käräjämäki A, et al. Novel subgroups of adult-onset diabetes and their association with outcomes: a data-driven cluster analysis of six variables. Lancet Diabetes Endocrinol 2018;6(5):361–9.
68. Dabelea D, Dolan LM, D'Agostino R Jr, et al. Association testing of TCF7L2 polymorphisms with type 2 diabetes in multi-ethnic youth. Diabetologia 2010;54(3): 535–9.
69. Mahmud FH, Elbarbary NS, Fröhlich-Reiterer E, et al. ISPAD Clinical Practice Consensus Guidelines 2018: other complications and associated conditions in children and adolescents with type 1 diabetes. Pediatr Diabetes 2018; 19(Suppl 27):275.
70. Donaghue KC, Marcovecchio ML, Wadwa RP, et al. ISPAD Clinical Practice Consensus Guidelines 2018: microvascular and macrovascular complications in children and adolescents. Pediatr Diabetes 2018;19:262.
71. Delamater AM, de Wit M, McDarby V, et al. ISPAD clinical practice consensus guidelines 2018: psychological care of children and adolescents with type 1 diabetes. Pediatr Diabetes 2018;19:237–49.
72. Goss P, Middlehurst A, Acerini C, et al. ISPAD Position statement on type 1 diabetes in schools. Pediatr Diabetes 2018;19(7):1338–41.
73. Hood KK, Peterson CM, Rohan JM, et al. Association between adherence and glycemic control in pediatric type 1 diabetes: a meta-analysis. Pediatrics 2009; 124(6):e1171–9.
74. Association AD. Professional Practice Committee: standards of medical care in diabetes—2018. Am Diabetes Assoc; 2018.
75. DeSalvo DJ, Miller KM, Hermann JM, et al. Continuous glucose monitoring (CGM) and glycemic control among youth with type 1 diabetes (T1D): international comparison from the T1D Exchange and DPV Initiative. Pediatr Diabetes 2018;19(7):1271–5.
76. 13. Children and Adolescents: Standards of Medical Care in Diabetes—2021. Diabetes Care 2021;44(Supplement 1):S180–99.
77. Danne T, Phillip M, Buckingham BA, et al. ISPAD Clinical Practice Consensus Guidelines 2018: insulin treatment in children and adolescents with diabetes. Pediatr Diabetes 2018;19:115–35.
78. Sherr JL, Tauschmann M, Battelino T, et al. ISPAD Clinical Practice Consensus Guidelines 2018: diabetes technologies. Pediatr Diabetes 2018;19:302–25.
79. Forlenza GP, Messer LH, Maahs DM, et al. Artificial Pancreas in Pediatrics. In: Sánchez-Peña RS, Cherňavvsky DR, editors. The Artificial Pancreas: Current Situation and Future Directions. Cambridge: Elsevier; 2019. p. 237-59.
80. Haidar A, Legault L, Matteau-Pelletier L, et al. Outpatient overnight glucose control with dual-hormone artificial pancreas, single-hormone artificial pancreas, or conventional insulin pump therapy in children and adolescents with type 1 diabetes: an open-label, randomised controlled trial. Lancet Diabetes Endocrinol 2015;3(8):595–604.

81. Russell SJ, Hillard MA, Balliro C, et al. Day and night glycaemic control with a bionic pancreas versus conventional insulin pump therapy in preadolescent children with type 1 diabetes: a randomised crossover trial. Lancet Diabetes Endocrinol 2016;4(3):233–43.

82. El-Khatib FH, Balliro C, Hillard MA, et al. Home use of a bihormonal bionic pancreas versus insulin pump therapy in adults with type 1 diabetes: a multicentre randomised crossover trial. Lancet 2017;389(10067):369–80.

83. Forlenza GP, Pinhas-Hamiel O, Liljenquist DR, et al. Safety evaluation of the MiniMed 670G system in children 7–13 years of age with type 1 diabetes. Diabetes Technol Ther 2019;21(1):11–9.

84. Breton MD, Kanapka LG, Beck RW, et al. A Randomized Trial of Closed-Loop Control in Children with Type 1 Diabetes. N Engl J Med 2020;383(9):836–45.

85. Adolfsson P, Riddell MC, Taplin CE, et al. ISPAD Clinical Practice Consensus Guidelines 2018: exercise in children and adolescents with diabetes. Pediatr Diabetes 2018;19:205–26.

86. Harris K, Boland C, Meade L, et al. Adjunctive therapy for glucose control in patients with type 1 diabetes. Diabetes Metab Syndr Obes Targets Ther 2018; 11:159.

87. Codner E, Acerini CL, Craig ME, et al. ISPAD clinical practice consensus guidelines 2018: limited care guidance appendix. Pediatr Diabetes 2018;19:328–38.

88. Ogle GD, von Oettingen JE, Middlehurst AC, et al. Levels of type 1 diabetes care in children and adolescents for countries at varying resource levels. Pediatr Diabetes 2019;20(1):93–8.

89. Zeitler P, Arslanian S, Fu J, et al. ISPAD clinical practice consensus guidelines 2018: type 2 diabetes mellitus in youth. Pediatr Diabetes 2018;19:28–46.

90. Spear BA, Barlow SE, Ervin C, et al. Recommendations for treatment of child and adolescent overweight and obesity. Pediatrics 2007;120(Supplement 4): S254–88.

91. Arslanian S, Bacha F, Grey M, et al. Evaluation and management of youth-onset type 2 diabetes: a position statement by the American Diabetes Association. Diabetes Care 2018;41(12):2648–68.

92. Inge TH, Courcoulas AP, Jenkins TM, et al. Weight loss and health status 3 years after bariatric surgery in adolescents. N Engl J Med 2016;374(2):113–23.

93. Petitti DB, Klingensmith GJ, Bell RA, et al. Glycemic control in youth with diabetes: the SEARCH for diabetes in Youth Study. J Pediatr 2009;155(5):668–72.

94. Miller KM, Foster NC, Beck RW, et al. Current state of type 1 diabetes treatment in the U.S.: updated data from the T1D Exchange clinic registry. Diabetes Care 2015;38(6):971–8.

95. Moore SM, Hackworth NJ, Hamilton VE, et al. Adolescents with type 1 diabetes: parental perceptions of child health and family functioning and their relationship to adolescent metabolic control. Health Qual Life Outcomes 2013;11:50.

96. Lawrence JM, Standiford DA, Loots B, et al. Prevalence and correlates of depressed mood among youth with diabetes: the SEARCH for Diabetes in Youth study. Pediatrics 2006;117(4):1348–58.

97. Pyatak EA, Sequeira P, Peters AL, et al. Disclosure of psychosocial stressors affecting diabetes care among uninsured young adults with Type 1 diabetes. Diabet Med 2013;30(9):1140–4.

98. Kahkoska AR, Shay CM, Crandell J, et al. Association of race and ethnicity with glycemic control and hemoglobin A1c levels in youth with type 1 diabetes. JAMA Netw open 2018;1(5):e181851.

99. Svoren BM, Volkening LK, Butler DA, et al. Temporal trends in the treatment of pediatric type 1 diabetes and impact on acute outcomes. J Pediatr 2007; 150(3):279–85.

100. Rosenbauer J, Dost A, Karges B, et al. Improved metabolic control in children and adolescents with type 1 diabetes: a trend analysis using prospective multi-center data from Germany and Austria. Diabetes Care 2012;35(1):80–6.

101. Bulsara MK, Holman CD, Davis EA, et al. The impact of a decade of changing treatment on rates of severe hypoglycemia in a population-based cohort of children with type 1 diabetes. Diabetes Care 2004;27(10):2293–8.

102. de Beaufort CE, Swift PG, Skinner CT, et al. Continuing stability of center differences in pediatric diabetes care: do advances in diabetes treatment improve outcome? The Hvidoere Study Group on Childhood Diabetes. Diabetes Care 2007;30(9):2245–50.

103. Foster NC, Beck RW, Miller KM, et al. State of type 1 diabetes management and outcomes from the T1D Exchange in 2016–2018. Diabetes Technol Ther 2019; 21(2):66–72.

104. Ogle G, Kim H, Middlehurst A, et al. Financial costs for families of children with type 1 diabetes in lower-income countries. Diabet Med 2016;33(6):820–6.

105. Sidibé A, Traore H, Liman-Ali I, et al. Le diabète juvénile au Mali. Rev Française Endocrinol Clin Nutr Métabol 1999;40(6):513–21.

106. Duarte Gómez E, Gregory GA, Castrati Nostas M, et al. Incidence and mortality rates and clinical characteristics of type 1 diabetes among children and young adults in Cochabamba, Bolivia. J Diabetes Res 2017;2017:8454757.

107. Pacaud D, Lemay JF, Richmond E, et al. Contribution of SWEET to improve paediatric diabetes care in developing countries. Pediatr Diabetes 2016;17:46–52.

108. The effect of intensive treatment of diabetes on the development and progression of long-term complications in insulin-dependent diabetes mellitus. The Diabetes Control and Complications Trial Research Group. N Engl J Med 1993; 329(14):977–86.

109. Nathan DM, Cleary PA, Backlund JY, et al. Intensive diabetes treatment and cardiovascular disease in patients with type 1 diabetes. N Engl J Med 2005; 353(25):2643–53.

110. Orchard TJ, Nathan DM, Zinman B, et al. Association between 7 years of intensive treatment of type 1 diabetes and long-term mortality. JAMA 2015;313(1): 45–53.

111. Dabelea D, Stafford JM, Mayer-Davis EJ, et al. Association of type 1 diabetes vs type 2 diabetes diagnosed during childhood and adolescence with complications during teenage years and young adulthood. JAMA 2017;317(8):825–35.

112. Sauder KA, Stafford JM, Mayer-Davis EJ, et al. Co-occurrence of early diabetes-related complications in adolescents and young adults with type 1 diabetes: an observational cohort study. Lancet Child Adolesc Health 2019;3(1):35–43.

113. Kahkoska AR, Nguyen CT, Adair LA, et al. Longitudinal phenotypes of type 1 diabetes in youth based on weight and glycemia and their association with complications. J Clin Endocrinol Metab 2019;104(12):6003–16.

114. Dahlquist G, Kallen B. Mortality in childhood-onset type 1 diabetes: a population-based study. Diabetes Care 2005;28(10):2384–7.

115. Corbin KD, Driscoll KA, Pratley RE, et al. Obesity in type 1 diabetes: pathophysiology, clinical impact, and mechanisms. Endocr Rev 2018;39(5):629–63.

116. Kamrath C, Mönkemöller K, Biester T, et al. Ketoacidosis in children and adolescents with newly diagnosed type 1 diabetes during the COVID-19 pandemic in Germany. JAMA 2020;324(8):801–4.

117. Palermo NE, Sadhu AR, McDonnell ME. Diabetic ketoacidosis in COVID-19: unique concerns and considerations. J Clin Endocrinol Metab 2020;105(8): 2819–29.

118. Reddy PK, Kuchay MS, Mehta Y, et al. Diabetic ketoacidosis precipitated by COVID-19: a report of two cases and review of literature. Diabetes Metab Syndr Clin Res Rev 2020;14(5):1459–62.

119. Herman WH. The economic costs of diabetes: is it time for a new treatment paradigm? Diabetes Care 2013;36(4):775–6.

120. Ford ES, Williamson DF, Liu SM. Weight change and diabetes incidence - findings from a national cohort of US adults. Am J Epidemiol 1997;146(3):214–22.

121. Colditz GA, Willett WC, Rotnitzky A, et al. Weight gain as a risk factor for clinical diabetes mellitus in women. Ann Intern Med 1995;122(7):481–6.

122. Cassano PA, Rosner B, Vokonas PS, et al. Obesity and body fat distribution in relation to the incidence of non-insulin-dependent diabetes mellitus: a prospective cohort study of men in the Normative Aging Study. Am J Epidemiol 1992; 136:1474–86.

123. Hazuda HP, Mitchell BD, Haffner SM, et al. Obesity in Mexican American subgroups: findings from the San Antonio Heart Study. Am J Clin Nutr 1991;53: 1529S–34S.

124. Feskens EJ, Kromhout D. Effects of body fat and its development over a ten-year period on glucose tolerance in euglycaemic men: the Zutphen Study. Int J Epidemiol 1989;18:368–73.

125. Lind PM, Lind L. Endocrine-disrupting chemicals and risk of diabetes: an evidence-based review. Diabetologia 2018;61(7):1495–502.

Emerging and Public Health Challenges Existing in Gestational Diabetes Mellitus and Diabetes in Pregnancy

Yamuna Ana, MPH[a], Shriyan Prafulla, MPH[a],
Ravi Deepa, PhD scholar[a], Giridhara R. Babu, PhD[b],*

KEYWORDS

- Gestational diabetes mellitus • Diabetes in pregnancy • Challenges • Screening
- Management • Prevention

KEY POINTS

- Diabetes in pregnancy and gestational diabetes mellitus adversely impact the health of mother and baby.
- There are several challenges owing to multiple screening tests and guidelines.
- Training health care providers regarding recent guidelines of the screening and management is essential.
- Diabetes in pregnancy and gestational diabetes in pregnancy can be prevented and well-controlled by adherence to the lifestyle interventions and reorienting public health systems to a life-course perspective.

INTRODUCTION

Diabetes in pregnancy (DIP) is a chronic, metabolic disease characterized by elevated blood glucose levels. The World Health Organization (WHO) criteria for DIP is when 1 or more of the criteria are met, such as when the fasting plasma glucose is 7.0 mmol/L or greater ($\geq$126 mg/dL), the 2-hour plasma glucose is 11.1 mmol/L or greater ($\geq$200 mg/dL) after a 75-g oral glucose load, and the random plasma glucose is 11.1 mmol/L of greater ($\geq$200 mg/dL) in the presence of diabetes symptoms.[1] Gestational diabetes mellitus (GDM) is defined as any degree of glucose intolerance with onset or first recognition during pregnancy.[2] GDM is diagnosed at any time in pregnancy if 1 or more of the criteria are met, such

a Public Health Foundation of India, IIPH-H, Bangalore Campus, SIHFW Premises, Beside Leprosy Hospital, 1st Cross, Magadi Road, Bangalore 560023, Karnataka, India; b Lifecourse Epidemiology, Public Health Foundation of India, IIPH-H, Bangalore Campus, SIHFW Premises, Beside Leprosy Hospital, 1st Cross, Magadi Road, Bangalore 560023, Karnataka, India
* Corresponding author. Public Health Foundation of India, IIPH-H, Bangalore Campus, SIHFW Premises, Beside Leprosy Hospital, 1st Cross, Magadi Road, Bangalore 560023, Karnataka, India.
E-mail address: giridhar@iiphh.org

Endocrinol Metab Clin N Am 50 (2021) 513–530
https://doi.org/10.1016/j.ecl.2021.05.008
0889-8529/21/© 2021 Elsevier Inc. All rights reserved.

as when the fasting plasma glucose measures 5.1 to 6.9 mmol/L (92–125 mg/dL), 1-hour plasma glucose is 10.0 mmol/L or greater (≥180 mg/dL), or the 2-hour plasma glucose is 8.5 to 11.0 mmol/L (153–199 mg/dL) after a 75-g oral glucose load.[3] In 2019, 1 in 6 births was affected by GDM across the world.[4] DIP is more severe and differs from GDM; the prognosis depends on the extent of preexisting diabetes, treatment and management aspects, and how well the woman adheres to her treatment protocol.

Risk factors for GDM include older age; overweight or obesity; a family history of diabetes; previously delivered an infant with overweight; hypothyroidism; women from ethnic groups as African American, American Indian, Asian American, Hispanic or Latino, or Pacific Islander; and impaired glucose tolerance.[5] The risk factors for DIP depends on the type of diabetes women who have had GDM in their previous pregnancy and those who have a family member with type 2 diabetes mellitus. Women bearing multiple pregnancies also are at a higher risk.

According to the International Diabetes Federation, about 20 million live births had some form of hyperglycemia in pregnancy and in which an estimated 84% were due to GDM. Worldwide, most GDM and DIP cases were in low- and middle-income countries and those countries, where access to maternal care is often inadequate. Both conditions are severe health problems that disproportionally affect minority populations, resulting in a higher prevalence, greater severity of complications, and higher mortality rate. Therefore, women with DIP or GDM should regularly assess their blood glucose levels to reduce the risk of adverse pregnancy outcomes with the support of family and health care providers.[4]

Globally, the South East Asia region has the highest prevalence of GDM and live births affected by GDM. Other regions, namely, North America and the Caribbean, Europe, South and Central America, and the Western pacific, had a GDM prevalence of higher than 10%; the lowest was seen in the Middle East and North Africa (**Table 1**). There is wide variation in the prevalence of GDM owing to the overall status of the country's socioeconomic condition, availability of health care facilities, screening criteria used, demographic factors, underlying challenges for the prevention and management of DIP and GDM.

CHALLENGES TO SCREENING

Screening tests for DIP and GDM varies depending on the country protocols, type of guidelines followed, type of the health care provider, and available resources

Table 1
Worldwide prevalence of GDM and live birth affected by GDM in 2019

Territory	Prevalence of GDM in 2019 (%)	Live Births Affected by GDM in 2019 (in 1 Million)	Proportion
South-East Asia	27	6594	6.6
North America and the Caribbean	20.8	1567	4.4
Europe	16.3	2002	3.0
South and Central America	13.5	1018	3.0
Western pacific	12.3	3822	2.2
Africa	9.6	3538	7.1
Middle East and North Africa	7.5	1871	4.4

(Table 2). Even though all the national guidelines suggest that risk factor assessment needs to be performed at every antenatal care visit, screening for risk assessment during an antenatal checkup is poor.[6] To identify those with GDM or DIP, pregnant women should undergo early testing in the antenatal care using the standard diagnostic approach as suggested by the WHO, International Diabetes Federation, and respective national guidelines. Women with severe obesity, who had GDM during a previous pregnancy, delivered a large for gestational age infant, the presence of

Table 2
Different GDM screening procedure adopted by developing and developed countries

Sr No	Country	Screening Method
1	South Africa	Random blood glucose and 50-g GCT[13]
		Fasting blood glucose and urine dipstick test[14]
		50-g GCT[15]
		75-g 1-h glucose[16] premeal and postmeal blood glucose level[17]
2	Bangladesh	Fasting blood glucose and1 hour 50-g OGCT[18]
		75-g OGTT
3	India	3-h 100-g glucose OGTT[19] universal 2-h 75-g OGCT(nonfasting)[20]
		Capillary blood glucose[21]
		1-h 50-g challenge test[22]
		2-h 75-g OGTT(fasting)[22]
		Fasting blood glucose[23]
4	Ethiopia	75-g OGTT(fasting and 2-h)[24]
		Random blood sugar and 3-h 100-g OGTT[25]
		2-h 75-g OGTT by capillary testing[26]
5	Kenya	Venous fasting blood glucose[27]
		1-h 50-g GCT
		2-h 75-g OGTT
		Venous HbA1C
6	Pakistan	75-g OGCT – nonfasting[28]
		75-g OGTT[29]
		100-g 3 hours OGTT[30]
7	Belgium	Fasting plasma glucose[31]
		75-g 1-h GCT
		100-g OGTT
		75-g OGTT
8	Germany	50-g GCT[32]
		75-g OGTT
		Fasting venous plasma[33]
		HbA1c
9	Italy	50-g GCT[34]
		100-g OGTT
		HbA1c[35]
		One step 75-g OGTT
10	United Kingdom	Fasting plasma glucose[36]
		2-h 75-g OGTT
		Random blood sugar[37]
		Standardized meal tolerance test
		Premeal and postmeal blood glucose test
		Glycosylated Hb measurement

Abbreviations: GCT, glucose concentration test; HbA1c, hemoglobin A1c; OGTT, oral glucose tolerance testing.

glycosuria, polycystic ovarian syndrome, and a family history of type 2 diabetes mellitus constitute the high-risk group. The feasibility of conducting the initial glucose challenge test and follow-up with glucose tolerance testing in early pregnancy is the most important determinant of effective screening.

There are multiple screening and diagnostic tests resulting in the practitioner's non-adherence to the guidelines. The data on adherence to guidelines for diagnosis and management of GDM varies across countries. In India, the practice of national guidelines for the diagnosis and management of GDM is unclear; only 46% of public health doctors used oral glucose tolerance testing for screening for GDM.[7] A cross-sectional survey conducted among doctors providing care to patients with GDM in low-income and lower-middle income countries shows that only 68% of the doctors reported practicing any guidelines in their settings.[8] A prospective study on adherence to clinical GDM guidelines carried out in Ghana shows 48% of providers adhere to the guidelines.[9,10] Some of the renowned screening criteria are issued by the WHO, International Federation of Gynecology and Obstetrics, the International Diabetes Federation, and The International Association of Diabetes and Pregnancy Study Groups. Selecting the best guideline for the diagnosis of GDM remains an area of debate. It is essential to match the acceptance of enhanced detection with the practicality of screening in large populations.[11] Neither of these guidelines have taken the realities of resource-poor countries into consideration. Although the International Association of Diabetes and Pregnancy Study Groups guidelines simplified the screening protocol and diagnostic requirements for GDM, these concepts are difficult to implement in low-resource settings. With the rising prevalence of GDM in developing countries, there seems to be an urgent need to establish a quick, feasible and easy to follow screening approach that can be used at the point of care in different settings.[12]

Screening for GDM is usually done at 24 to 28 weeks of gestation because insulin resistance increases during the second trimester, and glucose levels increase in women who cannot produce enough insulin to adopt this resistance. The American Diabetes Association states that there is no need to screen and are less likely to benefit from screening among low-risk women. These include women under 25 years of age, not a member of ethnic group, a body mass index of 25 kg/m^2 or less, no previous history of abnormal glucose tolerance or adverse obstetrics outcomes, and no known history of diabetes in first-degree relatives. However, the evidence suggests that universal screening, especially in Southeast Asian countries, would be beneficial.[38,39] Our recent study showed that Indian women in the younger age group (18–25 years) have a higher prevalence of GDM.[40]

In most of the circumstances, there is a delayed start of antenatal care. As a result, screening women for GDM in the 24- to 32-week range and timely risk factor assessment cannot be performed. GDM screening recommended by risk factor assessment is not always useful. With the risk factor screening, actual GDM cases could be missed. Evidence suggests that about 4% of the women with GDM will be missed if the selective screening recommendations are followed.[41] Considering age greater than 30 years as a risk factor might have resulted in 22% of missed cases of GDM.[42] Also, with the broader consideration of risk factors for screening, only 3% to 9% of the GDM cases would be missed.[41,43,44] Body mass index does not reflect the true risk of developing GDM. Most of the screening and diagnostic tests require pregnant women to be in a fasting, state but ensuring the women present in a fasting state test is challenging. All the gold standard screening and diagnostic tests are time consuming, depending on the tests; it may take up to 3 hours from fasting to last sample drawn. Also, women can experience nausea and vomiting associated with heavy glucose ingestion. Therefore, these tests need to be repeated from the beginning in such situations, and sometimes women do not report for the repeat tests. There could be a scarcity of test consumables in some health facilities and a lack of equipment and other logistics when the women arrive for the test.

Across the world, different guidelines are followed to screen and diagnose GDM and DIP at various laboratories and health care facilities. Fasting and nonfasting tests are carried out based on different guidelines, and have different cutoff points for diagnosis (**Table 3**). Therefore, the greatest challenge arises in terms of following the different guideline for the diagnosis and initiation of disease management.

CHALLENGES IN SELF-MANAGEMENT

The first line of GDM management includes complex self-care regimes, such as daily monitoring of blood glucose and dietary modification depending on the blood glucose level of the pregnant woman. Patients with diabetes need to be guided during treatment for self-monitoring of blood glucose levels. This practice will allow them to monitor treatment choice and help to improve diet and exercise. Patients using an intense insulin regimen are encouraged to track hypoglycemia and hyperglycemia by self-monitoring of blood glucose. The increased level of self-monitoring of blood glucose in a day helps to eliminate complications and keeps a check on glucose level. Integrating self-management education, along with continuous glucose monitoring, would be useful to decrease blood glucose levels.[47]

Issues such as lack of experience, physical health limitations, trust in treatment and self-efficacy, lack of support, and cultural influences[48] have been major factors affecting self-management. The provision of adequate information is essential for promoting self-management. Social support increases patients' trust. Good interactions between the provider and the patient enhance patient understanding and reinforce knowledge about the disease. It strengthens patients' trust and improves health outcomes.[49] Nutritional self-management is a crucial aspect, taking time to learn about nutritional values to make balanced and healthy meals is a major challenge for women. The diagnosed women have to plan an additional clinic visit to specialists and dieticians to manage their blood glucose levels.[50] Support from health care professionals and social support have shown to foster positive self-management. Targeted educational services and initiatives are needed to address the cultural context that affects self-management. This focused approach could affect diary management and helps to manage blood glucose. Therefore, good self-management is associated with a lower risk of severe pregnancy complications and fetal morbidity, decreasing the future risk of type 2 diabetes.[50]

The lack of adequate patient knowledge about GDM represents a major obstacle to its effective management. Compliance with diet, exercise, and medication is a major challenge for patients with GDM. Pregnant women's family and friends may confuse and affect the pregnant woman's decision to follow the health care advice. The lack of community awareness and cultural elements are the inhibitors to GDM treatment. Myths like "exercise hurts the baby" and "pregnant mothers have to eat food for two" have harmful impacts on pregnant women and prevent them from following the instructions of their doctor to exercise and follow a certain diet.[51,52] Poor communication with the health care delivery system cause misunderstandings. As a result, many women remain physically inactive during pregnancy, and the craving for such non-nutritious food items is a major barrier to adherence. The costs associated with managing GDM are an obstacle for pregnant women seeking medical advice and antenatal care. Equipment that includes glucometers and related products, medicines, and lifestyle changes cause financial strain. Low wages,

Table 3
Different criteria used in the screening and diagnosis of GDM

Method	Test	Cutoff Measurements	Challenges in Adherence
WHO	Fasting 75-g 2-h oral glucose tolerance test	FPG ≥126 mg/dL 2-h ≥140 mg/dL	Suppliers side Lack of infrastructure and human resource
American Diabetes Association	50-g GCT 3hours 100-g OGTT	GCT ≥140 mg/dL FPG ≥95 mg/dL 1-h ≥180 mg/dL	Lack of knowledge and training on GDM among health care provider
American Diabetes Association	75-g OGTT	2-h ≥155 mg/dL 3-h ≥140 mg/dL FPG ≥92 mg/dL 2-h ≥153 mg/dL	Lack of standard protocols for screening Repeated visits to hospital Repeated invasive sample collection[45]
International Federation of Gynecology and Obstetrics	Single-step 75-g OGTT	2-h plasma glucose >140 mg/dL	Unable to complete owing to vomiting and nausea Demand side
International Association of Diabetes and Pregnancy Study Groups	Fasting 2-h OGTT	FPG ≥92 mg/dL 2-h ≥153 mg/dL	Overnight fasting Women do not attend antenatal care clinic Lack of awareness on the importance of GDM testing Societal status Fear of consequences of results Access to health care in rural areas Lack of transport to reach facility Cost associated with the test Long waiting period for completion of test.[46]

Abbreviations: FPG, fasting plasma glucose; OGTT, oral glucose tolerance testing.

insufficient public health facilities, and routine follow-up visits contribute to financial constraints.[53]

CHALLENGES IN PROVIDER MANAGEMENT

In low- and middle-income countries, the challenges faced in provider management are the lack of qualified phlebotomists and standardized laboratories to measure blood glucose, the use of conflicting guidelines, and a pregnant woman's unwillingness to undergo GDM screening in a fasting state.[54] Despite the need for universal screening, some health care facilities do not conduct tests for all pregnant women. Hospital treatment for diabetes requires the provision of hospital services and quality assurance standards for ongoing improvement. In hospitals, treatment protocols and guidelines are implemented inconsistently. Well-qualified specialists can strengthen the management guidelines and improve health outcomes. Regular monitoring of blood glucose is required among those who take insulin by intravenous infusion.[55] The blood glucose monitoring device should be checked for its accuracy before use. Every hospital should implement a hypoglycemia management protocol, and a plan should be developed to prevent and treat hypoglycemia. To prevent possible hypoglycemia, the treatment regimen has to be checked and modified as required. Provision of proper durable medical instruments, materials, drugs, and appropriate education to be provided at discharge to prevent further complications.[56,57]

The lack of standardized training on GDM screening and diagnosis and[58] lack of trained health care providers are major barriers in GDM management in low- and middle-income countries.[59] In the absence of structured information and policies for screening and management of GDM, the information obtained by pregnant women gets implemented in different ways.[60] The field-based health care staff such as assistant nurse managers or accredited social health activists in the primary health care setting are the first line of interaction, but have been poorly equipped to provide information, counseling, referral, and follow-up services in GDM care in resource-poor settings.[61] Unmet training needs among nurses and other health care staff for GDM screening and management lead to a delay in the diagnosis of women who initially seek antenatal care services and end up misdiagnosed until late gestation.[62] There is a need for pre- and in-service training are the standard guidelines for first-line health care professionals to treat GDM women and provide quality treatment.[63]

The lack of awareness on GDM management protocols among health care providers is a challenge in the hospitals' GDM management. There is a need to strengthen health care practitioners' expertise and skills to understand and manage GDM.[64] Access to health care is identified as a screening and management challenge.[60] Many pregnant women either lack antenatal care or deliver without consultation. Wherever transportation is an obstacle, it is hard to ensure periodic follow-up visits for those obtaining insulin as a medication[58] The costs associated with access to medical care, including travel costs, spending on specific tests, procurement of test equipment and treatment, and hospitalization costs, have been described as key barriers to proper GDM management.[53] Inadequate availability of screening facilities at different levels across public institutions and a scarcity of endocrinologists and dieticians limit care standards in many low-income settings. The deficit of laboratory supplies and screening reagents, periodic glucometer calibration against laboratory parameters, and lack of insulin supplies hampers the treatment. The lack of multidisciplinary teams harms the efficient management of GDM.

CHALLENGES IN THE PREVENTION OF GESTATIONAL DIABETES MELLITUS AND DIABETES IN PREGNANCY AND TREATMENT

Challenges arise at each level of prevention, such as primordial, primary, secondary, and tertiary prevention of GDM and DIP (**Fig. 1**).

Lifestyle Changes

Unhealthy dietary practices and physical inactivity are the greatest challenges for the management of GDM. Optimal preconceptional care includes educating women with diabetes and providing effective birth control until they achieve good glycemic control; these challenges are inherent to the prevention of DIP.[65] Various factors act as barriers and facilitators for implementing a preventive intervention, such as family and friends, limited knowledge, economic factors, social support, and so on.[66] Physical activity is recommended for women with GDM because it improves glycemic control. The specific physical changes during pregnancy discourage many pregnant women from participating in physical activity.[67] Studies have shown that physical illness (nausea and vomiting) and lack of time are the biggest barriers to exercise. Many women do not know that physical inactivity increases the risk of diabetes and dietary factors are seen as the main cause.[68] In GDM management, medical nutritional therapy is

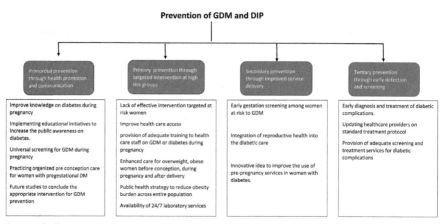

Fig. 1. Challenges arising during primordial, primary, secondary and tertiary prevention of GDM and DP.

essential. However, this services is affected by either a lack of dieticians or conflicting dietary advice for women with GDM. To achieve the treatment goal, the nutritional plan should be culturally appropriate and customized to the individual. Preparing a balanced meal is also a challenge owing to the costs and lack of awareness regarding nutritious foods.[69]

There are other barriers for compliance with treatment, including a lack of finances to buy insulin, glucometer, and testing strips; a lack of family or peer support; a complex therapeutic regimen (insulin storage, self-injection, and self-monitoring of blood glucose); religious and cultural factors on consulting traditional healers; and poor services at the treating hospitals.[70] Further, poor self-monitoring of blood glucose in women diagnosed with GDM results in delays in addressing complications.[69] Women under insulin treatment have higher fetal risk.[71] Most women with GDM remain in the home at 6 to 12 weeks postpartum. Scheduling postpartum screening is stressful owing to work constraints or a lack of childcare, and most of the women perceive themselves as healthy and think that postpartum screening is unnecessary.[72] Other challenges occur during the implementation of research activities hat are focused on GDM, the presence of other risk factors on further health outcomes, newborn outcomes, and so on (**Fig. 2**).

CHALLENGES IN THE TREATMENT OF GESTATIONAL DIABETES MELLITUS AND DIABETES IN PREGNANCY

The biggest obstacle is the lack of financial support, including problems with travel costs, consultant fees, and the higher prices for healthy food.[73] In adolescents, lower self-esteem, lower self-efficacy, greater depressive symptoms, and more binge eating are responsible for disparities in adherence to medical care.[74] The lack of community awareness and cultural elements are the inhibitors to GDM treatment. Myths like exercise hurt the baby and pregnant mothers have to eat food for two cause harmful impacts in pregnant women and prevent them from following the instructions of the doctor to exercise and follow a certain diet.[51,52] The lack of adequate patient knowledge about GDM represents a major obstacle to its effective management. The costs associated with equipment include glucometers and related products, medicines, and lifestyle changes that create financial strain. Low wages, insufficient public health

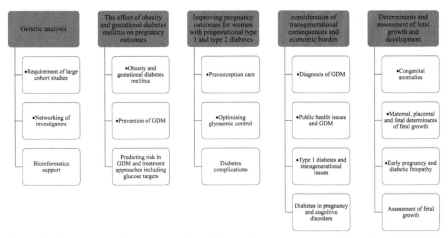

Fig. 2. Challenges at various aspects for diabetes in pregnancy and Gestational Diabetes Mellitus.

facilities, and routine follow-up visits contribute to financial constraints.[53] Access to health care is a challenge to screen and management because many patients come to antenatal care consultation late in their pregnancy or deliver without having had prenatal care. Wherever transportation is an obstacle, it is difficult to ensure regular follow-up visits among those who receive insulin as a treatment.[58] Inadequate cooperation between different experts and the lack of multidisciplinary teams is present. This could harm the efficient management of GDM. The time lag between a blood draw and its final examination in the laboratory triggers measurement errors, leading to incorrect results.[58] It is difficult for illiterate patients to monitor blood glucose by repeated pricking and venous puncture; often there is difficulty in obtaining a personal glucometer. Discontinuation of diet and an inability to comply with insulin administration owing to concerns regarding insulin administration concerns and its side effects are also of concern.[58]

INTERMEDIATE- AND LONG-TERM COMPLICATIONS OF GESTATIONAL DIABETES MELLITUS

Women who develop GDM are at risk for other health concerns. Similar to type 2 diabetes mellitus, GDM causes vascular damage and can cause adverse outcomes in neonates. More than two-thirds women with GDM will develop type 2 diabetes in the 2 decades after their pregnancy. The long-term risk of cardiovascular disease, including stroke, is significantly increased in women with GDM. Therefore, it is not just about blood sugar and managing one's blood sugar. Women must be monitored for all the other cardiovascular risks and their future implications. Women can decrease their risk by maintaining a healthy lifestyle that includes a diet rich in vegetables and fruits, whole grains, and lean proteins, along with regular exercise. There is an issue in tracking and following up with women with GDM. Even though clinical guidelines exist, postpartum glucose testing rates are exceedingly low. Studies recommended introducing routine screening for hyperglycemia during pregnancy and strategies for the follow-up to prevent GDM and DIP's long-term effects in women and their children. Patient barriers to postpartum glucose testing include low motivation for self-care, structural obstacles, and competing priorities. The prevention of early-onset disease has great potential for medical cost savings and improvements in quality of life. GDM is associated with multiple adverse pregnancy outcomes. Women with GDM are at subsequent high risk of type 2 diabetes, especially in the 3 to 6 years after delivery. Exposure to hyperglycemia in the womb predisposes children to an increased risk of becoming overweight or obese, which is associated with the development of type 2 diabetes. GDM is a severe and underrecognized threat to maternal and child health. Many women with GDM experience pregnancy-related complications, including high blood pressure, high birth weight babies, and obstructed labor. Approximately one-half of women with a history of GDM develop type 2 diabetes within 5 to 10 years after delivery. Women with GDM have a greater risk of developing diabetes in the future compared with those women who have normal glucose tolerance during pregnancy. Intervention in the form of counseling regarding exercise and a healthy, high-fiber, unrefined carbohydrate, low cholesterol diet, as well as advice regarding smoking cessation, together with weight monitoring, may prevent the onset of diabetes and its associated cerebrovascular and cardiovascular problems.[75] Women with GDM had a higher risk of composite adverse maternal outcome caesarean delivery, pregnancy-induced hypertension, premature rupture of membranes, antepartum hemorrhage, and postpartum hemorrhage compared with women without GDM.[76] Maternal complications include infections, polyhydramnios, preterm delivery, severe hypoglycemia, and diabetic ketoacidosis. Fetal complications include spontaneous abortion, malformations, unexplained stillbirths, macrosomia, altered fetal growth, respiratory distress syndrome, hypoglycemia, hypocalcemia, hyperbilirubinemia, and polycythemia, cardiomyopathy, long-term effects on cognitive development, and inheritance of diabetes.[77]

TACKLING THE CHALLENGES NECESSITATES ADAPTING A LIFE-COURSE PERSPECTIVE

GDM represents a transient and yet part of the continuum in terms of the life-course trajectory of overweight, obesity, and hyperglycemia. Therefore, a life-course approach involving the prevention and management of GDM should be adapted to prevent GDM. In utero exposure to maternal hyperglycemia results in fetal hyperinsulinemia, leading to increased fetal fat cells. This factor is a precursor for childhood adiposity and a continued trajectory leading to diabetes in later life, including hyperglycemia in pregnancy (**Fig. 3**). Therefore, interventions to prevent the development GDM should be initiated as early as during early childhood. The challenges at each phase through the life-course trajectory should be addressed including lack of knowledge, ignorance of potential risks, and myths among the community members.[51,52]

Failure in preventing or controlling glucose intolerance in young children, adolescent girls, and women during the preconceptual stage are windows of opportunities for intervention in a lifecycle that perpetuates the transgenerational transmission of glucose tolerance.[64,78] These deficiencies include a lack of organized preconception care for women with pregestational diabetes[79] and a lack of resources to encourage young children and adolescents to follow a healthy dietary pattern. There is a lack of high-quality, longitudinal studies to determine the appropriate intervention for the prevention of GDM.[80] Measures taken to decrease the disease-related burden, especially in this high-risk population, are generally unsuccessful.[80] Although the best time to prevent GDM is before pregnancy, the lack of public health strategies and focus on decreasing obesity in the entire population makes it challenging.[81,82] Tackling overweight, obesity, and hyperglycemia is not integrated into reproductive health or all women's diabetes care plans. The lack of innovative ideas to improve women's

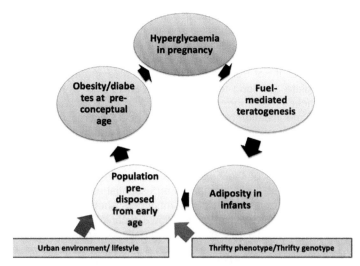

Fig. 3. Hyperglycemia in pregnancy and risk of chronic diseases: Life cycle.

pregnancy services has led to the current high burden of the DIP and GDM popula-tions.[83] This situation is further complicated by poor availability of guidance and adequate training to health care professionals in addressing overweight, obesity, and hyperglycemia,[58] the lack of enhanced care and infrastructure,[82] and the ineffec-tive screening initiatives for individuals with a high risk of diabetes.[81] Also, there are multiple challenges in tackling the disease during pregnancy. These include several screening tests to diagnose GDM,[53] the lack of effective nonpharmacologic interven-tions,[84,85] the poor impact of any exercise or dietary guidance during pregnancy,[86] and poor access to the health care system.[58] The control of GDM during pregnancy is affected by prolonged waiting for tests, vomiting induced by the test,[58] lack of trained phlebotomists and standardized laboratories, and the poor use of protocols.[54] Failure to recognize other GDM or diabetes-related medical problems during preg-nancy and treat them to mitigate diabetic complications is an important issue.[81] Inef-ficient care during pregnancy accelerates the risk of diabetes progression and intensifies the complications of diabetes mellitus.[87] The failure of early detection and treatment of diabetes leads to complications such as diabetic retinopathy, ne-phropathy, and cardiovascular and peripheral vascular disease.[81]

Building a more structured model for GDM/DP is essential. Integrating GDM man-agement in public health program could bring major benefits (**Box 1**). Universal screening for GDM should be implemented. Increasing knowledge and awareness

---

Box 1
Ways to integrate GDM management in public health

- Antenatal screening and treatment along with strict postpartum follow-up
- Integrating noncommunicable disease control programs with maternal and child health programs.
- Strengthening and using the existing health care system.
- Transgenerational prevention of diabetes.

among pregnant women, family, and health care professionals paves the way for better outcomes. Women should be counseled on healthy lifestyle behaviors, the need for health care-seeking behavior, self-care at home, the importance of follow-up, and the need for adherence to the advised treatment. Education should include the risk factors and the consequences if not treated for GDM, self-care, the importance of regular follow-up, intermediate and long-term complications for the mother and offspring, and so on. This practice may improve treatment compliance and confer better health outcomes. Lifestyle modification behaviors should include increased physical activity and a decreased consumption of sweetened beverages and high energy-dense food items.

Health care workers have to play a larger role in creating awareness of GDM among antenatal women. Training of the health care workers regarding updated national guidelines of management and treatment is an essential aspect. Accredited Social Health Activist workers or assistant nurse managers should regulate home visits and mobilize the GDM women for regular follow-up care. For screening, there is a need for practice that is both a cost-effective and patient-friendly approach. The Diabetes in Pregnancy Study Group of India criterion is a 1-step, cost-effective, evidence-based procedure to diagnose GDM in any socioeconomic setting.[53,88] Also, because social taboos and myths, especially in rural areas, exist, there is a pressing need for counseling and awareness to the public concerning disease prognosis.[89]

SUMMARY

Challenges occur at each phase of management and implementation of GDM and DIP services. They are based on different cultural and social levels, health system services, health care professionals, and patient or community needs.[90] Various studies have reported the many challenges related to screening and management from both the service provider side and the beneficiary side. Community awareness on DIP and GDM, the cost associated with the care and need for periodic follow-up visits and regular monitoring of blood glucose levels are the major highlighted problems. Underprivileged patients do suffer from additional challenges like cultural and language barriers owing to their migratory status. Adolescents mostly do not adhere to medical care owing to a lack of self-efficacy, self-esteem, higher depressive symptoms, and more binge eating. Patients are often unable to afford glucometer strips to track their blood glucose levels regularly, and the absence of endocrinologists and dieticians as well as a lack of a multidisciplinary team at the health facility are greatest challenges. Good communication between patients and doctors will ensure patients are advised well and follow medical advice. Improving overall the health care system is a solution to the challenge so that the noncommunicable disorders are integrated into the existing program framework. Health care providers, health care managers, public health experts, and policymakers need to understand and take these challenges and barriers into account and ensure that appropriate measures are placed to resolve this without hindrance.

CLINICS CARE POINTS

- For a diagnosis of GDM, point-of-care capillary maternal glucose tests were superior to routine laboratory practices and were found to have significant potential, predominantly in health care settings where facilities for phlebotomy are poor.[91]
- Point-of-care analysis is a feasible alternative for routine glucose analysis in GDM screening in resource poor settings.[27]

- The American Diabetes Association suggests point-of-care analysis venous oral glucose tolerance testing are feasible diagnostic alternatives for low-resource settings where laboratory infrastructure is not available.[92]

DISCLOSURE

This work was supported by the Wellcome Trust DBT India Alliance Fellowship (grant number: IA/CPHI/14/1/501499) to Giridhara R Babu.

REFERENCES

1. World Health Organization. WHO recommendation on the diagnosis of gestational diabetes in pregnancy 2018. Available at: https://extranet.who.int/rhl/topics/preconception-pregnancy-childbirth-and-postpartum-care/antenatal-care/who-recommendation-diagnosis-gestational-diabetes-pregnancy-0. Accessed December 19, 2020.
2. Metzger BE, Coustan DR, Committee O. Summary and recommendations of the fourth international workshop-conference on gestational diabetes mellitus. Diabetes care 1998;21:B161.
3. World Health Organization. Diagnostic criteria and classification of hyperglycaemia first detected in pregnancy. Geneva (Switzerland): World Health Organization; 2013.
4. Federation ID. Care & prevention: gestational diabetes 2020. Available at: https://www.idf.org/our-activities/care-prevention/gdm. Accessed September 19, 2020.
5. Dhanaraj B, Papanna MK, Adinarayanan S, et al. Prevalence and risk factors for adult pulmonary tuberculosis in a metropolitan city of South India. PLoS One 2015;10(4):e0124260.
6. Prual A, Toure A, Huguet D, et al. The quality of risk factor screening during antenatal consultations in Niger. Health Policy Plan 2000;15(1):11–6.
7. Babu GR, Tejaswi B, Kalavathi M, et al. Assessment of screening practices for gestational hyperglycaemia in public health facilities: a descriptive study in Bangalore, India. J Public Health Res 2015;4(1):448.
8. Utz B, Kolsteren P, De Brouwere V. A snapshot of current gestational diabetes management practices from 26 low-income and lower-middle-income countries. Int J Gynecol Obstet 2016;134(2):145–50.
9. Amoakoh-Coleman M, Agyepong IA, Zuithoff NP, et al. Client factors affect provider adherence to clinical guidelines during first antenatal care. PLoS One 2016;11(6):e0157542.
10. Amoakoh-Coleman M, Agyepong IA, Kayode GA, et al. Public health facility resource availability and provider adherence to first antenatal guidelines in a low resource setting in Accra, Ghana. BMC Health Serv Res 2016;16(1):505.
11. Jiang S, Rajagopal R, Simmons D. Continuing Challenges in the Medical Management of Gestational Diabetes Mellitus. EMJ Diabetes.
12. Nielsen KK, Courten Md, Kapur A. The urgent need for universally applicable simple screening procedures and diagnostic criteria for gestational diabetes mellitus–lessons from projects funded by the World Diabetes Foundation. Glob Health Action 2012;5(1):17277.
13. Abudu O, Kuti J. Screening for diabetes in pregnancy in a Nigerian population with a high perinatal mortality rate. Asia-Oceania J Obstet Gynaecol 1987;13(3):305–9.

14. Wokoma F, John CT, Enyindah C. Gestational diabetes mellitus in a Nigerian antenatal population. Trop J Obstet Gynaecol 2001;18(2):56–60.
15. Adegbola O, Ajayi G. Screening for Gestational Diabetes Mellitus in Nigerian Pregnant Women using fifty grams oral glucose challenge test. 2008.
16. Ranchod H, Vaughan J, Jarvis P. Incidence of gestational diabetes at Northdale Hospital, Pietermaritzburg. South Afr Med J 1991;80(1):14–6.
17. Basu JK, Jeketera CM, Basu D. Obesity and its outcomes among pregnant South African women. Int J Gynecol Obstet 2010;110(2):101–4.
18. Jesmin S, Akter S, Akashi H, et al. Screening for gestational diabetes mellitus and its prevalence in Bangladesh. Diabetes Res Clin Pract 2014;103(1):57–62.
19. O'sullivan JB. Criteria for the oral glucose tolerance test in pregnancy. Diabetes 1964;13:278–85.
20. Seshiah V, Balaji V, Balaji MS, et al. One step procedure for screening and diagnosis of gestational diabetes mellitus. Diabetes 2005;126:200.
21. Bhavadharini B, Mahalakshmi MM, Maheswarl K, et al. Use of capillary blood glucose for screening for gestational diabetes mellitus in resource-constrained settings. Acta Diabetol 2016;53(1):91–7.
22. Zargar AH, Sheikh MI, Bashir MI, et al. Prevalence of gestational diabetes mellitus in Kashmiri women from the Indian subcontinent. Diabetes Res Clin Pract 2004; 66(2):139–45.
23. Gopalakrishnan V, Singh R, Pradeep Y, et al. Evaluation of the prevalence of gestational diabetes mellitus in North Indians using the International Association of Diabetes and Pregnancy Study groups (IADPSG) criteria. J Postgrad Med 2015;61(3):155.
24. Seyoum B, Kiros K, Haileselase T, et al. Prevalence of gestational diabetes mellitus in rural pregnant mothers in northern Ethiopia. Diabetes Res Clin Pract 1999; 46(3):247–51.
25. Wakwoya EB, Amante TD, Tesema KF. Gestational diabetes mellitus is a risk for macrosomia: case-control study in Eastern Ethiopia. BioRxiv 2018;492355.
26. Muche AA, Olayemi OO, Gete YK. Predictors of postpartum glucose intolerance in women with gestational diabetes mellitus: a prospective cohort study in Ethiopia based on the updated diagnostic criteria. BMJ Open 2020;10(8): e036882.
27. Pastakia SD, Njuguna B, Ajwang'Onyango B, et al. Prevalence of gestational diabetes mellitus based on various screening strategies in western Kenya: a prospective comparison of point of care diagnostic methods. BMC Pregnancy Childbirth 2017;17(1):226.
28. Riaz M, Nawaz A, Masood SN, et al. Frequency of gestational diabetes mellitus using DIPSI criteria, a study from Pakistan. Clin Epidemiol Glob Health 2019; 7(2):218–21.
29. Zaman N, Taj N, Nazir S, et al. Gestational diabetes mellitus and obesity: an experience at a teaching hospital in Bahawalpur, Pakistan. Rawal Med J 2013;38(2): 165–8.
30. FAROUGH M, AHMAD I, AYAZ A, ALI BL. Maternal and neonatal outcomes in gestational diabetes mellitus. 2007. Available at: https://www.sid.ir/en/journal/ViewPaper.aspx?id=100914.
31. Benhalima K, Van Crombrugge P, Devlieger R, et al. Screening for pregestational and gestational diabetes in pregnancy: a survey of obstetrical centers in the northern part of Belgium. Diabetology Metab Syndr 2013;5(1):66.

32. Melchior H, Kurch-Bek D, Mund M. The prevalence of gestational diabetes: a population-based analysis of a nationwide screening program. Deutsches Ärzteblatt Int 2017;114(24):412.
33. Kleinwechter H, Schäfer-Graf U, Bührer C, et al. Gestational diabetes mellitus (GDM) diagnosis, therapy and follow-up care. Exp Clin Endocrinol Diabetes 2014;122(07):395–405.
34. Lapolla A, Dalfrà MG, Bonomo M, et al. Gestational diabetes mellitus in Italy: a multicenter study. Eur J Obstet Gynecol Reprod Biol 2009;145(2):149–53.
35. Vitacolonna E, Succurro E, Lapolla A, et al. Guidelines for the screening and diagnosis of gestational diabetes in Italy from 2010 to 2019: critical issues and the potential for improvement. Acta Diabetol 2019;56(11):1159–67.
36. Wagnild JM, Hinshaw K, Pollard TM. Associations of sedentary time and self-reported television time during pregnancy with incident gestational diabetes and plasma glucose levels in women at risk of gestational diabetes in the UK. BMC Public Health 2019;19(1):575.
37. Aldrich PM J, MDG Gillmer C. Screening for gestational diabetes in the United Kingdom: a national survey. J Obstet Gynaecol 1999;19(6):575–9.
38. Tariq H, Siraj A, Sarfraz T, et al. Universal vs selective screening of gestational diabetes mellitus by oral glucose tolerance test at 24-28 weeks pregnancy. Pakistan Armed Forces Med J 2019;69(4):795–800.
39. Jawad F, Ejaz K. Gestational diabetes mellitus in South Asia: epidemiology. J Pak Med Assoc 2016;66(9 Suppl 1):S5–7.
40. Babu GR, Deepa R, Lewis MG, et al. Do gestational obesity and gestational diabetes have an independent effect on neonatal adiposity? results of mediation analysis from a Cohort Study in South India. Clin Epidemiol 2019;11:1067.
41. Williams CB, Iqbal S, Zawacki CM, et al. Effect of selective screening for gestational diabetes. Diabetes care 1999;22(3):418–21.
42. Coustan DR, Nelson C, Carpenter MW, et al. Maternal age and screening for gestational diabetes: a population-based study. Obstet Gynecol 1989;73(4):557–61.
43. Moses RG, Moses J, Davis WS. Gestational diabetes: do lean young Caucasian women need to be tested? Diabetes Care 1998;21(11):1803–6.
44. Danilenko-Dixon DR, Van Winter JT, Nelson RL, et al. Universal versus selective gestational diabetes screening: application of 1997 American Diabetes Association recommendations. Am J Obstet Gynecol 1999;181(4):798–802.
45. Suganthi M. Comparison of one step glucose tolerance test (75 g GTT) and two step glucose tolerance test (100 g GTT) in screening and diagnosis of gestational diabetes mellitus. Int J Reprod Contraception, Obstet Gynecol 2018;7(12):4815.
46. Kragelund K. Review of projects addressing gestational diabetes mellitus supported by the World Diabetes Foundation in the period 2002-2010. Gestational diabetes mellitus. World Diabetes Foundation; 2011.
47. Association AD. 7. Diabetes technology: standards of medical care in diabetes—2019. Diabetes Care 2019;42(Supplement 1):S71–80.
48. Subarto C, Indriani S. Self-management on gestational diabetes mellitus: a systematic literature review. Paper presented at: Proceeding International Conference2019.
49. Xu Y, Toobert D, Savage C, et al. Factors influencing diabetes self-management in Chinese people with type 2 diabetes. Res Nurs Health 2008;31(6):613–25.
50. Carolan M, Gill GK, Steele C. Women's experiences of factors that facilitate or inhibit gestational diabetes self-management. BMC Pregnancy Childbirth 2012;12(1):99.

51. Ghaffari F, Salsali M, Rahnavard Z, et al. Compliance with treatment regimen in women with gestational diabetes: living with fear. Iranian J Nurs Midwifery Res 2014;19(7 Suppl1):S103.
52. Thara R, Padmavati R, Aynkran JR, et al. Community mental health in India: a rethink. Int J Ment Health Syst 2008;2(1):1–7.
53. Morampudi S, Balasubramanian G, Gowda A, et al. The challenges and recommendations for gestational diabetes mellitus care in India: a review. Front Endocrinol 2017;8:56.
54. Mohan V, Usha S, Uma R. Screening for gestational diabetes in India: where do we stand? J Postgrad Med 2015;61(3):151.
55. Cobaugh DJ, Maynard G, Cooper L, et al. Enhancing insulin-use safety in hospitals: practical recommendations from an ASHP Foundation expert consensus panel. Am J Health-System Pharm 2013;70(16):1404–13.
56. Garg R, Schuman B, Bader A, et al. Effect of preoperative diabetes management on glycemic control and clinical outcomes after elective surgery. Ann Surg 2018; 267(5):858–62.
57. Association AD. 15. Diabetes care in the hospital: standards of medical care in diabetes—2020. Diabetes Care 2020;43(Supplement 1):S193–202.
58. Utz B, De Brouwere V. "Why screen if we cannot follow-up and manage?" Challenges for gestational diabetes screening and management in low and lower-middle income countries: results of a cross-sectional survey. BMC Pregnancy Childbirth 2016;16(1):341.
59. Nielsen KK, de Courten M, Kapur A. Health system and societal barriers for gestational diabetes mellitus (GDM) services-lessons from World Diabetes Foundation supported GDM projects. BMC Int Health Hum Rights 2012;12(1):33.
60. Sahu B, Babu GR, Gurav KS, et al. Health care professionals' perspectives on screening and management of gestational diabetes mellitus in public hospitals of South India–a qualitative study. BMC Health Serv Res 2020;21(1):133.
61. Seetharam S, Channakeshavamurthy A, Holbrook K, et al. Addressing gestational diabetes mellitus: a reference manual for the grassroots. Swami Vivekananda Youth Movement; 2011.
62. Patel S, Vyas S. Evaluation of Training Program about Awareness of Gestational Diabetes Mellitus (GDM) among Health Care Workers of Ahmedabad Municipal Corporation. Natl J Community Med 2018;9(2):114–9.
63. Hewage SS, Singh SR, Chi C, et al. Health care providers' perceptions of responsibilities and resources to reduce type 2 diabetes risk after gestational diabetes mellitus. Clin Diabetes 2018;36(2):160–7.
64. Halim A, Abdullah ASM, Rahman F, et al. Exploring the perceptions, practices and challenges of gestational diabetes detection and management among health care providers in a district of Bangladesh. F1000Research 2020;9(189):189.
65. Mersereau P, Williams J, Collier SA, et al. Barriers to managing diabetes during pregnancy: the perceptions of health care practitioners. Birth 2011;38(2):142–9.
66. Kelly S, Martin S, Kuhn I, et al. Barriers and facilitators to the uptake and maintenance of healthy behaviours by people at mid-life: a rapid systematic review. PLoS One 2016;11(1):e0145074.
67. Downs DS, Hausenblas HA. Women's exercise beliefs and behaviors during their pregnancy and postpartum. J Midwifery women's Health 2004;49(2):138–44.
68. Downs DS, Ulbrecht JS. Understanding exercise beliefs and behaviors in women with gestational diabetes mellitus. Diabetes care 2006;29(2):236–40.

69. Goldschmidt VJ, Colletta B. The challenges of providing diabetes education in resource-limited settings to women with diabetes in pregnancy: perspectives of an educator. Diabetes Spectr 2016;29(2):101–4.
70. Mukona D, Munjanja SP, Zvinavashe M, et al. Barriers of adherence and possible solutions to nonadherence to antidiabetic therapy in women with diabetes in pregnancy: patients' perspective. J Diabetes Res 2017;2017:3578075.
71. Cundy T, Gamble G, Townend K, et al. Perinatal mortality in type 2 diabetes mellitus. Diabetic Med 2000;17(1):33–9.
72. Hamel MS, Werner EF. Interventions to improve rate of diabetes testing postpartum in women with gestational diabetes mellitus. Curr Diab Rep 2017;17(2):7.
73. Cardwell MS. Improving medical adherence in women with gestational diabetes through self-efficacy. Clin Diabetes 2013;31(3):110–5.
74. Littlefield CH, Craven JL, Rodin GM, et al. Relationship of self-efficacy and binging to adherence to diabetes regimen among adolescents. Diabetes care 1992;15(1):90–4.
75. Henry OA, Beischer NA. Long-term implications of gestational diabetes for the mother. Baillieres Clin Obstet Gynaecol 1991;5(2):461–83. https://doi.org/10.1016/s0950-3552(05)80107-5.
76. Muche AA, Olayemi OO, Gete YK. Effects of gestational diabetes mellitus on risk of adverse maternal outcomes: a prospective cohort study in Northwest Ethiopia. BMC Pregnancy Childbirth 2020;20(1):73.
77. Muhas C, Naseef P. A review article—gestational diabetes mellitus. Int J Curr Pharm Res 2017;9:1–5.
78. Seshiah V, Balaji V. Primordial prevention: maternal health and diabetes. Diabetes Management 2013;3(4):333.
79. Wahabi HA, Alzeidan RA, Esmaeil SA. Pre-pregnancy care for women with pregestational diabetes mellitus: a systematic review and meta-analysis. BMC Public health 2012;12(1):792.
80. Donazar-Ezcurra M, López-del Burgo C, Bes-Rastrollo M. Primary prevention of gestational diabetes mellitus through nutritional factors: a systematic review. BMC Pregnancy Childbirth 2017;17(1):30.
81. Dornhorst A, Merrin PK. Primary, secondary and tertiary prevention of non-insulin-dependent diabetes. Postgrad Med J 1994;70(826):529.
82. Ma RCW, Schmidt MI, Tam WH, et al. Clinical management of pregnancy in the obese mother: before conception, during pregnancy, and post partum. Lancet Diabetes Endocrinol 2016;4(12):1037–49.
83. Murphy H, Bell R, Dornhorst A, et al. Pregnancy in diabetes: challenges and opportunities for improving pregnancy outcomes. Diabetic Med 2018;35(3):292–9.
84. Tuomilehto J, Lindström J, Eriksson JG, et al. Prevention of type 2 diabetes mellitus by changes in lifestyle among subjects with impaired glucose tolerance. N Engl J Med 2001;344(18):1343–50.
85. Saaristo T, Moilanen L, Korpi-Hyövälti E, et al. Lifestyle intervention for prevention of type 2 diabetes in primary health care: one-year follow-up of the Finnish National Diabetes Prevention Program (FIN-D2D). Diabetes care 2010;33(10):2146–51.
86. Han S, Middleton P, Crowther CA. Exercise for pregnant women for preventing gestational diabetes mellitus. Cochrane Database Syst Rev 2012;(7):CD009021.
87. Erny-Albrecht K, Bywood PT, Oliver-Baxter J. The role of primary health care in primary and secondary prevention of diabetes. 2015. Available at: https://core.ac.uk/download/pdf/43335687.pdf.

88. Balaji V, Balaji M, Anjalakshi C, et al. Diagnosis of gestational diabetes mellitus in Asian-Indian women. Indian J Endocrinol Metab 2011;15(3):187.
89. Kayal A, Mohan V, Malanda B, et al. Women in India with Gestational Diabetes Mellitus Strategy (WINGS): methodology and development of model of care for gestational diabetes mellitus (WINGS 4). Indian J Endocrinol Metab 2016; 20(5):707.
90. Nielsen KK, Kapur A, Damm P, et al. From screening to postpartum follow-up–the determinants and barriers for gestational diabetes mellitus (GDM) services, a systematic review. BMC Pregnancy Childbirth 2014;14(1):41.
91. Daly N, Carroll C, Flynn I, et al. Evaluation of point-of-care maternal glucose measurements for the diagnosis of gestational diabetes mellitus. BJOG 2017;124(11): 1746–52.
92. Gallardo H, Lomelin-Gascon J, Martinez LA, et al. 1358-P: point of care OGTT for the screening of gestational diabetes: a feasible proposal for low-resource settings. Diabetes 2020;69(Supple):1358.

Characterizing Multimorbidity from Type 2 Diabetes

Insights from Clustering Approaches

Meryem Cicek, MPH[a],*,[1], James Buckley, MPH[b,c,1],
Jonathan Pearson-Stuttard, FRSPH[b,c], Edward W. Gregg, PhD[b,c]

KEYWORDS

- Type 2 diabetes mellitus • Multimorbidity • Clustering • Comorbidities
- Complications • Patterns • Population health • Risk stratification

KEY POINTS

- Patients with type 2 diabetes mellitus (T2DM) are at high risk of living with multiple co-occurring conditions.
- Clustering studies show common comorbidities in patients with T2DM are hypertension, lipid disorders, cardiovascular-related conditions (eg, coronary heart disease), microvascular conditions, and depression.
- Generally, individuals who are older, who are female, and who live in more deprived areas are at more risk of having T2DM-related multimorbidity.
- Applying clustering insights alongside other approaches can allow for risk stratification and guide implementation of interventions.
- Clinicians should consider the holistic health needs of individuals living with T2DM, particularly surrounding mental health.

INTRODUCTION
The Challenge of Type 2 Diabetes-Related Multimorbidity

Managing the rising prevalence of chronic conditions is a key challenge for health systems worldwide.[1] The co-occurrence of 2 or more chronic conditions is known as multimorbidity (**Box 1**) and is associated with reduced quality of life, impaired functional status, and increased burden on limited health care resources.[2,3] Multimorbidity is a

[a] Department of Primary Care and Public Health, School of Public Health, Imperial College London, Charing Cross Campus, Reynolds Building, St Dunstan's Road, London W6 8RP, UK;
[b] Department of Epidemiology and Biostatistics, School of Public Health, Imperial College London, Medical School Building, St Mary's Campus, Norfolk Place, London W2 1PG, UK; [c] MRC Centre for Environment and Health, School of Public Health, Imperial College London, Medical School Building, St Mary's Campus, Norfolk Place, London W2 1PG, UK
[1] Indicates joint first-authorship.
* Corresponding author.
E-mail address: meryem.cicek18@imperial.ac.uk

Endocrinol Metab Clin N Am 50 (2021) 531–558
https://doi.org/10.1016/j.ecl.2021.05.012 **endo.theclinics.com**
0889-8529/21/© 2021 The Authors. Published by Elsevier Inc. This is an open access article under the CC BY license (http://creativecommons.org/licenses/by/4.0/).

Box 1
Glossary of key terms

Comorbidity refers to a condition that co-occurs with another condition, with implied reference to an index condition.

Multimorbidity refers to the co-occurrence of 2 or more chronic conditions. The difference between comorbidity and multimorbidity is that the former requires an index condition to contextualize the condition, whereas the latter does not assign or differentiate importance on any 1 condition but considers the overall state of having multiple co-occurring conditions.

Concordant comorbidities are conditions that share a pathophysiologic pathway with the index condition of concern (eg, in the case of T2DM as an index condition, a concordant complication is chronic kidney disease or liver disease).

Discordant comorbidities are conditions that do not share a currently known pathophysiologic pathway with the index condition of concern (eg, in the case of T2DM as index condition, a discordant complication is osteoarthritis).

Cluster analyses are statistical approaches that aim to assign a set of objects (or data points) into a defined number of groups, known as clusters, so that objects in the same group possess more similar traits than other objects in other groups.

---

growing problem not only for high-income countries (HICs) but also for low- and middle-income countries (LMICs) who make up 77% of global deaths due to non-communicable diseases, of which 85% are premature deaths.[4] Some pooled prevalence estimates of global multimorbidity reveal that currently HICs have the highest prevalence (37.9%), whereas LMICs follow closely behind (29.7%)[5] and are expected to increase over the following years.[6] By 2035, approximately 17% of the UK population is projected to have 4 or more chronic conditions, almost double the prevalence (9.8%) in 2018.[7] Previous studies have revealed social inequalities in multimorbidity, demonstrating earlier onset of multiple chronic conditions in patients living in the most deprived areas compared with the most affluent.[8,9] This global progression in emerging multimorbidity will have widespread implications for patients, health systems, and governments.

Patients with diabetes are more likely to develop multiple conditions compared with those without diabetes.[10] This greater risk reflects the fundamental impact that extended exposure to elevated glucose and insulin resistance have on multiple organ systems, most notably through its effects on microvasculature, macrovasculature, and immune response. These effects in people with type 2 diabetes mellitus (T2DM) lead to an approximate doubling of risk for myocardial infarction, a 5-fold increased risk of renal failure, and more than a 10-fold increased risk of amputation and blindness.[11] However, the impact on multiple conditions is also partly due to declining mortalities, increased life expectancy, and differing trends in cause-specific mortality, leading to a diversification in cause of death and complications.[12] Thus, even in the face of declining risk of complications over time, people with T2DM live longer to experience more events and more conditions contributing to multimorbidity. The rising number of young people with T2DM is of particular concern, as earlier onset leads to a longer duration of disease and consequently more years lived with a greater risk for developing other conditions.[13] Early onset of T2DM can lead to a more disruptive natural history and worsened quality of life,[14] consequently, having adverse societal effects on labor markets and significant productivity losses.[15,16] This review aims to explore how the commonly reported clusters of T2DM-related multimorbidity are characterized in the current literature.

Shifting the Morbidity Discourse

Historically, health systems have viewed single conditions in siloes as opposed to focusing on the holistic health needs of patients. Similarly, research to identify risk factors and effective prevention and treatment approaches has generally focused on single disease processes, posing challenges in the areas of multimorbidity surveillance, effective interventions, and the interface between care pathways. Thus, most health systems are not fully designed nor sufficiently equipped to provide tailored care to patients with multiple conditions.[17] However, greater awareness and concern about multimorbidity have led to an emerging literature, moving away from simply counting conditions to instead measuring impact on patients and systems.[18,19] Therefore, it is essential that multimorbidity research aims to consider all stages of the life course and focus on complex health states where the burden of multiple conditions is greater than the sum of its parts.[20]

There are far-reaching impacts of T2DM-related multimorbidity, which have implications not only for patients but also for families, community, and the health system (**Fig. 1**). Multimorbidity leads to multifaceted demands at the health system level; increased and sustained interactions with health care providers,[3] adverse events owing to polypharmacy, and nonoptimally integrated care pathways all contribute to the complexity of planning care for multimorbid patients.[21] This complexity calls for a multitiered approach guided by research that first seeks to understand the patterns

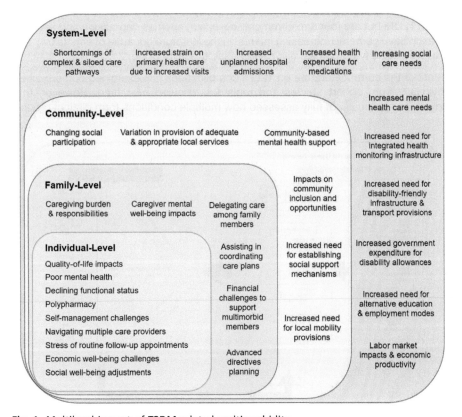

Fig. 1. Multilevel impact of T2DM-related multimorbidity.

of conditions that characterize multimorbidity, the implications for treatments, and how they change over time.

Development of Type 2 Diabetes Mellitus–Related Multimorbidity

Risk factors of T2DM are shared with other non-communicable diseases, such as vascular conditions and cancers, which can increase the risk of developing further comorbidities. For example, the overlap of risk factors, such as obesity and dyslipidemia, means individuals with T2DM are at higher risk for cardiovascular complications.[22–24] The progression to a multimorbid state is dependent on the contributions of many distal and proximal factors within the wider system context, which can occur at any stage and severity of T2DM (**Fig. 2**).

Comorbidities contributing to T2DM-related multimorbidity are both systemic yet heterogenous and can be classified as the following:

a. **Traditional** complications include microvascular (eg, retinopathy, nephropathy, neuropathy) and macrovascular (eg, heart disease, stroke, peripheral vascular disease) conditions.[25]
b. **Nontraditional** concordant comorbidities share common risk factors and pathophysiologic pathways but have not traditionally been considered part of T2DM sequelae, such as liver disease and cancers[10,26] (see **Box 1**), in part because they are less specific or have a lower magnitude of association with T2DM compared with traditional complications.
c. **Emerging discordant** comorbidities do not, at present, have a clear etiologic link with T2DM but are found to commonly co-occur, such as depression and asthma, which have garnered increasing interest in the literature because of effects on mortality, morbidity outcomes, and health-related quality of life.[26,27]

Most of the current literature on T2DM complications has examined comorbidities individually from cohort studies and registries followed over time. However, this body of literature has not fully assessed how multiple conditions form distinct groups

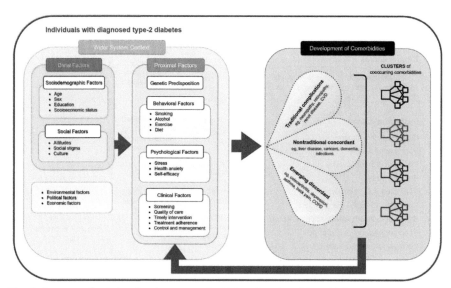

Fig. 2. Framework of the development of T2DM-related multimorbidity.

and patterns of co-occurrence, and over time. Thus, to inform this synthesis, the authors have conducted a systematic review of the selected studies that have examined the association of T2DM with clusters of multimorbidity. These patterns can be identified using population-based analytical approaches, such as cluster analyses (see **Box 1**), on T2DM patients.

METHODS

This review aimed to identify population-based observational studies with a focus on T2DM among adults as the index condition, and that produced some type of cluster or grouping in their results. The authors identified 1714 records from Ovid EMBASE, Ovid Medline, Ovid Global Health, Web of Science, and Cochrane databases from January 2000 to August 2020. Studies that simply listed a few limited preselected comorbidities without any indication of clustering or grouping were excluded. After multiple rounds of screening (**Fig. 3**), 91 studies were fully read, leaving 12 eligible studies.

RESULTS

The final 12 studies included came from varying HIC settings except for 2 conducted in China[28,29] and adopted a range of different methods that varied in analytical statistical

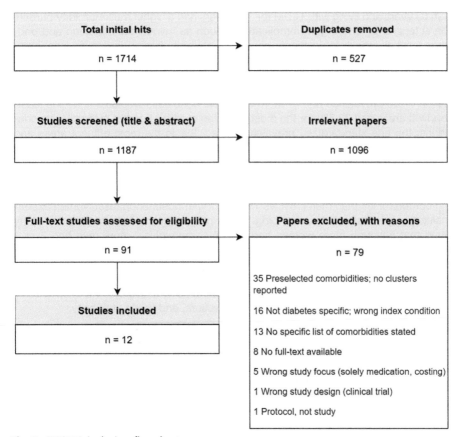

Fig. 3. PRISMA inclusion flowchart.

depth (**Table 1**). From the sample, the earliest study was conducted in 2012,[30] with most of the remaining studies produced after 2015.

As the format of the study results was heterogenous, owing to the varied methods used, the authors have summarized studies by 2 broad categories: (a) those employing combination groupings of co-occurring conditions (ie, pairs and triads) to define multimorbidity (**Table 2**); and (b) those studies of more complex statistical clustering methods (**Table 3**). The key clustering approaches used in the reviewed studies included agglomerative[24,31] and divisive[32] hierarchical clustering,[28] latent class analysis,[29,33] and graph theory,[34] all of which require substantially large health data sets. Moreover, novel machine learning approaches have been used to characterize and learn multimorbidity patterns,[35,36] but these methods are yet to be applied to T2DM specifically. Although the study approaches and settings were varied, predictors and predominant groups of conditions across clusters were identified and are discussed in the following sections.

Who Is at Risk of Type 2 Diabetes Mellitus–Related Multimorbidity?

Age and deprivation are the leading drivers of multimorbidity, as the prevalence and number of comorbidities increase with older age in patients with T2DM.[28,33,37] For example, the proportion of those with "complex" multimorbidity, defined as 4+ comorbidities, increases from 25% among persons less than 65 years to 42% among those aged 65 to 74 years, and 49% among those 75+ years of age.[37] Patients older than 65 years and living with T2DM for 10+ years had a higher multimorbidity burden, characterized by end-organ complications, such as myocardial infarction and end-stage renal disease.[33] Interestingly, clusters containing obesity were much more common in younger adults compared with those older than 65 years.[38] Increasing deprivation level was strongly and consistently associated with an increasing proportion of patients with T2DM and a greater number of concurrent comorbidities[31]; the age-standardized prevalence of 1 or more comorbid conditions was 33.3% for the least-deprived areas and 32.7% for the most-deprived areas.[24] For 4 or more chronic conditions, the age-standardized prevalence was 2.9% in the most affluent areas and 4.4% in the most deprived areas.[24]

Women have a proportionally greater burden of multimorbidity than their male counterparts in some studies,[24,29,31,33] although the magnitude of this association is modest and inconsistent. A greater proportion of women presented with 4+ co-occurring comorbidities than men (18% vs 15.9%),[31] with postmenopausal women experiencing the greatest risk of developing further comorbidities.[29] However, a US study found that although more women had 1 or 2 comorbidities, more men had 3 or 4 comorbidities.[37] In addition, there was little effect of sex on comorbidity number among patients aged 65+.[39]

Studies of T2DM-related multimorbidity clustering have not yet examined the relationship with common physiologic risk factors commonly associated with T2DM complications, such as elevated HbA1c, blood pressure, and levels of obesity.

How Are Type 2 Diabetes Mellitus–Related Multimorbidity Clusters Characterized?

Most reviewed studies were cross-sectional in nature, characterizing multimorbidity among patients at a specific point in time, with some studying patients with varying duration of T2DM. Across studies, 3 types of condition clusters appeared consistently, namely, (a) cardiometabolic precursor conditions, (b) vascular conditions, and (c) mental health conditions.

Across 6 diverse study settings, cardiometabolic precursor conditions, such as disorders of lipid metabolism, obesity, and hypertension, were the most common conditions at diagnosis.[24,32,37–39] Hypertension was consistently the most common condition in multimorbid combinations and clusters.[24,31,32,37–39] In individuals with 2 comorbid conditions in addition to T2DM, hypertension was commonly found alongside hyperlipidemia (67.5%),[37] arthritis (20%), and anxiety (6.8%).[37,39] Among individuals with 3 conditions in addition to T2DM, 51% had some combination of hypertension, hyperlipidemia, and obesity.[38]

The authors identified similar clusters of conditions that predominantly contained concordant cardiovascular and microvascular conditions usually associated with later-stage disease, such as coronary heart disease (CHD), stroke, atrial fibrillation, peripheral vascular disease (PVD), and chronic kidney disease (CKD).[24,28,29,31] Cardiovascular conditions were the most prevalent comorbidity type at diagnosis (64%)[30] and constituted the second most prevalent triad alongside hypertension.[39] These results were consistent across different clustering methodologies, with a study applying novel graph theory techniques to hospital admissions finding a distinct cluster of cardiovascular-related conditions, including cardiac arrythmias and CHD.[34] Three conditions, namely hypertension, CHD, and acute cerebrovascular disease, formed a comprehensive multimorbid web with T2DM.[28] These conditions were the most common comorbidities of T2DM, and conversely, the other way around whereby T2DM was also the most common comorbidity of each of these conditions.[28,30] This web demonstrates a bidirectional, mutually reinforcing association between these conditions and T2DM.

Several studies exhibited distinct clusters containing mainly mental health conditions.[24,31,33,34] In an English cohort, a cluster composed of depression, severe mental illness, chronic obstructive pulmonary disease, and asthma was observed regardless of duration lived with T2DM,[24] and with more prominent representation among women.[24,33] Specifically, Seng and colleagues[33] found that younger women formed a distinct cluster with high psychiatric disease burden, including anxiety, major depression, schizophrenia, and bipolar disorder, whereas an Australian study found a similar cluster predominantly containing conditions such as depression, psychoses, and substance abuse, along with liver disease.[34]

How Does Multimorbidity Vary According to Duration of Type 2 Diabetes Mellitus?

There was a clear lack of longitudinal cohort-based multimorbidity studies that tracked specific patients over time. Rather, the few studies that considered some element of time stratified patients by the duration lived of T2DM at the time of study. A cluster of older patients with moderate to long T2DM duration were found to have high disease burden with end-organ complications, for example, myocardial infarction, end-stage renal disease, stroke, and amputation.[33] This finding was consistent with findings by Gao and colleagues,[29] as longer T2DM duration and older age were associated with a higher prevalence of all comorbidities. Cluster analysis at 2, 5, and 9 years post-T2DM diagnosis revealed a diversification of conditions as T2DM progresses.[24] This finding was demonstrated by an increase in the number and heterogeneity of clusters formed, departing from the previously distinct body systems found in clusters of earlier duration, for example, closer clustering of depression and asthma at 9 years after diagnosis compared with at diagnosis.[24] Hypertension consistently appeared in the top combination duos of conditions at both 2 and 5 years after diagnosis of T2DM alongside CKD (15.4%, 17.8%), CHD (10.3%, 11.3%), atrial fibrillation (7.5%, 8.7%), stroke (6.9%, 8.0%), and across age stratifications (**Fig. 4**).[24] Interestingly, out of all the chronic comorbidities, hypertension had the highest incidence density in the year before T2DM diagnosis (75.2 new cases per 1000 patient-years), but decreased significantly at 5 years after diagnosis (42.6 new cases per 1000 patient-years).[30]

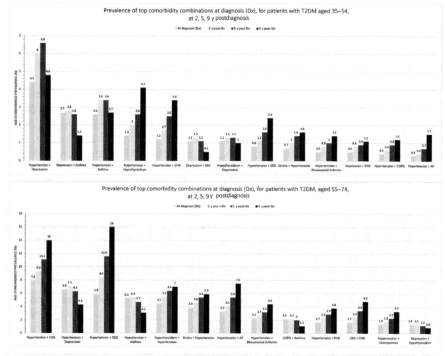

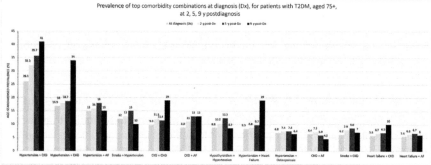

Fig. 4. Prevalence of top comorbidity combinations at diagnosis for patients with T2DM. Prevalence of top comorbidity combinations at diagnosis (Dx), for patients with T2DM at 2, 5, 9 years after diagnosis for 3 age bands. AF, atrial fibrillation; COPD, chronic obstructive pulmonary disease; SMI, severe mental illness. (*Adapted from* Nowakowska M, Zghebi SS, Ashcroft DM, et al. The comorbidity burden of type 2 diabetes mellitus: patterns, clusters and predictions from a large English primary care cohort. BMC Med 2019;17(1):145; with permission.)

What Is the Impact on Health Care Utilization?

Patients with diabetes have high rates of hospitalization, more complex hospital trajectories, with more transitions between other conditions, and double the number of "admission sequences" compared with patients without diabetes.[34] Moreover, rates of health care utilization are disproportionately higher in T2DM patients with mental health comorbidities than those without.[33,40] Seng and colleagues[33] found that the use of tertiary health care was highest among (a) "younger females with short to moderate T2DM duration and high psychiatric disease burden" and (b) "older patients with moderate to long T2DM duration and high disease burden with end-organ complications."[33] Compared with healthy patients, the risk of emergency department visits was 3.31 times higher for group (a) and 2.47 times higher for group (b).

Having a mental comorbidity was significantly and independently associated with a 1.25 times increased risk of being admitted to hospital, 1.30 times as likely to use emergency and specialist care, and 1.17 times as likely to visit the general practitioner compared with only having physical concordant comorbidities.[40] This finding highlights the amplified effect of mental comorbidities on health care utilization for multimorbid patients with T2DM.

Overall, the reviewed studies demonstrated that:

- The multimorbidity clusters were dominated by conditions directly related to T2DM pathogenesis, for example, hypertension, disorders of lipid metabolism, and obesity, often considered risk factors for other comorbidities.[24,28,31,32,37,38]
- Across several studies, concordant vascular-related conditions frequently appeared in clusters[24,28,29,31] and combination groupings,[30,37,38] such as CHD, PVD, stroke, and CKD.
- Four studies demonstrated distinct clusters of mental health comorbidities, such as depression and anxiety,[31,34] with particularly elevated prevalence among younger women.[24,33]
- As the duration of T2DM increases, clusters demonstrate increased heterogeneity departing from clusters previously belonging to distinct body systems, which indicates diversification of multimorbidity at progressive intervals.[24]
- Health care utilization rates are high among multimorbid patients with T2DM,[34] especially among those with mental health comorbidities.[33,40]

DISCUSSION

In this first-ever review of the findings of epidemiologic studies focusing on T2DM-related multimorbidity clustering, the authors found common comorbidities of T2DM to be hypertension, cardiovascular-related diseases, microvascular conditions, depression, and lipid disorders. Their findings indicate that generally T2DM individuals who are older, female, and more deprived are at a higher risk of having T2DM-related multimorbidity.

Concordant comorbidities, such as hypertension and cardiovascular and microvascular conditions, dominated clusters across the studies, agreeing with global trends in T2DM complications[27] and novel nonclustering studies.[41] Hypertension was the most central condition, indicating it was an important mediator of connections between other conditions, seen across various subgroups.[41] This finding is consistent with the long-standing literature that hypertension is the key driver in the development of cardiovascular and microvascular conditions. Given the highly prevalent co-occurrence of hypertension and other precursor conditions, such as obesity and lipid disorders, and their established roles as drivers of vascular morbidity and mortality, it is important to focus on these as key risk factors in the control and management of T2DM and related multimorbidity. In the case of PVD, prolonged time spent with hypertension can worsen downstream microvascular conditions, such as retinopathy and foot ulcers, which are often irreversible and should be the focus of secondary prevention programs.[28]

Although concordant comorbidities, such as hypertension and hyperlipidemia, are central to T2DM-related multimorbidity, discordant comorbidities, such as depression and osteoarthritis, can have a direct adverse effect on self-care behaviors.[26] Specifically, mental health disorders may have effects on T2DM self-management, quality of life, and subsequent control of overlapping risk factors, such as diet and physical activity.[42] As these findings indicate, depression is frequently associated with T2DM-related multimorbidity consistent with epidemiologic research that demonstrates the increasing prevalence of comorbid depression in T2DM populations globally.[27,43,44] The association of T2DM with depression is likely to be bidirectional and involving common hormonal and inflammatory pathways.[45] The concurrence of both physical conditions and mental health disorders has been associated with significantly worse health outcomes, compared with those without comorbid mental illness[42]; this indicates a need to adopt a more holistic approach to managing T2DM-related multimorbidity, such that deterioration in mental health can be detected early to prevent further morbidity burden.

Challenges Within the Field of Type 2 Diabetes Mellitus–Related Multimorbidity

The identification of multimorbidity clusters serves several purposes. First, it allows for the descriptive characterization of multimorbidity in populations in a way that takes into account a comprehensive spectrum of conditions; second, it identifies subsets of the population that may be driving demands on health systems; and third, it provides clues to the diverse etiologic pathways of T2DM-related morbidity. However, this review exposes several challenges and gaps in this rapidly evolving literature on T2DM-related multimorbidity.

First, the current literature does not provide clear distinction of the temporality or sequence of phenotypes of multimorbidity and clustering. Specific temporal trends in T2DM-related multimorbidity are yet to be studied in more population-based settings,[28] as reviewed studies were largely cross-sectional. In addition, concordant conditions are likely to have an inflated coprevalence with T2DM because of care-related factors; for example, clinicians will be more attentive for T2DM in a patient that has myocardial infarction.[30] Second, it is difficult to infer the magnitude of association and risk of different forms of multimorbidity. Traditional definitions of multimorbidity rely on counts of conditions[18] and do not normally consider important factors, such as the burden of the disease, severity, and the interaction between conditions, as this is reflected in most of the reviewed studies that predominantly report on counts or prevalence. Third, the heterogeneity of methodologic approaches, data inputs, and condition classifications makes comparisons across studies difficult. Cluster analysis itself is an exploratory classification method, and different algorithms can yield different results.[31] These limitations have made for difficult interpretation, and translation of findings into meaningful clinical applications.

Future Direction: Longitudinal Clustering

To make this literature more useful and interpretable for clinical and public health practice, adoption of specific reporting guidelines across cluster analyses[46]; the application of such techniques to a variety of low-income settings; and the advancement of clustering research toward more longitudinal progression-focused exploratory approaches utilizing the advances of machine learning should be considered.[35] A shift from a prevalence-based to an incidence-based epidemiologic approach guided by etiologic medical literature will reveal the trajectories of multimorbidity rather than patterns conflated by risk factors accrued earlier in the patient journey. Such approaches are crucial to reveal temporal associations, to estimate population preventable fractions, and to identify leverage points whereby an intervention can have a greater magnitude of effect in multimorbid patients compared to a more downstream intervention.

Clinical Applications: Stratification and Holistic Care

As further work identifies risk patterns for multimorbidity among subpopulation groups, T2DM populations could be stratified according to the risk of developing multimorbidity, dominant clusters of conditions in order to implement specific preventative measures. For instance, the authors' findings show it is important to prioritize dementia screening for patients with longer T2DM duration, and depression, specifically for younger women.[24,33] Alongside mental health conditions, identifying and managing other prominent comorbidities have the potential to reduce polypharmacy burden through control of common risk factors and to optimize treatment pathways via reductions in fragmented care.[10,40] Targeting central conditions (eg, hypertension and obesity), themselves risk factors for a host of other conditions, can realign care provisions beyond a traditional single disease focus.

SUMMARY

T2DM-related multimorbidity is complex and exhibits variation in different study populations. Common comorbidities in patients with T2DM are hypertension, lipid disorders, cardiovascular-related conditions (eg, CHD), microvascular conditions, and depression. Patients with T2DM that are older, female, and more deprived are generally at higher risk of developing multimorbidity. Clinicians should be increasingly aware of the more heterogeneous needs of individuals living with T2DM, particularly surrounding mental health. Future research is needed to explore more granular patient trajectories, their associated risk factors, and population-level temporal trends to further both clinical delivery and public health planning purposes.

CLINICS CARE POINTS

- *Patient stratification is key to tackling multimorbidity at the clinical level:* a preventative approach to detecting and monitoring specific comorbidities with high likelihood in particular demographic segments, for example, development of risk scores to guide timely intervention for delaying end-stage organ complications like renal failure or myocardial infarction in middle-aged patients with chronic kidney disease or cardiovascular disease, respectively.

- *Research to assess suitability of a depression and/or dementia screening program for patients with type 2 diabetes mellitus:* increased provision of screening for depression among younger adults, particularly women, and dementia for patients with longer type 2 diabetes mellitus duration is perhaps a crucial component in curbing the severity of type 2 diabetes mellitus–related multimorbidity.

- *Holistic and dynamic clinical treatment and management:* important to focus management of concordant type 2 diabetes mellitus comorbidities through common risk factors (eg, hypertension and hyperlipidemia) and account for patients' behavioral risk factors (eg, exercise, diet, smoking) and living contexts (eg, the effect of deprivation) for more holistic care.

DISCLOSURE

J. Pearson-Stuttard is vice-chairman of the Royal Society for Public Health and reports personal fees from Novo Nordisk A/S and Lane Clark & Peacock LLP outside of the submitted work. All other authors have nothing to disclose. This work has been funded by the Medical Research Council (MRC) UK, grant number MR/V005057/1.

Table 1
Characteristics of all included studies

Study Title	First Author, y	Study Design	Setting	n	Study Aim	Data Source	Measures/Outputs
Combination groupings							
Global health care use by patients with type 2 diabetes: does the type of comorbidity matter?	Calderón-Larrañaga et al,[40] 2015	Longitudinal retrospective cohort study; negative binomial regression	Spain	65,716	To identify patterns of health care use among T2DM patients with multimorbidities	Primary care EHRs and the Hospital Minimum Basic Dataset (CMBD in Spanish)	IRR for health care use outcomes for each level of care: primary (no. of visits), specialist (no. of visits, no. of specialities visited), hospital (total and unplanned admissions, length of stay), emergency (no. of visits, no. of priority visits)
Comorbidity Burden and Health Services Use in Community-Living Older Adults with Diabetes Mellitus: A Retrospective Cohort Study	Gruneir et al,[39] 2016	Retrospective cohort study	Canada	448,736	To examine comorbidity and its association with various health services among community-dwelling older adults with T2DM	Multiple linked population-based administrative databases (demographic, hospital, ambulatory, insurance, medication, home care)	Prevalence of number, type, and combinations (of 1, 2, 3) of comorbidities Frequencies of 1-y use of health services (physician visits, emergency department visits, inpatient hospital admissions, home care use, nursing home admissions)

Study	First author, year	Study design	Country	N	Objective	Data source	Outcomes
Prevalence and coprevalence of comorbidities among patients with type 2 diabetes mellitus	Iglay et al,[37] 2016	Retrospective cohort study	USA	1,389,016	To quantify the prevalence and coprevalence of comorbidities among T2DM patients	Quintiles electronic medical record	Prevalence and coprevalence of comorbidities
Multiple chronic conditions in type 2 diabetes mellitus: prevalence and consequences	Lin et al,[38] 2015	Cross-sectional study; logistic regression	USA	161,174	To examine multiple chronic comorbidity (MCC) patterns among T2DM patients and identify comorbidity clusters associated with poor patient outcomes	Deidentified EHRs dataset from health care informatics company, Optum Humedica	Prevalence of MCC clusters among younger and older than age 65 y; Predicted probabilities for diabetes outcomes (face-to-face visits, reaching glycated hemoglobin <8%) and health care outcomes (emergency visits, 30-d hospital readmission), for top 15 clusters
Prevalence and incidence density rates of chronic comorbidity in type 2 diabetes patients: an exploratory cohort study	Luijks,[30] 2012	Longitudinal exploratory cohort study	Netherlands	714	To establish comorbidity rates in a primary-care population of patients with T2DM	Primary-care network: Continuous Morbidity Registration	Prevalence and incidence density rates of comorbidities and their clusters before, during, and after diabetes diagnosis (post-1, 5, 10 y)

(continued on next page)

Table 1
(continued)

Study Title	First Author, y	Study Design	Setting	n	Study Aim	Data Source	Measures/Outputs
Statistical clustering							
Multimorbidity in people with type 2 diabetes in the Basque Country (Spain): prevalence, comorbidity clusters, and comparison with other chronic patients	Alonso-Morán et al,[31] 2015	Retrospective cohort study; agglomerative hierarchical clustering, logistic regression	Spain	1,473,937	To compare multimorbidity among patients with and without T2DM and identify disease clusters in T2DM patients	Primary care EHRs and the Hospital Minimum Basic Dataset (CMBD in Spanish)	Prevalence of no. of comorbidities and probabilities of having at least 1 comorbidity by age/sex/ deprivation OR of having each of 51 chronic comorbidities with T2DM, and morbidity clusters of concurrently occurring conditions
Comorbidity in Adult Patients Hospitalized with Type 2 Diabetes in Northeast China: An Analysis of Hospital Discharge Data from 2002 to 2013	Chen et al,[28] 2016	Longitudinal retrospective cohort study; hierarchical clustering	China	4,400,892	To evaluate comorbidity burden and patterns among hospitalized T2DM patients	EHR database	Prevalence of comorbidities by age/sex ACoR and RCoR of comorbidities co-occurring with T2DM. Clusters of comorbidities based on RCoRs
Latent class analysis suggests 4 classes of persons with type 2 diabetes mellitus based	Gao et al,[29] 2017	Cross-sectional study; latent class analysis, multinomial logistic regression	China	5500	To classify persons with T2DM based on complications and comorbidities	Structured questionnaire of patients across 10 hospitals	Predicted probabilities of T2DM complications and comorbidities, to produce 4 classes OR of the

Title	Author, Year	Study design	Country	Sample	Aim	Data source	Outcome
on complications and comorbidities in Tianjin, China: a cross-sectional analysis							association between class membership and various demographic factors, diabetes severity, and behavioral factors
Comorbidity network for chronic disease: a novel approach to understand type 2 diabetes progression	Khan et al,[34] 2018	Health informatics study; graph theory and social network analysis	Australia	749,000	To understand the comorbidity pattern of T2DM and develop a research framework to model chronic disease progression in terms of comorbidity	Administrative private health care dataset with ICD-10 diagnosis codes on hospital admission and discharge data	Modularity score and network node strength to produce comorbidity network of T2DM
The comorbidity burden of type 2 diabetes mellitus: patterns, clusters, and predictions from a large English primary care cohort	Nowakowska et al,[24] 2019	Longitudinal retrospective cohort study; agglomerative hierarchical clustering	England	102,394	To quantify comorbidity patterns in people with T2DM, to estimate the prevalence of 6 chronic conditions in 2027 and to identify clusters of similar conditions	UK Clinical Practice Research Datalink health dataset linked with Index of Multiple Deprivation data	Crude and age-standardized prevalence of comorbidities, and their clusters at T2DM diagnosis and 2, 5, 9 y after diagnosis, by sex and deprivation

(continued on next page)

Table 1
(continued)

Study Title	First Author, y	Study Design	Setting	n	Study Aim	Data Source	Measures/Outputs
Differential Health Care Use, Diabetes-Related Complications, and Mortality Among Five Unique Classes of Patients with Type 2 Diabetes in Singapore: A Latent Class Analysis of 71,125 Patients	Seng et al,[33] 2020 [32]	Retrospective cohort study; latent class analysis, negative binomial, and Cox regressions	Singapore	71,125	To segment T2DM patients into distinct classes and evaluate their differential health care use, complications, and mortality patterns	Ministry of Health administrative database	5 classes of patients produced Frequencies of comorbidities by demographic factors. IRR of complications, health care use outcomes, and 4-y all-cause mortality among the classes
Identifying Subgroups of Type II Diabetes Patients using Cluster Analysis	Solomon et al, 2017	Retrospective cohort study; hierarchical clustering using DIANA	USA	6250	To uncover correlations between demographic subgroups of T2DM patients and their comorbidities, among a predominantly African American population	Inpatient EHRs from Howard University	Comorbidity clusters of 2, 3, 4, 5 by distinct patient group characteristics based on sex and marital status

Abbreviations: ACoR, absolute co-occurrence risk; DIANA, divisive analysis; EHR, electronic health record; GP, general practice; ICD, *International Classification of Diseases;* ID, incidence density; IRR, incidence rate ratio; MCC, multiple chronic comorbidities; OR, odds ratio; RCoR, relative co-occurrence risk.

Table 2
Summary of results from studies adopting combination groupings

Study Title	First Author, y	Grouping Method	Grouping Pattern	Key Quantitative Outcomes
Global health care use by patients with type 2 diabetes: does the type of comorbidity matter?	Calderón-Larrañaga et al,[40] 2015	EDC used[a]	4 mutually exclusive groups: 1. Individuals with no chronic comorbidities 2. Individuals with only concordant comorbidities 3. Individuals with at least 1 discordant physical comorbidity excluding those with mental comorbidities 4. Individuals with at least 1 mental comorbidity	The mean number of chronic comorbidities was higher in patients with mental comorbidity (5.5) compared with those with discordant physical comorbidity (4.1) or only concordant comorbidity (1.7) Within the groups of patients with discordant and mental comorbidity, 85.3% and 87.1% had at least 1 concordant comorbidity and 2.8% and 1.3% had >3 concordant comorbidities, respectively
Comorbidity Burden and Health Services Use in Community-Living Older Adults with Diabetes Mellitus: A Retrospective Cohort Study	Gruneir et al,[39] 2016	EDC used[a]	Top 3 pairs of comorbid conditions: 1. Arthritis + hypertension (20.0%) 2. Other CVD conditions + hypertension (10.6%) 3. Disorders of lipid metabolism + hypertension (10.0%) Top 3 triads of comorbid conditions: 1. Arthritis + other CVD conditions + hypertension (9.9%), 2. Arthritis + disorders of lipid metabolism + hypertension (7.1%) 3. Arthritis + anxiety + hypertension (6.2%)	>90% of both men and women had at least 1 comorbid condition and more than 40% had 5+ conditions Hypertension was most common condition across all age groups, affecting 79.1% of the entire cohort. Arthritis affected 59.6% of the cohort, and other CVD conditions affected 59.3% 3 additional conditions affected more than one-third of the cohort: ischemic heart disease (37.6%), anxiety (36.9%), and disorders of lipid metabolism (33.7%)

(continued on next page)

Table 2
(continued)

Study Title	First Author, y	Grouping Method	Grouping Pattern	Key Quantitative Outcomes
Prevalence and co-prevalence of comorbidities among patients with type 2 diabetes mellitus	Iglay et al,[37] 2016	Ranking of prevalence and coprevalence of comorbidities, assessed using *ICD-9-CM*	Top 5 pairs of comorbid conditions: 1. Hypertension and hyperlipidemia (67.5%) 2. Obesity and hypertension (66.0%) 3. Obesity and hyperlipidemia (62.5%) 4. Hypertension and CKD (22.4%) 5. Hyperlipidemia and CKD (21.1%)	In those <65 y of age, only 12.4% of patients had CKD, but this increased to 27.7% in those 65–74 y and 43.2% in those 75+ y Due to the higher prevalence of obesity in those aged <65, obesity and hypertension (66.1%) were the most common comorbidity pair For patients aged 65+, the highest coprevalence was for the combination of hypertension and hyperlipidemia (65–74 y: 76.2%; 75+ y: 75.2%)
Multiple chronic conditions in type 2 diabetes mellitus: prevalence and consequences	Lin et al,[38] 2015	Prevalence-driven groupings: prevalence rate of each comorbid condition examined, and *t* tests used to compare prevalence between patients aged <65 and ≥65 y. For analysis of MCCs, the most prevalent comorbidities that affected ≥5% of the sample were prioritized	Ranked combinations: 1. Obesity-hyperlipidemia-hypertension (19%) 2. Hyperlipidemia-hypertension (17%) 3. Obesity-hyperlipidemia (4%) 4. Obes-hyperlipidemia-hypertension-CAD (2.5%) 5. Hyperlipidemia-hypertension-CAD (2.5%) 6. Obesity-hyperlipidemia-hypertension-COPD/asthma (1.5%) 7. Obesity-hyperlipidemia-hypertension-Arthritis (1.5%)	Overall, 51% had some combination of hypertension, hyperlipidemia and obesity Clusters including obesity were far more common among younger adults (aged <65 y); the leading MCC cluster was hypertension-hyperlipidemia-obesity (23%), whereas among older adults (aged ≥65 y), the most common cluster was hypertension and hyperlipidemia only (20%) 14% of younger patients had no diagnosed comorbidities, compared with 11% of older patients. Older patients exhibited greater cluster heterogeneity; the top 10 clusters accounted for a smaller proportion of older adults (66%) than younger adults (78%)

| Prevalence and incidence density rates of chronic comorbidity in type 2 diabetes patients: an exploratory cohort study | Luijks et al,[30] 2012 | Comorbid diseases were classified into clusters, according to the diagnostic chapters of ICPC-1 | Prevalent disease groups at T2DM diagnosis: Cardiovascular (64.0%) Musculoskeletal (31.1%) Mental (24.1%) Urogenital (15.4%) Respiratory (14.1%) Skin (9.9%) | 15.4% of patients did not have a chronic comorbidity at diabetes diagnosis. 27.2% had 3+ discordant comorbidities Ear and eye diseases (particularly cataract) had a high incident density rate after diabetes diagnosis compared with before diagnosis 46.9 per 1000 patient-years 26.4% of those without any chronic condition at time of diabetes diagnosis developed at least 1 comorbidity in the first subsequent year |

Abbreviations: CAD, coronary artery disease; COPD, chronic obstructive pulmonary disease; CVD, cardiovascular disease; EDC, expanded diagnostic clusters; ICD-9-CM, *International Classification of Diseases, Ninth Revision, Clinical Modification; ICPC-1, International Classification of Primary Care, First Version;* MCC, multiple chronic comorbidities.

ᵃ The EDC is internationally validated and groups *ICPC* and *ICD* codes into 260 clusters based on clinical, diagnostic, and therapeutic similarities.

Table 3
Summary of results from studies adopting statistical clustering

Study Title	First Author, y	Clustering Method	Clustering Pattern	Key Quantitative Outcomes
Multimorbidity in people with type 2 diabetes in the Basque Country(Spain): prevalence, comorbidity clusters and comparison with other chronic patients	Alonso-Morán et al,[31] 2015	Agglomerative hierarchical clustering (Ward's minimum-variance method)	Cluster A: concordant diseases directly T2DM-related (hypertension, IHD, AF, other chronic heart diseases, CKD, heart failure) Cluster B: mental illnesses (anxiety and depression) Cluster C: digestive, bone and joint diseases (dyspepsia, degenerative joint disease, low back pain, osteoporosis, diverticular intestine disease, rheumatoid arthritis, autoimmune and connective tissue diseases) Cluster D: vision diseases (glaucoma, blindness, low vision) Cluster E: respiratory diseases (asthma, emphysema, chronic bronchitis, COPD)	OR of the comorbidity co-occurrence with T2DM: PVD (2.24), heart failure (2.0), hypertension (1.97), CKD (1.83), transplant status (1.75), chronic liver disease (1.65) Prevalence of having: 1+ comorbidity (89.7% overall, [87.6% of men, 92% of women]); 3+ comorbidities (46.5%); 10+ comorbidities (1.7% of men, 1.9% of women)
Comorbidity in Adult Patients Hospitalized with Type 2 Diabetes in Northeast China: An Analysis of Hospital Discharge Data from 2002 to 2013	Chen et al,[28] 2016	Hierarchical clustering (Ward's minimum-variance method with Euclidean distance measure) ACoR[a] and RCoR[b] calculated for each condition. Major T2DM-related comorbidities were defined as having both ACoR >1% and RCoR >1 27 major comorbidities clustered into 3 categories with high,	a. High RCoR group: • Essential hypertension: peripheral & visceral atherosclerosis • Disorders of lipid metabolism: chronic renal failure • Occlusion or stenosis of precerebral artery: urinary tract infections	Overall, essential hypertension was the most common comorbidity with ACoR of 58.4%, whereas peripheral and visceral atherosclerosis had the strongest association with T2DM with RCoR of 4.206 Dyslipidemia was the second most severe comorbidity with RCoR of 3.447 (median RCoR: men [2.779],

medium, and low RCoRs with T2DM

- Other endocrine disorders: coronary atherosclerosis
- Other cerebrovascular diseases: acute myocardial infarction
- Other nutritional, endocrine, & metabolic disorders

b. Medium RCoR group
- Acute cerebrovascular disease: skin & subcutaneous tissue infection
- Other liver diseases: fluid & electrolyte disorders
- Conduction disorders: other upper respiratory infections
- Other lower respiratory disease: pneumonia
- Congestive heart failure: transient cerebral ischemia
- Acute bronchitis

c. Low RCoR group:
- Cardiac dysrhythmias: hyperplasia of prostate
- Noninfectious gastroenteritis: other eye disorders
- Thyroid disorders: biliary tract disease
- Other nervous system disorders: cataract

women [2.099]). Women had higher co-occurrence of chronic renal failure (RCoR 2.461) than men (RCoR 2.155) Older patients (aged 60–69) had the highest prevalence of comorbidities with hypertension (32.7%), CHD (28.5%), acute CVD (25.9%) being top conditions

(continued on next page)

Table 3
(continued)

Study Title	First Author, y	Clustering Method	Clustering Pattern	Key Quantitative Outcomes
Latent class analysis suggests 4 classes of persons with type 2 diabetes mellitus based on complications and comorbidities in Tianjin, China: a cross-sectional analysis	Gao et al,[29] 2017	LCA, multinomial logistic regression	Class 1: complications & comorbidities group (6.1%); high conditional probability of suffering from all complications and comorbidities. Highest age, family history, central obesity, and suburban residence Class 2: high risk of complications group (25.7%); diabetic peripheral neuropathy, retinopathy, and lower-limb vascular disease Class 3: high risk of comorbidities and CVD group (14.3%): hypertension, dyslipidemia and metabolic syndrome, and CVD Class 4: diabetes without complications & comorbidities group (53.9%): low conditional probabilities for all complications. Youngest of the groups, lowest family history, female proportion, and central obesity	Overweight (46.9%) and obesity (21.3%) were prevalent among T2DM patients. Patients with higher BMIs had higher odds of being in class 1 (OR 1.43) and class 3 (OR 1.45) Women aged <48.5 y had lower adjusted odds of being in class 2 (OR 0.59) and class 3 (OR 0.46), compared with men. However, women aged 48.5+ y had higher adjusted odds of being in class 3 (OR 1.40)
Comorbidity network for chronic disease: a novel approach to understand type 2 diabetes progression	Khan et al,[34] 2018	Network theory, social network analysis Disease networks created with directional edges based on admission sequence, with varying node strengths.[c] An overall comorbidity network created based on the trajectory of the population cohort over time, and the unique characteristics of progression toward T2DM vs non-T2DM patients. Generated by aggregating individual disease networks	Cluster 1: CVD-related diseases (hypertension, cardiac arrhythmias, presence of bypass grafts, COPD) along with cancer and anemia-related conditions Cluster 2: liver disease, long-term insulin use, behavioral disorders (depression, psychoses, drug abuse) Cluster 3: other heart-related comorbidities (congestive heart failure, coronary angioplasty implants) and pulmonary circulation disorders	The node strengths of top comorbidities and conditions in descending order are as follows: cardiac arrhythmias (1), long-term use of insulin (1), liver disease (0.35), cataract (0.25), valvular disease (0.15), uncomplicated hypertension (0.125), presence of aortocoronary bypass graft (0.125), presence of coronary angioplasty implant and graft (0.12), congestive heart failure (0.11), pulmonary circulation disorders (0.1)

| The comorbidity burden of type 2 diabetes mellitus: patterns, clusters, and predictions from a large English primary care cohort | Nowakowska et al,[24] 2019 | Agglomerative hierarchical clustering, prevalence at 0, 2, 5, 9 y after diagnosis of diabetes | At diagnosis:
 Cluster 1: PVD, CHD, stroke, atrial fibrillation, heart failure
 Cluster 2: cancer, hypertension, CKD
 Cluster 3: depression, SMI
 Cluster 4: COPD, asthma
 Cluster 5: hypothyroidism, rheumatoid arthritis, osteoporosis
 2-y after diagnosis:
 Cluster 1: hypertension, cancer, rheumatoid arthritis, osteoporosis, hypothyroidism
 Cluster 2: CKD, atrial fibrillation, heart failure, PVD, CHD, stroke, dementia
 Cluster 3: COPD, asthma, depression, SMI
 5-y after diagnosis:
 Cluster 1: hypothyroidism, osteoporosis, rheumatoid arthritis, dementia, stroke
 Cluster 2: CKD, hypertension, cancer
 Cluster 3: CHD, PVD, heart failure, atrial fibrillation
 Cluster 4: SMI, depression, asthma, COPD
 9-y after diagnosis: | Hypertension and CKD had the highest age-standardized coprevalence rate among all T2DM patients: 12.1% at the time of T2DM diagnosis, and 15.4%, 17.8%, and 21.5% after 2, 5, and 9 y after diagnosis. Overall, the second most coprevalent combination at diagnosis is hypertension and CHD at 9.3%. Depression prevalence increased over the study period for all T2DM patients. Age-standardized prevalence for women was higher than men at both time points in 2007 (women: 15.9%, men: 7%) and in 2016 (women: 21.5%, men: 10.4%) |

(continued on next page)

Table 3
(continued)

Study Title	First Author, y	Clustering Method	Clustering Pattern	Key Quantitative Outcomes
			Cluster 1: CHD, atrial fibrillation, heart failure, PVD, COPD Cluster 2: SMI, depression, asthma Cluster 3: hypothyroidism, rheumatoid arthritis, osteoporosis Cluster 4: hypertension, CKD, cancer, stroke, dementia	
Differential Health Care Use, Diabetes-Related Complications, and Mortality Among Five Unique Classes of Patients With Type 2 Diabetes in Singapore: A Latent Class Analysis of 71,125 Patients	Seng et al,[33] 2020	LCA used to derive groups of homogenous individuals by age (ie, less than [younger] and >65 [older]), ethnicity, duration of diabetes, and comorbidities. Cox regression models used to ascertain the relationship between class membership and risk of complications	Class 1: younger patients with short T2DM duration and "relatively healthy" (15.7%) Class 2: younger patients with short to moderate T2DM duration and moderate disease burden without end-organ complications (34.5%) Class 3: younger women with short to moderate T2DM duration and high psychiatric and neurologic disease burden (1.58%) Class 4: older patients with moderate T2DM duration and moderate disease burden (36.9%) Class 5: older patients with moderate to long T2DM duration, with depression, dementia, and high disease burden with end-organ complications (11.3%) *T2DM duration: short (<5 y), moderate (5–10 y), long (>10 y)*	Prevalence of key conditions are expressed as bands, mapped by class >100% prevalence: Class 3: anxiety, general anxiety disorder, major depression, schizophrenia, bipolar disorder, hemorrhagic stroke, dementia Class 5: major depression, CHD, previous MI, coronary artery bypass graft, PCI, heart failure, ESRD, kidney transplant, stroke, dementia, PVD, LEA >50%–100% prevalence: Class 4: dementia 25% ≤ 50% prevalence: Class 1: kidney transplant Class 3: stroke, ischemic stroke
Identifying Subgroups of Type II Diabetes	Solomon et al,[32] 2017	Hierarchical clustering using DIANA to produce clusters of 2, 3, 4, and 5, by sample subgroups	For clusters of 5 (ie, considers all the patient segments in the sample): Cluster 1: (single, male): hypertension, hyperlipidemia,	The top conditions across all the clusters and subgroups for both sexes were hypertension, hyperlipidemia, and

| Patients using Cluster Analysis | tobacco use disorder, onychomycosis, cholesterolemia, dehydration

Cluster 2: (nonsingle, male): hyperlipidemia, hypertension, onychomycosis, cholesterolemia, malignant neoplasm of prostate, benign neoplasm of colon

Cluster 3: (single, female): hypertension, hyperlipidemia, cholesterolemia, onychomycosis, tobacco use disorder, benign neoplasm of colon

Cluster 4: (nonsingle, female): hyperlipidemia, hypertension, cholesterolemia, benign neoplasm of colon, onychomycosis, acquired hypothyroidism

Cluster 5: (married, both sexes): hypertension, hyperlipidemia, benign neoplasm of colon, cholesterolemia, ergosterol deficiency, onychomycosis | cholesterolemia, with similar prevalence

Hypertension: prevalence in single men (9.6%), nonsingle men (10.4%), single women (9%), nonsingle women (9.6%), married both (11.6%)

Hyperlipidemia: prevalence in single men (8.7%), nonsingle men (11.2%), single women (8.6%), nonsingle women (9.8%), married both (8.96%)

Cholesterolemia: prevalence in single men (3.7%), nonsingle men (4.3%), single women (4.6%), nonsingle women (5.3%), married both (4.5%) |

Abbreviations: AF, atrial fibrillation; BMI, body mass index; ESRD, end-stage renal disease; IHD, ischemic heart disease; LCA, latent class analysis; LEA, lower-extremity amputation; MI, myocardial infarction; PCI, percutaneous coronary intervention; SMI, severe mental illness.

[a] ACoR (%) was calculated as a proportion of the occurrence of a comorbidity over the total occurrence of both the comorbidity and T2DM in the population.

[b] RCoR was calculated as the ratio of the occurrence of a comorbidity in those with T2DM over occurrence in those without T2DM, in the population.

[c] Node strength shows relative attribution of the comorbidity/condition for the most hospital admissions for diabetic patients in the final comorbidity network constructed.

REFERENCES

1. Pearson-Stuttard J, Ezzati M, Gregg EW. Multimorbidity - a defining challenge for health systems. Lancet Public Health 2019;4(12):e599–600.
2. Salive ME. Multimorbidity in older adults. Epidemiol Rev 2013;35(1):75–83.
3. Glynn LG, Valderas JM, Healy P, et al. The prevalence of multimorbidity in primary care and its effect on health care utilization and cost. Fam Pract 2011;28(5): 516–23.
4. World Health Organisation (WHO). Noncommunicable diseases. 2018. Available at: https://www.who.int/news-room/fact-sheets/detail/noncommunicable-diseases. Accessed October 8, 2020.
5. Nguyen H, Manolova G, Daskalopoulou G, et al. Prevalence of multimorbidity in community settings: a systematic review and meta-analysis of observational studies. J Comorbidity 2019;9. 2235042X19870934.
6. Xu X, Mishra GD, Jones M. Mapping the global research landscape and knowledge gaps on multimorbidity: a bibliometric study. J Glob Health 2017;7(1): 010414.
7. Kingston A, Robinson L, Booth H, et al. Projections of multi-morbidity in the older population in England to 2035: estimates from the Population Ageing and Care Simulation (PACSim) model. Age and Ageing 2018;47(3):374–80.
8. Barnett K, Mercer SW, Norbury M, et al. Epidemiology of multimorbidity and implications for health care, research, and medical education: a cross-sectional study. Lancet 2012;380(9836):37–43.
9. Tetzlaff J, Epping J, Sperlich S, et al. Widening inequalities in multimorbidity? Time trends among the working population between 2005 and 2015 based on German health insurance data. Int J equity Health 2018;17(1):103.
10. Piette JD, Kerr EA. The impact of comorbid chronic conditions on diabetes care. Diabetes Care 2006;29(3):725–31.
11. Gregg EW, Li Y, Wang J, et al. Changes in diabetes-related complications in the United States, 1990–2010. N Engl J Med 2014;370(16):1514–23.
12. Pearson-Stuttard J, Bennett J, Cheng YJ, et al. Trends in predominant causes of death in individuals with and without diabetes in England from 2001 to 2018: an epidemiological analysis of linked primary care records. Lancet Diabetes Endocrinol 2021;9(3):165–73.
13. Lascar N, Brown J, Pattison H, et al. Type 2 diabetes in adolescents and young adults. Lancet Diabetes Endocrinol 2018;6(1):69–80.
14. Copeland KC, Silverstein J, Moore KR, et al. Management of newly diagnosed type 2 diabetes mellitus (T2DM) in children and adolescents. Pediatrics 2013; 131(2):364–82.
15. Pedron S, Emmert-Fees K, Laxy M, et al. The impact of diabetes on labour market participation: a systematic review of results and methods. BMC Public Health 2019;19(1):25.
16. Wang L, Si L, Cocker F, et al. A systematic review of cost-of-illness studies of multimorbidity. Appl Health Econ Health Policy 2018;16(1):15–29.
17. Chiolero A, Rodondi N, Santschi V. High-value, data-informed, and team-based care for multimorbidity. Lancet Public Health 2020;5(2):e84.
18. Stirland LE, González-Saavedra L, Mullin DS, et al. Measuring multimorbidity beyond counting diseases: systematic review of community and population studies and guide to index choice. BMJ 2020;368:m160.
19. Sciences AoM. Multimorbidity: a priority for global health research. London: The Academy of Medical Sciences; 2018. p. 1–140.

20. NIHR. National Institute for Health Research: strategic framework for multiple long-term conditions. Multimorbidity 2020. Available at: https://www.nihr.ac.uk/documents/research-on-multiple-long-term-conditions-multimorbidity-mltc-m/24639. Accessed October 8, 2020.

21. Boyd CM, Fortin M. Future of multimorbidity research: how should understanding of multimorbidity inform health system design? Public Health Rev 2010;32(2):451–74.

22. van Dieren S, Beulens JWJ, van der Schouw YT, et al. The global burden of diabetes and its complications: an emerging pandemic. Eur J Cardiovasc Prev Rehabil 2010;17(1_suppl):s3–8.

23. Petrie JR, Guzik TJ, Touyz RM. Diabetes, hypertension, and cardiovascular disease: clinical insights and vascular mechanisms. Can J Cardiol 2018;34(5):575–84.

24. Nowakowska M, Zghebi SS, Ashcroft DM, et al. The comorbidity burden of type 2 diabetes mellitus: patterns, clusters and predictions from a large English primary care cohort. BMC Med 2019;17(1):145.

25. Corriere M, Rooparinesingh N, Kalyani RR. Epidemiology of diabetes and diabetes complications in the elderly: an emerging public health burden. Curr Diab Rep 2013;13(6):805–13.

26. Aga F, Dunbar SB, Kebede T, et al. The role of concordant and discordant comorbidities on performance of self-care behaviors in adults with type 2 diabetes: a systematic review. Diabetes Metab Syndr Obes 2019;12:333–56.

27. Harding JL, Pavkov ME, Magliano DJ, et al. Global trends in diabetes complications: a review of current evidence. Diabetologia 2019;62(1):3–16.

28. Chen H, Zhang Y, Wu D, et al. Comorbidity in adult patients hospitalized with type 2 diabetes in Northeast China: an analysis of hospital discharge data from 2002 to 2013. Biomed Res Int 2016;2016:9.

29. Gao F, Chen J, Liu X, et al. Latent class analysis suggests four classes of persons with type 2 diabetes mellitus based on complications and comorbidities in Tianjin, China: a cross-sectional analysis. Endocr J 2017;64(10):1007–16.

30. Luijks H, Schermer T, Bor H, et al. Prevalence and incidence density rates of chronic comorbidity in type 2 diabetes patients: an exploratory cohort study. BMC Med 2012;10:128.

31. Alonso-Moran E, Orueta JF, Esteban JIF, et al. Multimorbidity in people with type 2 diabetes in the Basque Country (Spain): prevalence, comorbidity clusters and comparison with other chronic patients. Eur J Intern Med 2015;26(3):197–202.

32. Solomon TK, Rwebangira M, Kurban G, et al. identifying subgroups of type II diabetes patients using cluster analysis. 4th Annual Conference on Computational Science & Computational Intelligence (CSCI'17). Las Vegas, Nevada, December 14-16, 2017.

33. Seng JJB, Kwan YH, Lee VSY, et al. Differential health care use, diabetes-related complications, and mortality among five unique classes of patients with type 2 diabetes in Singapore: a latent class analysis of 71,125 patients. Diabetes Care 2020;43(5):1048–56.

34. Khan A, Uddin S, Srinivasan U. Comorbidity network for chronic disease: a novel approach to understand type 2 diabetes progression. Int J Med Inform 2018;115:1–9.

35. Hassaine A, Salimi-Khorshidi G, Canoy D, et al. Untangling the complexity of multimorbidity with machine learning. Mech Ageing Dev 2020;190:111325.

36. Hassaine A, Canoy D, Solares J, et al. Learning multimorbidity patterns from electronic health records using non-negative matrix factorisation. J Biomed Inform 2019;112:103606.

37. Iglay K, Hannachi H, Joseph Howie P, et al. Prevalence and co-prevalence of comorbidities among patients with type 2 diabetes mellitus. Curr Med Res Opin 2016;32(7):1243–52.

38. Lin PJ, Kent D, Winn A, et al. Multiple chronic conditions in type 2 diabetes mellitus: prevalence and consequences. Am J Manag Care 2015;21(1):e23–34.

39. Gruneir A, Markle-Reid M, Fisher K, et al. Comorbidity burden and health services use in community-living older adults with diabetes mellitus: a retrospective cohort study. Can J Diabetes 2016;40(1):35–42.

40. Calderón-Larrañaga A, Abad-Díez JM, Gimeno-Feliu LA, et al. Global health care use by patients with type-2 diabetes: does the type of comorbidity matter? Eur J Intern Med 2015;26(3):203–10.

41. Aguado A, Moratalla-Navarro F, López-Simarro F, et al. MorbiNet: multimorbidity networks in adult general population. Analysis of type 2 diabetes mellitus comorbidity. Sci Rep 2020;10(1):2416.

42. Bădescu SV, Tătaru C, Kobylinska L, et al. The association between diabetes mellitus and depression. J Med Life 2016;9(2):120–5.

43. Lopez-de-Andrés A, Jiménez-Trujillo I, Hernández-Barrera V, et al. Trends in the prevalence of depression in hospitalized patients with type 2 diabetes in Spain: analysis of hospital discharge data from 2001 to 2011. PLoS One 2015;10(2):e0117346.

44. Manderbacka K, Sund R, Koski S, et al. Diabetes and depression? Secular trends in the use of antidepressants among persons with diabetes in Finland in 1997-2007. Pharmacoepidemiol Drug Saf 2011;20(4):338–43.

45. Berge LI, Riise T. Comorbidity between type 2 diabetes and depression in the adult population: directions of the association and its possible pathophysiological mechanisms. Int J Endocrinol 2015;2015:164760.

46. Sounderajah V, Ashrafian H, Aggarwal R, et al. Developing specific reporting guidelines for diagnostic accuracy studies assessing AI interventions: the STARD-AI Steering Group. Nat Med 2020;26(6):807–8.

Anticipation of Precision Diabetes and Promise of Integrative Multi-Omics

Chang Liu, MPH[a], Yan V. Sun, PhD[a,b],*

KEYWORDS

- Precision medicine • Heterogeneity • Type 2 diabetes • GWAS • EWAS
- Multi-omics • Cluster

KEY POINTS

- Type 2 diabetes is a complex disease caused by both genetic and environmental factors and expresses heterogeneous phenotypes. Recent studies demonstrated subgroups of patients with type 2 diabetes with distinctive clusters of clinical and molecular profiles and differential outcomes.
- Hundreds of genetic loci from genome-wide association studies illustrate a complex genetic susceptibility of type 2 diabetes. These findings have revealed complex disease mechanisms and can assist in predicting risk of type 2 diabetes.
- Epigenomics, metabolomics, and other omics can complement the genomic to capture both genomic and environmental factors causing type 2 diabetes.
- The integrative multiomics approach at the population level will provide systems level understanding of the disease heterogeneity and contribute to the implementation of precision diabetes, which holds the promise of improved diagnosis, treatment, and management of diabetes and diabetic complications.

INTRODUCTION

Diabetes is a complex disease that presents multiple symptoms, results in hyperglycemia, and affects numerous systems. Based on the National Diabetes Statistics Report, there has been an increasing diabetes prevalence for the past 2 decades, with age-adjusted prevalence of 9.5% in 1999 to 2002 and 12% in 2013 to 2016 among US adults. In 2018, the overall diabetes prevalence among US adults was 13% (34.1 million people).[1] Diabetes causes complications in multiple organs and is

---

[a] Department of Epidemiology, Emory University Rollins School of Public Health, 1518 Clifton Road Northeast, Atlanta, GA 30322, USA; [b] Atlanta VA Healthcare System, 1670 Clairmont Road, Decatur, GA 30033, USA
* Corresponding author. Department of Epidemiology, Emory University, 1518 Clifton Road Northeast #3049, Atlanta, GA 30322.
E-mail address: yan.v.sun@emory.edu

Endocrinol Metab Clin N Am 50 (2021) 559–574
https://doi.org/10.1016/j.ecl.2021.05.011   endo.theclinics.com
0889-8529/21/© 2021 Elsevier Inc. All rights reserved.

the seventh leading cause of death.[2] Diabetes is categorized into 4 main types, including type 1 diabetes mellitus, which is caused by autoimmune β-cell destruction; type 2 diabetes mellitus (T2DM), which is caused by progressive loss of adequate β-cell insulin secretion, usually accompanied by insulin resistance; gestational diabetes mellitus; and other types of diabetes due to specific causes.[3] This paper focuses on T2DM, which is the most common type that accounts for more than 90% of diabetes cases.[4] Several known risk factors that affect β-cell function and insulin action are associated with T2DM, such as high body mass index (BMI), physical inactivity, poor diet, smoking, alcohol consumption, genetic predisposition, and other molecular markers. Poor glycemic control over time may lead to serious complications, such as cardiovascular disease, renal disease, retinopathy, and neuropathy.[5] Although T2DM is a growing public health burden globally, the prevention, management, and control of T2DM and its complications are not satisfying, partially attributable to heterogeneous risk profiles, causes, and mechanisms in the population. Precision medicine is an appealing approach for disease treatment and prevention that takes into account individual variability in genetic, environmental, lifestyle, and physiologic factors for each person. The emerging precision medicine approach may hold the promise to address the heterogeneity among patients with T2DM and ultimately improve the health outcomes. Since the American Diabetes Association launched the Precision Medicine in Diabetes Initiative in 2018, ongoing researches have been conducted to gather evidence and fill knowledge gaps, aiming at developing clinical guidelines in the next few years and eventually lead to clinical implementations. In light of recent development of multiomics technologies,[6] the authors reviewed recent genomic, epigenomic, and multiomic applications and discoveries in T2DM and discussed the opportunities and challenges in precision diabetes.

HETEROGENEITY AND SUBGROUPS OF TYPE 2 DIABETES MELLITUS

T2DM is a multifactorial disease that involves genetic susceptibility and many environmental factors.[7] The clinical implementation of precision medicine in T2DM relies on understanding the heterogeneity of T2DM subtypes with regard to genomics and environmental exposures, in addition to traditional risk factors with the ultimate goal of effective treatment.[8] The striking heterogeneity of T2DM risk, cause, and outcomes have inspired recent studies in search for subgroups of patients with T2DM. Rapidly evolving analytical algorithms and tool sets have been applied to investigate T2DM subtypes. Recent studies of T2DM subtypes and clustering analyses are summarized in **Table 1**. In a study of newly diagnosed patients with diabetes from the Swedish All New Diabetics in Scania cohort, a data-driven analysis of k-means and hierarchical clustering showed 5 distinct diabetes subtypes, including severe autoimmune diabetes, severe insulin-deficient diabetes, severe insulin-resistant diabetes, mild obesity-related diabetes, and mild age-related diabetes. The clusters of severe insulin-deficient diabetes and severe insulin-resistant diabetes represent 2 different subtypes of T2DM that are susceptible to higher risk of retinopathy and diabetic renal disease, respectively.[9] In another study using genotype data and high dimension electronic medical records data among 11,210 subjects, the researchers used topology-based approach to identify 3 subtypes of T2DM with distinct enrichment of T2DM complications and other multifactorial diseases: a subtype with complications of diabetic nephropathy and retinopathy; a subtype with cancer malignancy and cardiovascular diseases; and another subtype characterized by cardiovascular and neurologic diseases, allergies, and human immunodeficiency virus (HIV) infections.[10] Bayesian nonnegative matrix factorization clustering was conducted using the established T2DM genetic variants and relevant

Table 1
Studies of type 2 diabetes mellitus subtypes and cluster analysis

First Author, Year	Sample Size	Race/Ethnicity	Method
Li et al,[10] 2015	2551 cases, 8659 controls	Hispanic, African American, European	Topological approach
Amato et al,[83] 2016	96 cases	European	Hierarchical clustering
Ahlqvist et al,[9] 2018	Discovery: 8980 cases Replication: 5795 cases	European	Hierarchical clustering, k-means
Karpati et al,[84] 2018	60,423 cases	Israeli	K-means
Safai et al,[85] 2018	2290 cases	European	K-means, principal component analysis
Udler et al,[11] 2018	17,874 cases	European	Bayesian nonnegative matrix factorization clustering
Christiaens et al,[12] 2019	147 cases	European	Latent profile analysis
Dennis et al,[86] 2019	Discovery: 4351 cases Replication: 4447 cases	European	K-means
Zou et al,[87] 2019	3001 cases	Chinese, European, African American, Mexican American	K-means
Zaharia et al,[88] 2019	1105 cases	European	Hierarchical clustering
Kahkoska et al,[89] 2020	20,274 cases	Multiethnic	Hierarchical clustering
Tanabe et al,[90] 2020	1520 cases	East Asian	Hierarchical clustering, k-means

traits and resulted in clusters that featured different T2D mechanistic pathways of insulin deficiency and resistance.[11] Among patients with T2DM aged 75 years and older, latent profile analysis was performed to reveal 6 groups of subjects that need different glucose-lowering therapies, given the differences of T2DM diagnose age, β-cell function, and insulin sensitivity between profiles.[12] In addition, continuous glucose monitoring has been used to study the individual patterns of glucose elevation and classify subjects into specific "glucotypes.".[13] These studies shed light on the clinical application of optimal treatment selection, and future studies are needed to investigate whether there is differential treatment response between the T2DM subtypes. Previous studies have mainly focused on the European ancestry in developed countries (see **Table 1**). Coordinated efforts and resources are needed to expand the research to diverse global populations, particularly those with high burden of T2DM and underrepresented in current research (eg, South Asians). Although the heterogeneity of T2DM can be unpacked by the clustering analysis, omics-based studies are revealing the cause of T2DM on a molecular basis.

GENETIC SUSCEPTIBILITY OF TYPE 2 DIABETES MELLITUS

Genome-wide association studies (GWAS) are designed to identify genetic loci associated with disease and traits by surveying genome-wide single nucleotide polymorphisms (SNPs). Since the completion of the Human Genome Project and the International HapMap Project, researchers have been investigating the distribution of a large number of SNPs across populations with various characteristics in disease status, race/ethnicity, and demographic background and successfully identified numerous T2DM-associated loci. A summary of the GWAS of T2DM are shown in **Table 2**. A variant in the transcription factor 7-like 2 gene (*TCF7L2*) was strongly associated with T2DM across various ancestries,[14–20] and the mechanism of this genetic susceptibility is possibly due to impaired insulin secretion, incretin effects, and enhanced rate of hepatic glucose production.[21,22] In addition, other loci such as *KCNQ1*,[23–26] *CDKAL1*,[14,23,26,27] and *PAX4*[28–30] were also identified across studies and ancestries. The rapidly evolving statistical computing tools allow incorporation of more individual GWAS, larger sample size, and improved power for identifying novel T2DM variants with moderate effect sizes and low minor allele frequency (MAF). A meta-analysis combining 32 studies that include 898,130 subjects from the European ancestry tested 27 million variants (21 million rare variants of MAF <5%) and identified 135 novel loci that mapped outside previously reported T2DM regions, with 15 rare variants of MAF <5%.[23]

Most large-scale GWAS studies were conducted among European ancestry, whereas other populations are underrepresented, but there has been increasing efforts of investigation in non-European populations. T2DM is highly prevalent in people of African ancestry; however, there are a small number of published T2D GWAS reports with limited sample sizes, which restricted the GWAS discovery. A meta-analysis on T2DM in 23,827 African Americans discovered 2 novel susceptibility loci, and many previously reported loci are transferable to African Americans.[31] Sample sizes and number of variants identified are also growing in studies of other genetic ancestries such as South Asians[32–34] and East Asians.[28,35,36] Recent transethnic GWAS demonstrated to be fruitful in discovering genetic susceptibility of T2DM. A meta-analysis of 1.4 million multiethnic participants discovered total of 568 loci, including 318 new risk loci for T2DM and related vascular outcomes.[37] By investigating more than 56,000 African American participants, the number of significant T2DM loci in African ancestry was doubled compared with previous T2DM GWAS of African ancestry. Significant gene-diabetes interactions indicate that the genetic variants of T2DM can partially explain the diabetic complications of vascular outcomes, retinopathy, and chronic kidney disease.

Genetic risk scores (GRS) and polygenic risk scores (PRS) summarize the genetic effects of many individual variants and improve the prediction of disease risk over individual genetic variants. Based on results of large GWAS of T2DM, GRS and PRS have been developed to predict genetic susceptibility of T2DM,[38–40] as well as microvascular (eg, retinopathy, chronic kidney disease, and neuropathy) and macrovascular complications (eg, peripheral vascular disease, coronary heart disease, and ischemic stroke).[37] The T2DM PRS can be used to identify high-risk individuals based on estimated genetic susceptibility for prevention and accurate prognosis to reduce diabetic complication, both of which are the key components of precision diabetes. More evidence in the clinical utilities of the PRS is warranted to fully evaluate and implement the application of precision T2DM, particularly from large multiethnic studies.

EPIGENETIC, METABOLOMICS, AND MULTIOMIC MARKERS OF TYPE 2 DIABETES MELLITUS

Genetic susceptibility is an important risk factor of T2DM, indicated by a moderate heritability in various populations.[41] On the other end, environmental factors have

Table 2
Published genome-wide association studies of type 2 diabetes mellitus

First Author, Year	Sample Size	Race/Ethnicity	New/ Total Loci
Saxena et al,[91] 2007	Discovery: 1464 cases, 1467 controls Replication: 5065 cases, 5785 controls	European	3/8
Scott et al,[92] 2007	Stage 1: 1161 cases, 1174 controls Stage 2: 1215 cases, 1258 controls Stage 3: 14,586 cases, 17,968 controls	European	5/10
Sladek et al,[93] 2007	Stage 1: 694 cases, 669 controls Stage 2: 2617 cases, 2894 controls	European	4/5
Zeggini et al,[94] 2008	Stage 1: 4549 cases, 5579 controls Stage 2: 10,037 cases, 12,389 controls Stage 3: 14,157 cases, 43,209 controls	European	6/6
Yasuda et al,[95] 2008	Stage 1: 1612 cases, 1424 controls Stage 2: 9569 cases, 10,361 controls	Discovery: Japanese Replication: Korean, Chinese, European, Japanese	1/1
Tsai et al,[96] 2010	Stage 1: 995 cases, 894 controls Stage 2: 1803 cases, 1473 controls	Han Chinese	2/3
Voight et al,[97] 2010	Stage 1: 8130 cases, 38,987 controls Stage 2: 34,412 cases, 59,925 controls	European	12/14
Qi et al,[98] 2010	Discovery: 2591 cases, 3052 controls Replication: 10,870 cases, 73,735 controls	European	1/2
Yamauchi et al,[99] 2010	Stage 1: 4470 cases, 3071 controls Stage 2: 2886 cases, 3087 controls Stage 3: 3622 cases, 2356 controls	Japanese	2/7
Shu et al,[100] 2010	Discovery: 1019 T2D cases and 1710 controls Replication 1: 5643 cases, 7940 controls Replication 2: 3132 cases, 4965 controls	Discovery: Chinese Replication 1: European Americans, Koreans, Singapore Chinese Replication 2: Chinese	1/3

(continued on next page)

Table 2
(continued)

First Author, Year	Sample Size	Race/Ethnicity	New/Total Loci
Sim et al,[101] 2011	3781 cases, 4354 controls	Chinese, Malays, Asian Indians	6/6
Cho et al,[102] 2011	Stage 1: 6952 cases, 11,865 controls Stage 2: 5843 cases, 4574 controls Stage 3: 12,284 cases, 13,172 controls	East Asian	8/38
Palmer et al,[103] 2012	Discovery: 965 cases, 1029 controls Replication: 3132 cases, 3317 controls	African-American	1/1
Imamura et al,[104] 2012	Stage 1: 4470 cases, 3071controls Stage 2: 7605 cases, 3534 controls	Japanese	1/2
Li et al,[105] 2013	Stage 1: 1999 cases, 1976 controls Stage 2: 6570 cases, 6947 controls Stage 3: 3410 cases, 3412 controls	Han Chinese	2/9
Kooner et al,[106] 2013	Discovery: 5561 cases, 14,458 controls Replication: 13,170 cases, 25,398 controls	South Asian	6/7
Ng et al,[31] 2014	Stage 1: 8284 cases, 15,543 controls Stage 2a: 6061 cases, 5483 controls Stage 2b: 8130 cases, 38,987 controls	Stage 1 and 2a: African American Stage 2b: European	2/5
Hara et al,[107] 2014	Stage 1: 5976 cases, 20,829 controls Stage 2: 30,392 cases, 34,814 controls	East Asian	3/3
Mahajan et al,[108] 2014	Discovery: 26,488 cases, 83,964 controls Replication: 21,491 cases, 55,647 controls	Discovery: European, East Asian, south Asian, Mexican, Mexican American Replication: European	7/7
Williams et al,[25] 2014	Discovery: 3848 cases, 4366 controls Replication: ~22,000 subjects	Discovery: Mexican, other Latin American Replication: multiethnic	1/3
Imamura et al,[109] 2016	Discovery: 23,399 cases, 31,722 controls Replication: 65,936 cases, 158,030 controls	Discovery: Japanese Replication: East Asian, European, South Asian, Mexican/Latino	7/7

(continued on next page)

Table 2
(continued)

First Author, Year	Sample Size	Race/Ethnicity	New/ Total Loci
Scott et al,[110] 2017	Stage 1: 26,676 cases, 132,532 controls Stage 2: 14,545 T2D cases, 38,994 controls	European	13/82
Xue et al,[111] 2018	62,892 cases, 596,424 controls	European	39/139
Kwak et al,[36] 2018	Stage 1: 619 cases, 298 controls Stage 2: 2013 cases, 1013 controls Stage 3: 5218 cases, 7904 controls	East Asian	2/2
Mahajan et al,[23] 2018	74,124 cases, 824,006 controls	European	135/243
Suzuki et al,[30] 2019	36,614 cases, 155,150 controls	Japanese	28/88
Chen et al,[112] 2019	2633 cases, 1714 controls	African	1/2
Spracklen et al,[28] 2020	77,418 cases, 356,122 controls	East Asian	51/183
Vujkovic et al,[37] 2020	228,499 cases, 1,178,783 controls	European, African American, Hispanic, South Asian, East Asian	318/568

made a considerable contribution to the development to T2DM. Several molecular layers, including the epigenome, metabolome, and transcriptome, are influenced by exogenous and endogenous environment and can provide improved measurements of the changing environmental factors and biological responses to these factors.[6]

Epigenetic modifications can capture environmental exposures without changing the DNA sequence and play a critical role in mediation of the environmental risk and the pathogenesis of T2DM. Epigenome-wide association study (EWAS) is an examination of epigenome-wide markers in many individuals to scan for any epigenetic marker associated with a trait. Current EWAS in human populations are all based on genome-wide measurement of DNA methylation on cytosine (Sun YV 2014). Several EWAS have been conducted to discover the cytosine-guanine dinucleotide (CpG) sites associated with T2DM,[41–49] which help characterize populations at risk as well as shed light on potential therapeutic targets. Among identified genes from recent EWAS of T2DM (summarized in **Table 3**), the thioredoxin interacting protein (*TXNIP*) gene plays a role in glucose homeostasis,[50] and its association with T2DM was identified in studies across multiancestries.[42,45–47] A large study with 8 years of follow-up among more than 20,000 South Asian and European participants identified robust associations between DNA methylation sites and incident T2DM.[42] Further, there are growing efforts for research in underrepresented populations and populations with preexisting conditions. A study among sub-Saharan African subjects reported replication of known T2DM loci and a novel locus.[44] Another

Table 3
Published epigenome-wide association studies of type 2 diabetes mellitus

First Author, Year	Sample Size	Race/Ethnicity	Sites Identified
[a]Volkmar et al,[113] 2012	5 cases, 11 controls	European	276 (at P<.01)
Kulkarni et al,[47] 2015	174 cases, 676 controls	Mexican-American	51
Chambers et al,[42] 2015	Discovery: 1608 cases, 11,927 controls Replication: 306 cases, 6760 controls	Discovery: Indian Asian Replication: European	5
Florath et al,[45] 0216	Discovery: 153 cases, 835 controls Replication: 87 cases, 440 controls	European	1
Soriano-Tárraga et al,[46] 2016	Discovery: 151 cases, 204 controls Replication 1: 59 cases, 108 controls Replication 2: 63 cases, 582 controls	European	1
[a]Volkov et al,[114] 2017	6 cases, 8 controls	European	25,820 (at absolute methylation difference≥5%)
Cardona et al,[43] 2019	Discovery: 563 cases, 701 controls Replication 1: 1074 cases, 1590 controls Replication 2: 403 cases, 2204 controls	Discovery: European Replication 1: Indian Asian Replication 2: European	18
Meeks et al,[44] 2019	256 cases, 457 controls	Sub-Saharan African	4
Mathur et al,[51] 2019	156 cases, 525 controls	Multiethnic	6

[a] Studies of DNA methylation profiling in pancreatic islets from donors.

study showed that the associations of established T2DM CpG sites in *TXNIP*, *SOCS3*, and *PROC* hold among subjects with HIV infection, as well as some suggestive novel loci and interactions with HIV infection.[51] In addition, several studies have investigated T2DM-related traits, including fasting glucose, glucose metabolism, insulin resistance, and HbA1c levels.[41,52–55] Further, a recent epigenomic study investigated the response to antidiabetic medication and the side effect, which can contribute to the implementation of precision diabetes. This EWAS of Metformin treatment identified 11 and 4 CpG sites associated with metformin responsiveness and intolerance, respectively. The combined methylation risk scores of individual CpG sites achieved a robust prediction of the metformin responsiveness and intolerance.[56]

The metabolome is a global collection of small molecules and provides a functional readout of cellular activity reflecting the combined effects of inherited, acquired, and environmental factors. Recent advances make metabolome-wide association studies feasible as a powerful way to investigate complex biological questions.[57–59] Several mass spectrometry–based metabolome-wide association studies have identified novel metabolic markers associated with T2DM. Several studies have reported reproducible associations between amino acids and T2DM.[60–67] A meta-analysis estimated the pooled risk ratio of incidence T2DM for isoleucine (1.36, 95% confidence interval [CI] 1.24–1.48), leucine (1.36, 95% CI 1.17–1.58), and valine (1.35, 95% CI 1.19–1.53).[68] These findings highlight the potential of using amino acids as biomarkers in T2DM risk assessment, pathogenesis, and treatment.[69–72] A study among 629 Caucasian women also identified several metabolites that predicted incident T2DM, including sorbitol, galacticol, mannose, galactose, uric acid, oxalic acid, glucaric acid-1, 4-lactone, 3-methyl-2-oxopentanoic acid, and 2-hydroxybutyric acid. The optimal prediction was achieved with combination of traditional T2DM traits and these metabolic biomarkers.[73]

The emerging multiomic approach integrates multiple layers of high-throughput molecular markers to investigate the independent and interconnected associations for a disease. Such multiomic study of T2DM can reveal complex mechanisms and molecular systems underlying T2DM to have a more wholistic understanding of the disease pathophysiology. An EWAS of 4808 nondiabetic subjects of European ancestry identified CpG sites in relation to fasting insulin and glucose. The cross-omics analyses of epigenetics, genomics, and gene expression revealed that DNA methylation contributes substantially to the association between obesity and insulin metabolism, which highlights the role of DNA methylation in the development and progression of T2DM.[74] In another study, the integration of immunoglobulin G glycosylation profiling and GWAS enhanced the prediction of increased fasting plasma glucose among 511 Chinese subjects.[75] A longitudinal study with 8 years of follow-up among a T2DM risk cohort incorporated multilayers of big data including genome, immunome, transcriptome, proteome, metabolome, and microbiome; identified distinct molecular mechanisms such as weight gain leading to insulin resistance; delayed insulin secretion; and impaired β-cell sensitivity. These characterizations may explain the different T2DM pathogenesis between individuals.[76]

ANALYTICAL IMPLEMENTATION CHALLENGES IN PRECISION TYPE 2 DIABETES MELLITUS

Advanced technologies, instruments, and analytical methods now allow us to obtain several omics data from population sample more efficiently and accurately. The challenges in processing, managing, and analyzing such multiomic data have stimulated rapid growth in new analytical approaches and computationally efficient methods.[6] Machine learning and deep learning techniques have been adopted to construct prediction models using multiomic data, including genomics, transcriptomics, epigenomics, proteomics, and metabolomics.[77,78] The implementation of artificial intelligence opens up new opportunities in the research of precision medicine.[79] The translational and applied research in precision T2DM is still lacking, partially due to the complex and pervasive risk factors of T2DM, many of which showed relatively small effects.[80,81] Longitudinal deep phenotyping and exposome studies that embrace as many comorbidities and exposures as possible, coupled with advanced biostatistical algorithms, are anticipated to model and disentangle the complexity of T2DM. Integration of multiple layers of omics data in large populations will require sophisticated approaches and implementations in data collection, data processing, quality control, data management and integration, as well as efficient analytical tools. Ultimately, a close collaboration of experts from transdisciplinary fields holds the key to empower the advancement of precision T2DM.

SUMMARY

Precision medicine requires identification of distinct profiles of key characteristics that can define accurate diagnosis, select efficacious treatment, and reduce adverse effects of medication. T2DM is a very complex disease with a range of phenotypic manifestations and hundreds of known genetic loci and can cause complications in multiple organs systems. The effect of traditional risk factors such as obesity and BMI vary across ethnicities. Even at a normal range of BMI (ie, nonobese), some racial groups have a higher risk of T2DM compared with the European ancestry.[82] Such findings emphasize the importance of additional research on tailored screening guidelines and treatment regimen. Current methodologies and researches toward precision medicine in T2DM have been promising. Multiomic markers can characterize patients with T2DM into subgroups based on their different molecular profiles related to T2DM risk and cause, and identification of T2DM subtypes may potentially optimize treatment options. The exploration of diverse sources of clinical and molecular data revealed novel perspectives of T2DM biological mechanisms and possibilities of tailoring therapeutic targets on an individual basis. However, we just started to incorporate multiomic data in the research of T2DM, leaving many open questions and opportunities in clinical and public health utilities and applications. Research in diverse populations, particularly those underrepresented in previous omics studies of T2MD, are critical to evaluate and implement precision medicine approaches and address the health disparity. Although multiomic markers are not currently ready for routine clinical care of T2DM, the evidence from ongoing multiomic studies will be systematically evaluated for clinical validity to eventually realize clinical applications. We are at the beginning of an exciting era of precision diabetes, which will lead to improved diagnosis, treatment, and management of diabetes and diabetic complications.

CLINICS CARE POINTS

- The exploration of diverse sources of clinical and molecular data revealed novel perspectives of type 2 diabetes biological mechanisms and possibilities of tailoring therapeutic targets on an individual basis.
- The clinical implementation of precision medicine in type 2 diabetes relies on understanding the heterogeneity of type 2 diabetes subtypes in addition to the current understanding of traditional risk factors. Future studies are needed to investigate whether there is differential treatment response between the type 2 diabetes subtypes.
- Type 2 diabetes omics studies are being conducted to gather evidence and fill knowledge gaps, aiming at developing clinical guidelines in the next few years and eventually lead to clinical implementations.
- The evidence from ongoing multiomic studies of type 2 diabetes will be systematically evaluated for clinical validity to eventually realize clinical applications.

DISCLOSURE

The authors have nothing to disclose.

REFERENCES

1. Prevention, C.f.D.C.a.. National diabetes statistics report, 2020. Atlanta, GA: Centers for Disease Control and Prevention, U.S. Dept of Health and Human Services; 2020.

2. Xu J, et al. Mortality in the United States, 2018. NCHS Data Brief 2020;(355):1–8.
3. American Diabetes, A.. 2. classification and diagnosis of diabetes: standards of medical care in diabetes-2020. Diabetes Care 2020;43(Suppl 1):S14–31.
4. DeFronzo RA, et al. Type 2 diabetes mellitus. Nat Rev Dis Primers 2015;1:15019.
5. Zheng Y, Ley SH, Hu FB. Global aetiology and epidemiology of type 2 diabetes mellitus and its complications. Nat Rev Endocrinol 2018;14(2):88–98.
6. Sun YV, Hu YJ. Integrative analysis of multi-omics data for discovery and functional studies of complex human diseases. Adv Genet 2016;93:147–90.
7. Redondo MJ, et al. The clinical consequences of heterogeneity within and between different diabetes types. Diabetologia 2020;63(10):2040–8.
8. Philipson LH. Harnessing heterogeneity in type 2 diabetes mellitus. Nat Rev Endocrinol 2020;16(2):79–80.
9. Ahlqvist E, et al. Novel subgroups of adult-onset diabetes and their association with outcomes: a data-driven cluster analysis of six variables. Lancet Diabetes Endocrinol 2018;6(5):361–9.
10. Li L, et al. Identification of type 2 diabetes subgroups through topological analysis of patient similarity. Sci Transl Med 2015;7(311):311ra174.
11. Udler MS, et al. Type 2 diabetes genetic loci informed by multi-trait associations point to disease mechanisms and subtypes: a soft clustering analysis. PLoS Med 2018;15(9):e1002654.
12. Christiaens A, et al. Distinction of cardiometabolic profiles among people >/=75 years with type 2 diabetes: a latent profile analysis. BMC Endocr Disord 2019; 19(1):85.
13. Hall H, et al. Glucotypes reveal new patterns of glucose dysregulation. PLoS Biol 2018;16(7):e2005143.
14. Steinthorsdottir V, et al. A variant in CDKAL1 influences insulin response and risk of type 2 diabetes. Nat Genet 2007;39(6):770–5.
15. Damcott CM, et al. Polymorphisms in the transcription factor 7-like 2 (TCF7L2) gene are associated with type 2 diabetes in the Amish: replication and evidence for a role in both insulin secretion and insulin resistance. Diabetes 2006;55(9): 2654–9.
16. Ng MC, et al. Replication and identification of novel variants at TCF7L2 associated with type 2 diabetes in Hong Kong Chinese. J Clin Endocrinol Metab 2007; 92(9):3733–7.
17. Elbein SC, et al. Transcription factor 7-like 2 polymorphisms and type 2 diabetes, glucose homeostasis traits and gene expression in US participants of European and African descent. Diabetologia 2007;50(8):1621–30.
18. Tong Y, et al. Association between TCF7L2 gene polymorphisms and susceptibility to type 2 diabetes mellitus: a large Human Genome Epidemiology (HuGE) review and meta-analysis. BMC Med Genet 2009;10:15.
19. Lyssenko V. The transcription factor 7-like 2 gene and increased risk of type 2 diabetes: an update. Curr Opin Clin Nutr Metab Care 2008;11(4):385–92.
20. Cauchi S, et al. TCF7L2 is reproducibly associated with type 2 diabetes in various ethnic groups: a global meta-analysis. J Mol Med (Berl) 2007;85(7): 777–82.
21. Lyssenko V, et al. Mechanisms by which common variants in the TCF7L2 gene increase risk of type 2 diabetes. J Clin Invest 2007;117(8):2155–63.
22. Villareal DT, et al. TCF7L2 variant rs7903146 affects the risk of type 2 diabetes by modulating incretin action. Diabetes 2010;59(2):479–85.

23. Mahajan A, et al. Fine-mapping type 2 diabetes loci to single-variant resolution using high-density imputation and islet-specific epigenome maps. Nat Genet 2018;50(11):1505–13.

24. Hanson RL, et al. A genome-wide association study in American Indians implicates DNER as a susceptibility locus for type 2 diabetes. Diabetes 2014;63(1): 369–76.

25. Consortium STD, et al. Sequence variants in SLC16A11 are a common risk factor for type 2 diabetes in Mexico. Nature 2014;506(7486):97–101.

26. Flannick J, et al. Exome sequencing of 20,791 cases of type 2 diabetes and 24,440 controls. Nature 2019;570(7759):71–6.

27. Kim J, et al. Interaction of iron status with single nucleotide polymorphisms on incidence of type 2 diabetes. PLoS One 2017;12(4):e0175681.

28. Spracklen CN, et al. Identification of type 2 diabetes loci in 433,540 East Asian individuals. Nature 2020;582(7811):240–5.

29. Mahajan A, et al. Refining the accuracy of validated target identification through coding variant fine-mapping in type 2 diabetes. Nat Genet 2018;50(4):559–71.

30. Suzuki K, et al. Identification of 28 new susceptibility loci for type 2 diabetes in the Japanese population. Nat Genet 2019;51(3):379–86.

31. Ng MC, et al. Meta-analysis of genome-wide association studies in African Americans provides insights into the genetic architecture of type 2 diabetes. PLoS Genet 2014;10(8):e1004517.

32. Chowdhury R, et al. Genetic studies of type 2 diabetes in South Asians: a systematic overview. Curr Diabetes Rev 2014;10(4):258–74.

33. Khan IA, et al. Type 2 diabetes mellitus and the association of candidate genes in Asian Indian population from Hyderabad, India. J Clin Diagn Res 2015;9(11): GC01–5.

34. Khan IA, et al. Genetic confirmation of T2DM meta-analysis variants studied in gestational diabetes mellitus in an Indian population. Diabetes Metab Syndr 2019;13(1):688–94.

35. Zhang S, et al. East Asian Genome-wide association study derived loci in relation to type 2 diabetes in the Han Chinese population. Acta Biochim Pol 2019; 66(2):159–65.

36. Kwak SH, et al. Nonsynonymous variants in PAX4 and GLP1R are associated with type 2 diabetes in an East Asian Population. Diabetes 2018;67(9): 1892–902.

37. Vujkovic M, et al. Discovery of 318 new risk loci for type 2 diabetes and related vascular outcomes among 1.4 million participants in a multi-ancestry meta-analysis. Nat Genet 2020;52(7):680–91.

38. Udler MS, et al. Genetic risk scores for diabetes diagnosis and precision medicine. Endocr Rev 2019;40(6):1500–20.

39. Hivert MF, et al. Updated genetic score based on 34 confirmed type 2 diabetes Loci is associated with diabetes incidence and regression to normoglycemia in the diabetes prevention program. Diabetes 2011;60(4):1340–8.

40. Lall K, et al. Personalized risk prediction for type 2 diabetes: the potential of genetic risk scores. Genet Med 2017;19(3):322–9.

41. Walaszczyk E, et al. DNA methylation markers associated with type 2 diabetes, fasting glucose and HbA1c levels: a systematic review and replication in a case-control sample of the lifelines study. Diabetologia 2018;61(2):354–68.

42. Chambers JC, et al. Epigenome-wide association of DNA methylation markers in peripheral blood from Indian Asians and Europeans with incident type 2

diabetes: a nested case-control study. Lancet Diabetes Endocrinol 2015;3(7): 526–34.

43. Cardona A, et al. Epigenome-wide association study of incident type 2 diabetes in a British Population: EPIC-Norfolk Study. Diabetes 2019;68(12):2315–26.

44. Meeks KAC, et al. Epigenome-wide association study in whole blood on type 2 diabetes among sub-Saharan African individuals: findings from the RODAM study. Int J Epidemiol 2019;48(1):58–70.

45. Florath I, et al. Type 2 diabetes and leucocyte DNA methylation: an epigenome-wide association study in over 1,500 older adults. Diabetologia 2016;59(1): 130–8.

46. Soriano-Tarraga C, et al. Epigenome-wide association study identifies TXNIP gene associated with type 2 diabetes mellitus and sustained hyperglycemia. Hum Mol Genet 2016;25(3):609–19.

47. Kulkarni H, et al. Novel epigenetic determinants of type 2 diabetes in Mexican-American families. Hum Mol Genet 2015;24(18):5330–44.

48. Dziewulska A, Dobosz AM, Dobrzyn A. High-throughput approaches onto uncover (Epi)Genomic architecture of type 2 diabetes. Genes (Basel) 2018; 9(8):374.

49. Dhawan S, Natarajan R. Epigenetics and Type 2 diabetes risk. Curr Diab Rep 2019;19(8):47.

50. Parikh H, et al. TXNIP regulates peripheral glucose metabolism in humans. PLoS Med 2007;4(5):e158.

51. Mathur R, et al. DNA methylation markers of type 2 diabetes mellitus among male veterans with or without human immunodeficiency virus infection. J Infect Dis 2019;219(12):1959–62.

52. Hidalgo B, et al. Epigenome-wide association study of fasting measures of glucose, insulin, and HOMA-IR in the Genetics of Lipid Lowering Drugs and Diet Network study. Diabetes 2014;63(2):801–7.

53. Kriebel J, et al. Association between DNA Methylation in Whole Blood and Measures of Glucose Metabolism: KORA F4 Study. PLoS One 2016;11(3):e0152314.

54. Arpon A, et al. Epigenome-wide association study in peripheral white blood cells involving insulin resistance. Sci Rep 2019;9(1):2445.

55. Dayeh T, et al. Genome-wide DNA methylation analysis of human pancreatic islets from type 2 diabetic and non-diabetic donors identifies candidate genes that influence insulin secretion. PLoS Genet 2014;10(3):e1004160.

56. Garcia-Calzon S, et al. Epigenetic markers associated with metformin response and intolerance in drug-naive patients with type 2 diabetes. Sci Transl Med 2020;12(561):eaaz1803.

57. Kaddurah-Daouk R, Kristal BS, Weinshilboum RM. Metabolomics: a global biochemical approach to drug response and disease. Annu Rev Pharmacol Toxicol 2008;48:653–83.

58. Jones DP, Park Y, Ziegler TR. Nutritional metabolomics: progress in addressing complexity in diet and health. Annu Rev Nutr 2012;32:183–202.

59. Patti GJ, Yanes O, Siuzdak G. Innovation: metabolomics: the apogee of the omics trilogy. Nat Rev Mol Cell Biol 2012;13(4):263–9.

60. Wang TJ, et al. Metabolite profiles and the risk of developing diabetes. Nat Med 2011;17(4):448–53.

61. Floegel A, et al. Identification of serum metabolites associated with risk of type 2 diabetes using a targeted metabolomic approach. Diabetes 2013;62(2):639–48.

62. Stancakova A, et al. Hyperglycemia and a common variant of GCKR are associated with the levels of eight amino acids in 9,369 Finnish men. Diabetes 2012; 61(7):1895–902.
63. Ferrannini E, et al. Early metabolic markers of the development of dysglycemia and type 2 diabetes and their physiological significance. Diabetes 2013;62(5): 1730–7.
64. Wang-Sattler R, et al. Novel biomarkers for pre-diabetes identified by metabolomics. Mol Syst Biol 2012;8:615.
65. Cheng S, et al. Metabolite profiling identifies pathways associated with metabolic risk in humans. Circulation 2012;125(18):2222–31.
66. Palmer ND, et al. Metabolomic profile associated with insulin resistance and conversion to diabetes in the Insulin Resistance Atherosclerosis Study. J Clin Endocrinol Metab 2015;100(3):E463–8.
67. Tillin T, et al. Diabetes risk and amino acid profiles: cross-sectional and prospective analyses of ethnicity, amino acids and diabetes in a South Asian and European cohort from the SABRE (Southall And Brent REvisited) Study. Diabetologia 2015;58(5):968–79.
68. Guasch-Ferre M, et al. Metabolomics in prediabetes and diabetes: a systematic review and meta-analysis. Diabetes Care 2016;39(5):833–46.
69. Welsh P, et al. Circulating amino acids and the risk of macrovascular, microvascular and mortality outcomes in individuals with type 2 diabetes: results from the ADVANCE trial. Diabetologia 2018;61(7):1581–91.
70. Kahl S, Roden M. Amino acids - lifesaver or killer in patients with diabetes? Nat Rev Endocrinol 2018;14(8):449–51.
71. Bi X, Henry CJ. Plasma-free amino acid profiles are predictors of cancer and diabetes development. Nutr Diabetes 2017;7(3):e249.
72. Nagao K, Yamakado M. The role of amino acid profiles in diabetes risk assessment. Curr Opin Clin Nutr Metab Care 2016;19(5):328–35.
73. Savolainen O, et al. Biomarkers for predicting type 2 diabetes development-Can metabolomics improve on existing biomarkers? PLoS One 2017;12(7): e0177738.
74. Liu J, et al. An integrative cross-omics analysis of DNA methylation sites of glucose and insulin homeostasis. Nat Commun 2019;10(1):2581.
75. Ge S, et al. Type 2 diabetes mellitus: integrative analysis of multiomics data for biomarker discovery. OMICS 2018;22(7):514–23.
76. Schussler-Fiorenza Rose SM, et al. A longitudinal big data approach for precision health. Nat Med 2019;25(5):792–804.
77. Martorell-Marugan J, et al. Deep learning in omics data analysis and precision medicine. In: Husi H, editor. Computational biology. Brisbane (AU): 2019.
78. Grapov D, et al. Rise of deep learning for genomic, proteomic, and metabolomic data integration in precision medicine. OMICS 2018;22(10):630–6.
79. Hamamoto R, et al. Epigenetics analysis and integrated analysis of multiomics data, including epigenetic data, using artificial intelligence in the era of precision medicine. Biomolecules 2019;10(1):62.
80. Fuchsberger C, et al. The genetic architecture of type 2 diabetes. Nature 2016; 536(7614):41–7.
81. McCarthy MI. Painting a new picture of personalised medicine for diabetes. Diabetologia 2017;60(5):793–9.
82. Gujral UP, Narayan KMV. Diabetes in normal-weight individuals: high susceptibility in nonwhite populations. Diabetes Care 2019;42(12):2164–6.

83. Amato MC, et al. Phenotyping of type 2 diabetes mellitus at onset on the basis of fasting incretin tone: results of a two-step cluster analysis. J Diabetes Investig 2016;7(2):219–25.

84. Karpati T, et al. Patient clusters based on HbA1c trajectories: a step toward individualized medicine in type 2 diabetes. PLoS One 2018;13(11):e0207096.

85. Safai N, et al. Stratification of type 2 diabetes based on routine clinical markers. Diabetes Res Clin Pract 2018;141:275–83.

86. Dennis JM, et al. Disease progression and treatment response in data-driven subgroups of type 2 diabetes compared with models based on simple clinical features: an analysis using clinical trial data. Lancet Diabetes Endocrinol 2019;7(6):442–51.

87. Zou X, et al. Novel subgroups of patients with adult-onset diabetes in Chinese and US populations. Lancet Diabetes Endocrinol 2019;7(1):9–11.

88. Zaharia OP, et al. Risk of diabetes-associated diseases in subgroups of patients with recent-onset diabetes: a 5-year follow-up study. Lancet Diabetes Endocrinol 2019;7(9):684–94.

89. Kahkoska AR, et al. Validation of distinct type 2 diabetes clusters and their association with diabetes complications in the DEVOTE, LEADER and SUSTAIN-6 cardiovascular outcomes trials. Diabetes Obes Metab 2020;22(9):1537–47.

90. Tanabe H, et al. Factors associated with risk of diabetic complications in novel cluster-based diabetes subgroups: a Japanese Retrospective Cohort Study. J Clin Med 2020;9(7):2083.

91. Diabetes Genetics Initiative of Broad Institute of, H, et al. Genome-wide association analysis identifies loci for type 2 diabetes and triglyceride levels. Science 2007;316(5829):1331–6.

92. Scott LJ, et al. A genome-wide association study of type 2 diabetes in Finns detects multiple susceptibility variants. Science 2007;316(5829):1341–5.

93. Sladek R, et al. A genome-wide association study identifies novel risk loci for type 2 diabetes. Nature 2007;445(7130):881–5.

94. Zeggini E, et al. Meta-analysis of genome-wide association data and large-scale replication identifies additional susceptibility loci for type 2 diabetes. Nat Genet 2008;40(5):638–45.

95. Yasuda K, et al. Variants in KCNQ1 are associated with susceptibility to type 2 diabetes mellitus. Nat Genet 2008;40(9):1092–7.

96. Tsai FJ, et al. A genome-wide association study identifies susceptibility variants for type 2 diabetes in Han Chinese. PLoS Genet 2010;6(2):e1000847.

97. Voight BF, et al. Twelve type 2 diabetes susceptibility loci identified through large-scale association analysis. Nat Genet 2010;42(7):579–89.

98. Qi L, et al. Genetic variants at 2q24 are associated with susceptibility to type 2 diabetes. Hum Mol Genet 2010;19(13):2706–15.

99. Yamauchi T, et al. A genome-wide association study in the Japanese population identifies susceptibility loci for type 2 diabetes at UBE2E2 and C2CD4A-C2CD4B. Nat Genet 2010;42(10):864–8.

100. Shu XO, et al. Identification of new genetic risk variants for type 2 diabetes. PLoS Genet 2010;6(9):e1001127.

101. Sim X, et al. Transferability of type 2 diabetes implicated loci in multi-ethnic cohorts from Southeast Asia. PLoS Genet 2011;7(4):e1001363.

102. Cho YS, et al. Meta-analysis of genome-wide association studies identifies eight new loci for type 2 diabetes in East Asians. Nat Genet 2011;44(1):67–72.

103. Palmer ND, et al. A genome-wide association search for type 2 diabetes genes in African Americans. PLoS One 2012;7(1):e29202.

104. Imamura M, et al. A single-nucleotide polymorphism in ANK1 is associated with susceptibility to type 2 diabetes in Japanese populations. Hum Mol Genet 2012; 21(13):3042–9.
105. Li H, et al. A genome-wide association study identifies GRK5 and RASGRP1 as type 2 diabetes loci in Chinese Hans. Diabetes 2013;62(1):291–8.
106. Kooner JS, et al. Genome-wide association study in individuals of South Asian ancestry identifies six new type 2 diabetes susceptibility loci. Nat Genet 2011; 43(10):984–9.
107. Hara K, et al. Genome-wide association study identifies three novel loci for type 2 diabetes. Hum Mol Genet 2014;23(1):239–46.
108. Replication DIG, et al. Genome-wide trans-ancestry meta-analysis provides insight into the genetic architecture of type 2 diabetes susceptibility. Nat Genet 2014;46(3):234–44.
109. Imamura M, et al. Genome-wide association studies in the Japanese population identify seven novel loci for type 2 diabetes. Nat Commun 2016;7:10531.
110. Scott RA, et al. An expanded genome-wide association study of type 2 diabetes in Europeans. Diabetes 2017;66(11):2888–902.
111. Xue A, et al. Genome-wide association analyses identify 143 risk variants and putative regulatory mechanisms for type 2 diabetes. Nat Commun 2018;9(1): 2941.
112. Chen J, et al. Genome-wide association study of type 2 diabetes in Africa. Diabetologia 2019;62(7):1204–11.
113. Volkmar M, et al. DNA methylation profiling identifies epigenetic dysregulation in pancreatic islets from type 2 diabetic patients. EMBO J 2012;31(6):1405–26.
114. Volkov P, et al. Whole-genome bisulfite sequencing of human pancreatic islets reveals novel differentially methylated regions in type 2 diabetes pathogenesis. Diabetes 2017;66(4):1074–85.

Moving?

Make sure your subscription moves with you!

To notify us of your new address, find your **Clinics Account Number** (located on your mailing label above your name), and contact customer service at:

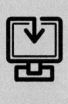

Email: journalscustomerservice-usa@elsevier.com

800-654-2452 (subscribers in the U.S. & Canada)
314-447-8871 (subscribers outside of the U.S. & Canada)

Fax number: 314-447-8029

Elsevier Health Sciences Division
Subscription Customer Service
3251 Riverport Lane
Maryland Heights, MO 63043

*To ensure uninterrupted delivery of your subscription, please notify us at least 4 weeks in advance of move.

Printed and bound by CPI Group (UK) Ltd, Croydon, CR0 4YY

08/05/2025

01864697-0004